D0513709

DISPOSED OF
BY LIBRARY
HOUSE OF LORDS

LAW REFORM AND HUMAN REPRODUCTION

Titles in the series:

All titles are provisional

LAW REFORM AND HUMAN REPRODUCTION

Edited by
SHEILA A.M. McLEAN

Dartmouth
Aldershot ● Brookfield USA ● Hong Kong ● Singapore ● Sydney

© Sheila A.M. McLean 1992

All rights reserved. No part of this publication may be reproduced,
stored in a retrieval system, or transmitted in any form or by any
means, electronic, mechanical, photocopying, recording, or
otherwise without the prior permission of the publisher.

Published by
Dartmouth Publishing Company Limited
Gower House
Croft Road
Aldershot
Hants GU11 3HR
England

Dartmouth Publishing Company Limited
Distributed in the United States by Ashgate Publishing Company
Old Post Road
Brookfield
Vermont 05036
USA

A CIP catalogue record for this book is available from the British
Library

Library of Congress Cataloging-in-Publication Data
Law reform and human reproduction/edited by Sheila A.M. McLean
      p.   cm. — (Medico-legal series)
   Includes bibliographical references and index.
   1. Human reproduction–Law and legislation. 2. Law reform.
I. McLean, Sheila. II. Series.
K2000.L39   1991
344'.0419—dc20
[342.4419]   91–23172
                                              CIP

ISBN 1 85521 026 6

Printed and bound in Great Britain by
Billing and Sons Ltd, Worcester

Contents

Contributors

Christian Byk is Special Adviser for Bioethics, Council of Europe, Strasbourg, France.

R. Alta Charo is Assistant Professor of Law and Medical Law at the University of Wisconsin-Madison, USA.

Bernard Dickens is Professor of Law at the University of Toronto, Canada.

Ann E. Fink is a Social Anthropologist and a Visiting Research Fellow at the University of Tel Aviv, Israel.

Michael D.A. Freeman is Professor of English Law at University College London, UK.

Anne Griffiths is Lecturer in Law at Edinburgh University, Edinburgh, Scotland.

Jiří Haderka is Judge and Associated Professor of Law at the Palacký University in Olomouc, Czechoslovakia.

Mark Henaghan is Senior Lecturer in Law at the University of Otago, Dunedin, New Zealand.

Kenneth McK. Norrie is Lecturer in Law at the University of Strathclyde, UK.

Louis Waller is Sir Leo Cussen Professor of Law at Monash University, Victoria, Australia.

Preface

The fact that this series, in common with many other individual contributions to the area of medical law and ethics, has produced a number of books concentrating on human reproduction shows the extent to which reproductive technologies have stimulated excitement, controversy and legal and ethical debate. Few issues are of such importance to individuals and societies as the continuation of the species, and current capacity to circumvent nature's problems or shortcomings is a matter of profound interest to all of us.

Because this book aims to bring together disparate views on reproduction and its associated technologies, in two principal ways, it has been divided into two Parts. Part One provides a review of the legislative and social response to technology in a number of different jurisdictions and seeks to analyse both why and in what way certain areas have been regulated. Part Two explores individual issues which tend to form a less common aspect of the debate — in this case, egg donation and the consequences of reproduction and related policies in the developing world.

In preparing this collection, it must be said, the law constantly outstripped my editorial speed in a number of jurisdictions, and I am most grateful to those authors who were asked, and kindly agreed, to update their contribution to take account of this. It is no easy task to comment on these matters, since public and governmental action are apparently constant and the variation apparently limitless. However, this book also shows the extent to which some countries have acted relatively quickly and directively whilst others have adopted a more *laissez-faire* attitude.

In the preparation of this manuscript a number of people merit thanks: my family and friends for putting up with my bad humour every time yet another legal change was instituted somewhere in the world, Allan and Cara for their constant support; and, of course, the staff at Dartmouth who were, as ever, unfailingly kind and cooperative. All of the contributors have worked hard and enthusiastically on their chapters and I am very grateful to them. I must also express my thanks to Professor Douglas Cusine of Aberdeen University, who – although not a contributor to this volume – nonetheless invested a great deal of time and effort in this manuscript.

Sheila A.M. McLean
Glasgow University,
March 1991

List of Abbreviations

ACT   Australian Capital Territories
AI   artificial insemination
AID   artificial insemination by donor
AIDS   acquired immunodeficiency syndrome
AIH   artificial insemination by husband
CECOS   Centre d'Etude et de Conservation des Oeufs et du Sperme
DI   donor insemination
ER   embryonic re-implantation
ET   embryonic transfer
GIFT   gamete intrafallopian transfer
HIV   human immunodeficiency virus
IPPF   International Planned Parenthood Federation
IUD   intrauterine device
IVF   *in vitro* fertilization
LH   luteinizing hormone
OLRC   Ontario Law Reform Commission
OTA   Congressional Office of Technology Assessment
PKU   phenylketonuria
PRL   plasma prolactin
PROST   pronuclear surgical transfer
TDI   therapeutic donor insemination
UNFPA   United Nations Fund for Population Activities
WHO   World Health Organization
ZIFT   zygote intrafallopian transfer

PART ONE

1 Responding to the Reproduction Revolution: Law Reform – Dilemmas and Difficulties

MICHAEL D.A. FREEMAN

When the 'reproduction revolution'[1] began depends very much on one's definition of it. The oft-cited Biblical examples of surrogacy may be discounted and, though important, developments in donor insemination or AID may be ignored. The 'revolution', then, is seen to start with the birth of the first 'test-tube' baby, Louise Brown, in 1978.[2]

It is commonplace to castigate the law for being in arrears of social change – for what W. F. Ogburn called 'cultural lag'[3] – and there are many examples where such censure is well placed. But, in general, the 'reproduction revolution' is not one of them. The law, both in its legislative and judicial forms, has, in most relevant countries, responded with some rapidity and vigour to the new territory explored by the exponents of assisted conception.

Although legal systems could not anticipate the advances of biotechnology, they have not been, on the whole, resistant to change.[4] The legal process must be seen as part of the total culture and, under normal circumstances, it can only respond to demands levelled at it. The delays or hesitancies that have occurred can be explained as a hiatus in which issues have been defined, alternative solutions posed and interest groups have bargained for favourable formulations of the law.[5]

The essays in this volume illustrate the problem, the dilemmas and the difficulties. The debates unite much of the developed world (even where putative solutions divide it), but the concerns are unique to the 'North', as the chapter by Griffiths and Fink illustrates. The 'South' also continues to undergo its reproduction revolution, but it deals not in the language of IVF or GIFT but in the harsh realities of population control through one-child family policies, semi-voluntary sterilization programmes and debates about the value of lactation, family planning and infanticide. Griffiths and Fink's essay (Chapter 10) is a salutary reminder to those of us who see the reproduction revolution in terms of enhancing fertility. It also demonstrates two other points which concern, or should concern, those in more developed countries whose legislatures grapple with the problems thrown up by biomedical advances. First, there is the importance of social norms and the resistance of society to legislation which confronts or undermines custom. We are in an area of life, graphically depicted by the Israeli sociologist, Dror,[6] as 'expressive', which is strongly resistant to social engineering. Second, the interests of men and women are not necessarily congruent. It took the feminist movement some time to develop a response to new ways of making babies and the implications of these for women. Early commissions of enquiry, such as the Warnock Committee and the Ontario Law Reform Commission, were singularly uninformed by a feminist perspective or even, dare it be said, female insight. But feminists have now joined the debate and offered a different (sometimes a series of different) perspectives on the problems, the techniques and, indeed, on whether or not the whole revolution should continue.[7]

WHY LAWS?

In any area, but especially one in which new problems have been catapulted into the public arena by medical or technological development, the first question that the potential law reformer needs to ask him or herself is whether law is needed or is desirable at all. Justifying one's existence is a form of soul-searching and is, not surprisingly, rarely indulged in. A 'shoot first, ask questions later' approach is all too common, especially in cases where legislation is a panicked response to a barely understood phenomenon, as was all too clearly the case when the United Kingdom passed its Surrogacy Arrangements Act in 1985, in the wake of the 'Baby Cotton' affair.[8] As Cusine notes, this Act has consequently failed to be particularly successful. In nearly five years of its operation there have been no prosecutions and over 60 surrogate births. An organization to bring together potential surrogates and infertile couples (COTS) has emerged: it does not (cannot) charge for its services but neither does it screen, thus leaving scope for the lurking suspicion that better (whatever this might mean) arrangements may have been negotiated by the very agencies targeted by the legislation.

One response to surrogacy, as Charo reminds us, is static. This would emphasize the biological relationship and stress that this alone should continue to be the key to parenthood and all its accompanying rights and duties. Essentially conservative, this approach, by attempting to uphold traditional family configurations, would meet the approval of the Mary-Beth Whiteheads of this world[9] and, as Charo notes, might put a brake on surrogacy. However, it rests on the underlying assumption that surrogacy is not considered as a legitimate infertility service, whereas the essays in this volume remind us that opinions as to the propriety of surrogacy are divided. Nonetheless, the static approach has severe drawbacks, not least of which is the elusiveness and uncertainty of the law on so many of the questions upon which this volume focuses.

The static approach has another drawback which becomes clearer in other areas of assisted conception. In surrogacy the only 'third party' whose activities it might be thought desirable to control are commercial agencies. Even in the most unacceptable of capitalist systems, 'baby-selling' may be considered the unacceptable face of capitalism.[10] Surrogacy does not require highly developed medical technology: NID will do as well as DI.

However, where medical intervention is essential, the desire to control 'those who would be God' means that the status quo approach fails. And, although medical practitioners can be trusted not to create hybrids and carry out other unacceptable, undesirable experiments with human life (just as we can be trusted not to murder, rape and burgle), it is often towards experiments lying 'beyond the pale' that legislation is directed. As Hart reminds us,[11] sanctions are created to ensure that those of us who obey voluntarily are not sacrificed to those of us who do not.

To consider legislation as a method of control is to adopt only one perspective, namely that of looking at law as a way of circumscribing activities. Nevertheless, it is frequently doctors themselves who want the legislation. The game cannot be played without an 'offside' or a 'no-ball' rule. Law, as Waller points out, is a way of giving 'democratic legitimacy' to medical experimentation. In the last decade doctors have gained scientific power over human reproduction. But power is only one mode of reasoning. Legislation legitimates activity in order to give it authority:[12] power itself cannot confer authority, although leading jurists such as John Austin[13] and Hans Kelsen[14] may be read as arguing that it does.

The static approach fails for a further reason. Whether or not legislation is passed to deal with new reproductive techniques, such innovations are still governed by the law. Whether law contains 'the answer' or even the 'right answer' may be doubted, but it certainly contains concepts and principles of general application which may hinder, rather than help, the resolution of problems associated with the new techniques considered in this volume. The legal problems which these create do not exist in a vacuum: there is an existing, but perhaps incomplete, structure adopted in the past to resolve unrelated problems. The predicament is at its most acute in civilian codified systems of law. This is illustrated by the provision in the French Civil Code (Art. 1128), to which Byk refers constantly and which states: 'contracts may only deal with things which can be the subject of trade' and by the experiences in Czechoslavakia, particularly the difficulties this country experiences in changing provisions in its code. Of course, as Byk acknowledges, the fact that Art. 1128 dates from 1804 does not preclude its creative interpretation, in conjunction with other principles of the French system, to tackle new problems. It is not surprising that French lawyers have interpreted 'things' so as not to include the human body.

Common law systems also experience these difficulties, as is all too apparent from the essays in the volume. Courts find themselves constricted by policies, concepts and categories invented to deal with the issues of another age. To take one obvious example, raised by a number of the contributors to this volume, the payment of a fee to a surrogate mother inevitably runs up against the prohibition of passing money during the adoption process.[15] But in all the systems which contain such a prohibition, no one had the problem of surrogacy in mind at its inception. It is therefore not surprising that an English court[16] has already separated the two processes of surrogacy and adoption in order to allow commissioning parents to regularize their relationship with their child. But, as Norrie points out, this is no guarantee that a similar conclusion will be reached in another case for, though a precedent, the case was clearly decided on its own special merits and, on any view, is a most liberal construction of the statute.

INTERPRETATIONAL PROBLEMS

Even the passing of laws specifically to tackle new biotechnology is no guarantee that interpretive doubts will disappear. All legislation requires interpretation no matter how clearly drafted and whatever the interpretational aids. Is linoleum 'furniture'?[17] Does a man who is murdered meet with an 'accident'?[18] The questions are endless and the answers depend on what the interpreter is looking for, and on values. Should legislation be interpreted literally or purposefully? Is one looking for legislative intent (if so, is there one and can it be found?)[19] or the meaning to be attached to the words? Intent is static: meaning changes. The UK Parliament in 1920 clearly did not intend a woman who lived with a man (a cohabitant in today's language –

a mistress in that of 1920) to be regarded as a member of his 'family' and therefore able to succeed to a tenancy on his death, but in 1975 the Court of Appeal in England was prepared to hold that the meaning of 'family' had changed[20] (although not, apparently, to embrace a lesbian couple).[21] Here, the judges took account of common parlance, as they did also in 1948 when they had to consider whether a marriage could be said to be consummated when a contraceptive sheath was used.[22]

These are areas where common parlance may assist. But, in the example used by Waller,[23] the problem magnifies and common parlance or public opinion is no guide at all. Legislation in the state of Victoria, Australia, defines an 'experimental procedure' as involving the carying out of research on 'an embryo of a kind that would cause damage to the embryo'. Is an experimental procedure involving the microinjection of a single sperm into an ovum research on an embryo? It is not surprising that the Standing Review and Advisory Committee on Infertility in Victoria was evenly divided on whether to allow this procedure to proceed. Half the Committee was of the opinion that there was no entity separate and distinct from the two pronuclei: the other half took the view that fertilization began and the embryo came into being with the entry of the sperm into the ovum. Those who took the latter view were, according to Waller, interpreting the terms in the legislation according to their 'common meaning'. But this is to stretch consensus since it may be doubted whether there is really a 'common meaning' at all. That there was a body to enable informed debate to take place is what really matters since, as a result, amending legislation was swiftly passed to carry out the original intentions of the legislature — to encourage endeavours to enable infertile couples to overcome infertility and establish families.

This example was worth detailed examination because the problems posed are neither unique to one state in Australia nor to the problem of defining an 'embryo'. The dilemma posed by the selective reduction of foetuses[24] (or foeticide, depending on the ideological stance taken) is yet another. Foetuses are neither 'lives in being' nor 'infants' — so neither the law of murder nor the Infant Life Preservation Act 1929 is applicable. Nor had the technique yet been developed when the Abortion Act was passed in 1967. Common parlance or 'common meaning' might even designate such a practice as 'abortion'. Legal opinion does not see it in this way: pregnancy has not been terminated. Opinion has been divided as to how morally acceptable is selective reduction. This debate continues; although the law seems to be settled in the UK by the Human Fertilization and Embryology Act 1990.[25] In terms of current discussion, it is also worth noting that the Act regulates treatment services which employ *in vitro* fertilization, but not certain forms of GIFT[26] – a strange omission, given how common, and how relatively success-ful, the technique has become.

WHAT KIND OF LAW?

Law can be reformed in a number of ways. In systems in which the judge occupies a central role (broadly speaking those of the common law, as opposed to civilian legal systems) much law reform is undertaken by the judges. This is not to say that judges in civilian systems are not also creative: anyone who looks at the provisions on *délit* in the French Civil Code (five articles framed pre-industrial revolution) could hardly think anything to the contrary. But in a system which puts its judges on a pedestal, which is pragmatic, inductive and incremental, and in which precedent plays such a major role, more authority attaches to judicial rulings.

To some extent law reform in the assisted conception area has been left to judges and, not surprisingly, rulings have been contro-versial – the *Baby M* saga in New Jersey being only the most notorious of the controversies. From what has been said so far, it will be apparent that leaving law reform to the judges, even in a common law system, has limited utility. But even if judges were capable of creating regulatory structures and developing the concepts to tackle the problems, there would be doubt over the moral propriety of entrusting lawmaking to the judiciary.

The dilemmas involved were seized upon by Ronald Dworkin.[27] As he points out, judicial lawmaking is anti-democratic in the sense that judges are not elected, are unrepresentative and are not answer-able; it operates retrospectively so as to create obligations *ex post facto*. Additionally, it is no respecter of minority rights and thus is an example of what Mill called the 'tyranny of the majority'.[28] Judges called upon to create law must, Dworkin believes, inevitably bow to the sentiments of the majority.[29]

Of these objections, the third is, I believe, the most severe. The anti-democratic argument has to contend with ambiguities inherent in democracy, as well as with the ubiquity of anti-democratic ele-ments within the legal process (observe how much law today is made by rules, regulations, circulars, directives and orders over which parliamentary control is minimal and scrutiny by the elector-ate non-existent).[30] At least when judges make new law they are required to give reasons which need to pass the muster of 'significant others'.[31]

The argument which points to the retrospective nature of judicial lawmaking is also less convincing than it initially seems. Judicial lawmaking is rarely totally unpredictable and the activities of those held to be unlawful or to create obligations are often the sort of hazardous activity which, it might reasonably be predicted, could lead to an unfavourable judicial response. Can those who skate on thin ice really expect to be told the exact spot at which they will fall in?

Dworkin argues that his own 'rights thesis' transcends these objections. There is a 'right answer' and judicial decisions are 'characteristically generated by principle'[32] and 'enforce existing political rights',[33] so that litigants are 'entitled' to the judge's 'best judgement about what their rights are'.[34] But we only need to look at some of the issues discussed in this volume to appreciate the problematic nature of this analysis. How is the judge to decide between the competing 'rights' of the surrogate and the commissioning couple?[35] Or between the pregnant woman who wants an abortion and the 'father' who wishes the pregnancy to continue?[36] Do embryos have rights?[37] Is there a right to reproduce and, if so, in what does it consist?[38] Dworkin tells us that when his superhuman judge (Hercules) 'relies on his own conception of dignity . . . he is still relying on his own sense of what the community's morality provides'.[39] It is surprising that Dworkin should use a phrase like 'the community's morality'. It assumes consensus, where there is rarely one. It leaves him a hostage to legal moralism.[40] Moreover, it leaves him open to the very objection to judicial lawmaking which is at the root of his thesis: community morality is no respecter of minority rights. This, as I have indicated, is a major objection to 'leaving it to the judges', particularly in a subject area where majority opinion can so easily be manufactured by lobbies which are sometimes prepared to engineer panics by methods which border on the unscrupulous.[41]

Whatever one makes of Dworkin's objections, the case against judicial lawmaking, particularly in areas outside what Lord Reid called 'lawyers' law',[42] is substantial. An examination of what is involved in adjudication, of the judicial office and role shows this.[43] A judge cannot act on his own initiative: he must wait for a case to be submitted to him for adjudication. Once seised of a *lis* he has to reach a decision: he cannot put off 'the evil day', he cannot compromise, he must pronounce. Hard cases make bad law, we are constantly told. But no decision at all is far from a satisfactory alternative.

Not only must a judge act: he is further circumscribed by the techniques available to him. When Parliament decides that something ought to be the law, it can consider the different ways of achieving that goal. For example, as Dickens and Charo indicate in Chapters 3 and 8 respectively, there are different approaches that can be adopted towards surrogacy. One of them, described by both and favoured by some,[44] is the regulatory approach. A legislature which believed this to be the best way of responding to surrogacy could establish regulatory bodies — organizations such as adoption agencies. Courts cannot do this. They can only act when a surrogacy dispute is brought for resolution and then only in limited ways, and they can only use judicial techniques (awards of damages, injunctions, declarations and so on). Without the institutional machinery, which a legislature can establish, the steps they can undertake are constricted.

Fuller, in his *Anatomy of the Law*,[45] brings out a further distinction. The judge, he argues, is always

> ...confronted by a *problem of system*. The rules applied to the decision of individual controversies cannot simply be isolated exercises of judicial wisdom. They must be brought into, and maintained in, some systematic inter-relationship; they must display some coherent internal structure.

Parliament is not similarly constrained: there is no logical necessity for a legislature to relate any statute to any other, although, of course, one which passed contradictory statutes is unlikely to survive for long[46] — or so conventional wisdom indicates!

It may be that the root of this difference lies in the fact that judges are expected (and are able) to act in this way because they are confronted with real human problems. Who keeps the child? Can the alleged father stop an abortion? Can a mentally handicapped woman be involuntarily sterilized? Legislatures, by contrast, perceive an issue in an abstract, generalized fashion. Because of pressure on time, they know that they are unlikely to be able to consider the question thoroughly again for a number of years. The rapid return, by the legislature in Victoria, to the subject of embryo experimentation to amend recently passed law is an egregious exception — but an exception nonetheless. Judges, on the other hand, can take minor steps which elicit new information and allow them to pull back 'without excessive loss if the new information indicates unexpected trouble'.[47] As Aubert put it: 'The safest strategy for the judge is to hide some of his footprints, so as not to commit himself and other judges beyond the minimum necessary.'[48] A judge can do this because he knows that, in due course, new problems similar to the first will arise and he or other judges will be able to test the formulated rule against new facts.

It may be thought that some of this applies with equal force to the solution of some of the problems which arise in the assisted reproduction field. And there may be some truth in this. But the basic frameworks, the underlying principles, cannot await litigation and cannot be constructed in the course of it. 'Trouble cases', to use Llewellyn's expression,[49] will inevitably arise, but one of the basic functions of law, the same jurist reminds us, is 'preventive channelling'[50] of conduct and expectations in order to avoid trouble in the first place.

Legislation then must remain the primary lawmaking instrument in this area. But how is the legislation to be formulated? To what extent can lawmaking powers devolve upon subsidiary institutions? The establishment of such institutions seems essential, but what powers are they to be given? Is their role to be the application of principle or its formulation? Take a problem, which is considered in Chapter 9 – that of egg donation between close relatives. Legislation could ban this, but should it choose, rather, to caution against it and therefore allow it in 'exceptional circumstances' (or for other limited reasons), should it attempt to spell these circumstances out or leave it to a regulatory body to formulate detailed principles or even to examine each case on its merits, or should the clinical judgment of each IVF clinic dictate decisionmaking in the individual case? The advantage of leaving the development of principles to the regulatory body is that this will consist of a body of experts drawn from different disciplines so that decisionmaking should result from the interplay of different knowledge bases and ethical positions. It has expertise and experience which a legislature lacks: it also has a degree of objectivity which may be lacking from the medical practitioners intimately connected with the infertility problems of their patients. This suggests that a regulatory body may be the optimum decisionmaker both at the level of principles (which are the exceptional cases?) and of the individual case (is this a case which calls for dispensation?)[51]

The courts will still have a role to play. In the United Kingdom the role of the courts in relation to medical decisionmaking (at least at the level of resource allocation) is in its infancy. Some reference may be made to the *Hincks*[52] and *Harriott*[53] cases. There are also the *Baby Barber*[54] and *Collier*[55] cases. The true question, applying administrative law principles, is whether statutory power has been abused. As Wade puts it:

> Statutory power conferred for public purposes is conferred as it were upon trust, not absolutely . . . . The real question is whether the discretion is wide or narrow, and where the legal line is to be drawn. A public authority . . . [is] obliged to act reasonably and in good faith and upon lawful and relevant grounds of public interest.[56]

An IVF clinic which denies treatment to an ex-prostitute is acting reasonably:[57] one which denies treatment to blacks or Jews is introducing unlawful and irrelevant considerations.[58] But where is the line to be drawn? The so-called *Wednesbury* principles,[59] formulated in England in 1948, allow a decision to be challenged if 'no reasonable authority' could have come to it. Would a 'reasonable' IVF clinic assist two lesbians to create a family or allow the conception of a child of mixed race to be assisted?[60] Are these matters of principle upon which the legislature should pronounce? Or should they be left to regulatory bodies or clinics and then ultimately to the courts? 'Courts of law', Wade reminds us, 'have nothing directly to do with mere [sic] decisions of policy. . . .'[61] The role of the courts is thus necessarily limited – at least that must be the case for the foreseeable future. However, with the pace of public law developments in the last quarter of a century, it would be foolhardy to predict the scope of judicial review 25 years on from now.

CONCLUSIONS: SOME LESSONS FROM THE FIRST DECADE

When historians come to observe the first decade of the 'reproduction revolution' and societal responses to it, what will they note, and what lessons can we learn?

They will see examples of 'moral panic'. As in the past, for example with food and drugs legislation[62] or measures to protect against child abuse,[63] they will observe how 'scandal' acts as a catalyst for law reform. But, whereas a French *cause célèbre*[64] prompted the French government to set up a commission with legislation to follow, in the United Kingdom after *Baby Cotton*[65] there was a helter-skelter rush into legislation. The contrast is not dissimilar from the 'rush to judgment' (as Kennedy and Lee called it)[66] in the 'Jeanette' sterilization case in England[67] and the measured and carefully constructed response of the Canadian Supreme Court in *Re Eve*.[68] In neither of the examples quoted can the UK response be said to have been successful: criminalizing commercial surrogacy solved very little, and upholding the involuntary sterilization of a minor led almost immediately to a batch of cases dealing with mentally handicapped adults.[69]

They will also observe debates which were shot through with conflicting values. It was the interests of the infertile which initially dominated debate in the 'reproduction revolution'. Only gradually, as Dickens observes, did the interests of the end-product, the child, come to assume the major importance. The shift in ruling in the *Baby M* case from trial to appellate court mirrors this conflict and reflects the trend towards an emphasis on the paramountcy of the child's welfare. The conflicts between utilitarian and deontological approaches, as in the Warnock Report,[70] were sometimes fought also in the legislative arena, as the debate in the British Parliament over embryo research reveals all too clearly. These debates will continue, not least because they are all-too-rarely formulated distinctly enough. If there are 'rights' in contention at all, at root it is the 'right to reproduce' which deserves attention. But what does this embrace? Does it also include a right not to reproduce? What does this say about abortion laws, and about the availability of contraceptives? Does the right to reproduce entail also the right (and/or duty) to bring up the child? If not, was William Stern (the father in the *Baby M* case) deprived of anything? The debates were culturally biased, as Charo's essay (Chapter 8) makes abundantly plain, and are also lacking in feminist input, as readers of any of the major reports discussed in this book will soon observe. There now exist feminist responses, but they are by way of critique rather than formulation of policy.

It will be all too clear how important Commissions of experts have been. This is forcefully illustrated by the French experience and by the importance attached to the work of Commissions in Victoria and Ontario. In France and in Victoria the role played by structured public opinion (a rare input into the legislative process) is a lesson for law reformers in other areas of law as well. Commissions of Inquiry will continue to have important work to do, as the Victorian experience illustrates. One of the lessons of the first decade of this revolution is the need constantly to examine the implications of new techniques, to think through the problems and to consider different approaches to legislation. This cannot be done by a legislature itself; it lies within the province of a Standing Commission established to examine and re-examine issues as they arise.

The authority to be set up in the United Kingdom by the 1990 Act is to be given a more limited (licensing) role. One of the lessons to be learnt from other countries is that consideration should be given to expanding its functions so that it becomes a Standing Commission with a brief to consider the medical, legal, social and ethical implications of developments in embryology and assisted fertilization.

NOTES

1   See Singer, P. and Wells, D. (1984), *The Reproduction Revolution: new ways of making babies*, Oxford: Oxford University Press.
2   Edwards, R.G. and Steptoe, P.C. *A Matter of Life*, London: Hutchinson; more personally, see Brown, L. and Brown, J. and Freeman, S. (1979), *Our Miracle Called Louise*, London: Paddington Press.

3 Ogburn, W.F. (1950), *Social Change with Respect to Culture and Original Nature*, (new edn), Vintage Books.
4 Responses to artificial insemination by donor are the exception; see Cusine, D.J. (1988), *New Reproductive Techniques: a legal perspective*, Aldershot: Dartmouth.
5 Friedman, L. and Ladinsky, J. (1967), 'Social change and the law of industrial accidents', *Columbia LR*, **67**, 50.
6 Dror, Y. (1959), 'Law and social change', *Tulane LR*, **33**, 787.
7 See, in particular, Corea, G. (1985), *The Mother Machine*, London: Harper and Rowe (Women's Press, 1988) and Spillane, P. (1989), *Beyond Conception*, London: Macmillan.
8 See Dyer, C. (1985), 'Baby Cotton and the birth of a moral panic', *The Guardian*, 15 January; Hutchinson, A. and Morgan, D. (1985), 'A Bill born from panic', *The Guardian*, 12 July. But 'it was not as a result of the Baby Cotton case that this Bill came forward' *per* The Earl of Caithness, *Hansard*, HL, vol. 465, col. 925.
9 In the 'Baby M' case: 217 NJ Super. 313, 525 A. 2d 128(1987); modified, 109 NJ 396, 537 A 2d. 1227 (1988).
10 See David Amess M. P., *Hansard*, HC, vol. 77, col. 46: 'the unacceptable face of capitalism' achieved 'its ultimate meaning in the buying and selling of a human being, which is a most degrading concept'.
11 Hart, H.L.A. (1961), *The Concept of Law*, Oxford: Clarendon Press, p. 193.
12 See Weber, M. (1978), *Economy and Society* (eds G. Roth and C. Wittich) Berkeley: University of California Press.
13 Austin, J. (1954), *The Province of Jurisprudence Determined*, London: Weidenfeld and Nicolson.
14 Kelsen, H. (1967), *The Pure Theory of Law*, Berkeley: University of California Press.
15 Adoption Act 1950, s.50 and Children Act 1975, s.22(5).
16 Re *Adoption Application No. 212/86* [1987] 2 FLR 191.
17 *Wilkes* v. *Goodwin* [1923] 2 KB 86.
18 *Trim School Board* v. *Kelly* [1914] AC 667.
19 See McCallum, G. in Summers, R. (ed.) (1968), *Essays In Legal Philosophy*, p. 237, originally in (1966), *Yale LJ*, **75**, 754.
20 *Dyson Holdings* v. *Fox* [1975] 3 All ER 1030.
21 *Harrogate B. C.* v. *Simpson* [1986] 2 FLR 91.
22 *Baxter* v. *Baxter* [1948] AC 174.
23 See Chapter 2, pp. 15–39 (1987).
24 See Keown, J. (1987), 'Selective reduction of multiple pregnancy', *NLJ*, **137**, 1165; see also Craft, I. (1987), *The Times*, 24 September.
25 S. 37(5).
26 For discussion, see Morgan, D. and Lee, R.G. (1991), *Blackstone's Guide to the Human Fertilization and Embryology Act*, London: Blackstone Press.
27 Dworkin, R. (1978), *Taking Rights Seriously*, (rev. edn.), London: Duckworth; see also Dworkin, R. (1986), *Law's Empire*, London: Fontana.
28 Mill, J.S. (1859), *On Liberty*.
29 Dworkin, R. (1971), 'Philosophy and the critique of law', in R. Wolff (ed.), *The Rule of Law*, New York: Simon and Schuster, p. 147 at 158–9; see also Cotterrell, R. (1989), *The Politics of Jurisprudence*, London: Butterworths, p. 167.
30 There are over 70 examples in the Children Act 1989 where gaps, often major ones, remain to be filled by rules or regulations or orders.
31 *Per* Becker, H. (1963), *Outsiders*, London: Free Press.
32 Dworkin (1978) op.cit., p. 97.

33   Ibid., p. 87.

34   Ibid., p. 104.

35   The problem may be that both parties have rights and that their rights conflict. As MacCormick puts it in Cohen, M. (1984), *Ronald Dworkin and Contemporary Jurisprudence*, London: Duckworth, p. 192, 'this is exactly what makes hard cases hard'. He thinks it better to refer to each having *'prima facie* rights'.

36   Cf. *Paton v. British Pregnancy Advisory Service Trustees* [1979] 2 All ER 987 and *C v. S* [1987] 1 All ER 1230. A foetus cannot be warded (see *Re F* [1988] 2 All ER 193).

37   Hursthouse, R. (1987), *Beginning Lives*, Oxford: Basil Blackwell; Baruch, E.H. *et al.* (1988), *Embryos, Ethics and Women's Rights*, Harrington Park Press; Fleming, L. (1987), 'The moral status of the foetus: a reappraisal' *Bioethics*, **1**, 15.

38   See McLean, S. (1986), 'The Right to Reproduce' in Campbell, T. *et al.* (eds), *Human Rights — From Rhetoric to Reality*, Oxford: Blackwell, p. 99. In the context of the right not to reproduce see Gordon, L. (1977), *Woman's Body, Woman's Right*, Harmondsworth: Penguin. In the context of sterilization see Trombley, S. (1988), *The Right to Reproduce*, London: Weidenfeld and Nicolson. On IVF and the right to reproduce see Uniacke, S. (1987), *Bioethics*, **1**, 241.

39   Dworkin (1978), p. 321.

40   See Devlin, P. (1965), *The Enforcement of Morals*, Oxford: Oxford University Press, attacked by Dworkin in *Taking Rights Seriously*, Oxford: op. cit., ch. 10.

41   See the description in Francome, C. (1984) *Abortion Freedom*, London: Allen & Unwin, p. 165 *et seq.*

42   See *Pettitt v. Pettitt* [1970] AC 777, 794–795.

43   See Freeman, M.D.A. (1973), 'Standards of adjudication', *Current Legal Problems*, **26**, 166; see also Fuller, L. (1963), 'Collective bargaining and the arbitrator', in *Wisconsin LR*, 3.

44   Including two dissentients to the Warnock Report (Wendy Greengross and David Davies). The latter expressed his views also in *The Times*, 19 July 1984. See also Freeman, M.D.A. (1986), 'After Warnock — whither the law?', *Current Legal Problems*, **39**, 33, pp. 45–8.

45   Fuller, L. (1971), *Anatomy of the Law*, Harmondsworth: Penguin, p. 134.

46   As in Lon Fuller's parable in chapter 1 of *The Morality of Law*, Harvard University Press, 1964.

47   *Per* Shapiro, M. (1965), *Law in Transition*, **2**, 134, 140.

48   Aubert, V. (1963), in *Legal Essays to Castberg*, Oslo: Universitets forlaget, p. 41 at p. 45.

49   Llewellyn, K. (1940), 'The normative, the legal and the law-jobs', *Yale LJ*, **49**, 1355.

50   Ibid.

51   Regulation is indeed the approach adopted — the Human Fertilization and Embryology Act, 1990.

52   (1979) 123 Sol. Jo. 436. The Court of Appeal judgement is unreported but see Finch, J.D. (1980), *Health Services Law*, Sweet and Maxwell, pp. 38–9.

53   [1988] 1 FLR 512.

54   *The Times*, 26 November 1987,

55   *The Times*, 6 January 1988.

56   (1986), *Administrative Law* (6th edn), Oxford: Clarendon Press, p. 391.

57   So it was held in the *Harriott* case (above). The social services department had refused to consider her for adoption. Her convictions for prostitution were 20 years earlier.

58 So the court said in *Harriott* (see pp. 518–19).
59 See Lord Greene, M.R. in *Associated Provincial Picture Houses* v. *Wednesbury Corp.* [1948] 1 KB 223, 230.
60 Cf. the recent controversial adoption case of *Re P* [1990] 1 FLR 96.
61 *Administrative Law*, op. cit., p. 176. As I write there is an attempted judicial review of the NHS reforms. I agree with Diana Brahams, *Law Soc. Gazette*, 20 December 1989, p. 19, that it is unlikely to succeed.
62 Particularly in the USA after the publication of Upton Sinclair's *The Jungle* (see Friedman, L.M. and Macaulay, S. (1969), *Law and The Behavioral Sciences*, New York: Bobbs Merrill).
63 See Parton, N. (1985), *The Politics of Child Abuse*, London: Macmillan, and the reassessment in The Violence Against Children Study Group (1990) *Taking Child Abuse Seriously*, London: Unwin Hyman.
64 'L'Enfant impossible de Corinne', *Le Point*, no. 617, 16 July 1984, p. 47.
65 *Re C* [1985] FLR 846.
66 *The Times*, 1 April 1987.
67 *Re B* [1987] 2 All ER 206, discussed by Freeman, M.D.A. (1988), 'Sterilising the mentally handicapped', in M.D.A. Freeman (ed.), *Medicine, Ethics and the Law*, London: Stevens, p. 55.
68 (1986) 31 DLR (4th edn), 1.
69 *T* v. *T* [1988] 2 WLR 189; *Re X, The Times*, 4 June 1987; *Re T* (an unreported case decided by Latey, J. on 14 May 1987); *Re F* [1989] 2 FLR, 376.
70 I refer to these conflicts in Freeman, op. cit., note 44, pp. 33–7.

2 Australia: The Law and Infertility – the Victorian Experience*

LOUIS WALLER

On 20 November 1984, the Governor of Victoria, Australia, assented to what was to be Act No. 10163. The long title of that statute, which had made its way through the Legislative Council and the Legislative Assembly of Victoria, is:

An Act relating to the regulation of certain procedures for the alleviation of infertility or to assist conception, to amend the *Human Tissue Act* 1982 and the *Freedom of Information Act* 1982, to prohibit agreements relating to surrogate motherhood and for other purposes.

Its short title is the Infertility (Medical Procedures) Act 1984, and it is an enactment which has achieved a large measure of recognition in the Victorian community, and beyond. At the time it was acclaimed as both novel and unique; today those claims cannot be sustained. The original Bill for the Act was introduced in the Legislative Council by the Attorney-General in March 1984,[1] together with a companion measure which became the Status of Children (Amendment) Act 1984.[2] That latter enactment passed the final stage in the legislative process on 15 May 1984 and was proclaimed on 1 August 1984, less than three months later.

The Infertility (Medical Procedures) Act 1984 was proclaimed in stages. Sections 1, 2 and 29 came into force on 14 May 1985. Section 1 provides for the short title; section 2 provides for the Act, or any or several of its provisions, to come into operation on those days

This is an amended text of the C. J. La Trobe Memorial Lecture delivered at La Trobe University, Melbourne on 27 October 1988.

fixed by the government, by proclamations published in the *Government Gazette*; however, section 29 provides for the establishment, and sets out the functions, of the Standing Review and Advisory Committee on Infertility.[3] Shortly after that first proclamation, the Committee was appointed and had its first meeting in October 1985. Its role in the implementation of the rest of the Act will be mentioned later.[4] A further group of sections was proclaimed to come into operation on 10 August 1986,[5] and the final stage was reached on 1 July 1988 when the remaining sections, including several new provisions introduced by the Infertility (Medical Procedures) (Amendment) Act 1987, came into force.[6]

The pioneering legislation of 1984 was the principal, but not the sole, outcome of the work of the Committee to Consider the Social, Ethical and Legal Issues Arising from *In Vitro* Fertilization. Its work contributed in no small measure to informed, sustained debate on the range of questions suggested by its title, both in Victoria and elsewhere. The Committee was established by the Attorney-General and the Minister of Health in the Thompson Liberal government, in March 1982, and I was appointed as its Chairman.[7] The remaining eight members were all appointed by the Cain Labour government, which was elected in April 1982.[8] The Committee consisted of five men and four women. Three were from the profession of medicine, two from the law, two were ordained Christian clergymen with special training and scholarship in theology, one was a social worker, and another a trained primary schoolteacher with interests and involvement in multicultural affairs in Victoria. Its terms of reference were broad.[9] Why a Committee?

My dear colleague, Rev. Dr Frank Harman – a member of the IVF Committee and of the Standing Review and Advisory Committee – once said that 'God so loved the world that he did *not* give it a Committee . . .'. However, it has become a well established practice for governments to seek answers – if not *the* answer – to serious questions of the day by soliciting the opinions, views and recommendations of selected groups of people drawn from specific areas, or constituencies, within the particular community. Cynics may opine that the appointment of a committee (by whatever name) is a government's sure way of postponing for an uncertain (but always lengthy) period its own hour of decision. But in a modern democratic society, 'the Committee on', or 'the Commission for', may provide government with advice which does bring the views and attitudes of that community from which the members are drawn into the clearest, and sharpest, of focuses. Whether any action and, if any, what action is taken as a result depends on a variety of considerations and circumstances, some of which will be revealed by the account that follows.

THE VICTORIAN IVF COMMITTEE

By the end of 1981 the phenomenon then usually labelled, in a plethora of media reports, comments, accounts and speculations, as 'the test-tube baby' was the subject of serious questions canvassed in the councils of the major Christian denominations in Victoria, and in other groups in the community.[10] Some of these questions had been raised by religious and secular groups nearly a decade earlier on the publication of the first reports of successful laboratory fertilizations of mammalian gametes and the development of mammalian embryos, and the birth, after transfer, of healthy mice, followed by calves, lambs or kids.[11] Dr Paul Ramsey, a renowned American ethicist, had argued that since there could be no certainty that *in vitro* fertilization would result in no harm whatever to a child born from its employment, it should never be done.[12] Other commentators contended that the translation of scientific discoveries into clinical practice in animal husbandry should not be followed by unnatural intervention in the marriage relationship.[13] Then the first IVF baby, Louise Brown, was born in Oldham, Great Britain, on 25 July 1978. The first Australian test-tube baby, Candice Reid, was born in Melbourne on 23 June 1980. These births and the publicity which followed them[14] – and the publicity which followed further successful live births in Melbourne in 1981[15] – raised the issue of laboratory fertilization high into the public consciousness. In November 1981, however, the Roman Catholic Archbishop of Melbourne sent this telegram to the Prime Minister, following a report that the National Health and Medical Research Council had made a large grant to support a research project on human embryos developed in Petri dishes in the laboratory of a Melbourne hospital.[16]

> Respectfully request review of grant being used for such callous immoral experimentation on living human beings.[17]

In January 1982, both Sir Frank Little and the Anglican Primate of Australia, Sir Marcus Loane, publicly voiced general and wide-ranging concerns about 'the test-tube baby programme'.[18] Other members of the Victorian community asked: 'How would IVF children cope with the knowledge of how they were conceived?'[19] Professor Carl Wood, the acknowledged pioneer of the use of IVF in the treatment of infertile couples in Victoria, responded to these statements, which appeared in local papers in the first month of that year, by calling, not for the first time, for the establishment of a government enquiry into 'test-tube ethics'.[20]

Side by side with the critics and the questioners of the new birth technologies were those who advocated their sustained and expanded employment: many infertile couples, their families and their friends. *In vitro* fertilization had enabled some infertile couples — especially where tubal disease in the wife was the clear explanation for failure to conceive — to establish a family of their own. Others had been given hope. All these views found a place in the generous language of the IVF Committee's terms of reference.

The Committee fulfilled its obligation to complete an Interim Report within three months of starting its enquiries. Between June and September 1982 it held nine meetings, interviewing a number of experts in the area of reproductive medicine, infertility counselling, moral philosophy and child psychiatry. It also solicited submissions from the community, collected and read material from a variety of sources and held a public hearing. The introductory statement to its Interim Report that 'Infertility affects the lives of some 250,000 couples in Australia, that is, about 10% of the married population. For many of them it is a serious, even tragic, deprivation'[21] set the context. The Committee's central recommendation focused on the most common situation, where a husband and wife supply their own gametes for the production in the laboratory of an embryo or embryos, to be inserted into the uterus of the wife with the aim of a subsequent successful implantation and pregnancy (at least).[22] It was its unanimous view that this form of the procedure was acceptable to the Victorian community, and that it ought to be recognized in those terms.[23]

The Committee, recognizing the grave concerns (some of which have been mentioned) about the procedure and its outcomes went on immediately to propose that legislation be enacted to provide a system for the approval or licensing of hospitals to undertake IVF programmes, and imposing conditions in relation to such approvals.[24] Counselling for infertile couples admitted to an IVF programme was to be a core condition.[25] Comprehensive information for would-be participants, including information about risks, success rates (and thereby disappointment rates) was to be provided, so that 'each couple [will be able] to express in writing their free and informed consent to participate . . .'.[26]

The call for legislation[27] was not supported by, nor was it the result of, any examination of other modes of regulation. The view that there should be a statute was reached swiftly, unanimously and without equivocation.

The Committee published its second report, *Report on Donor Gametes in IVF*, in August 1983. Its third and final report, *Report on the Disposition of Embryos produced by In Vitro Fertilization*, appeared in August 1984. Throughout its work, the IVF Committee solicited public comments and submissions,[28] and made the community aware of the questions it was asking by publishing, in April 1983, an *Issues Paper on Donor Gametes in IVF*.

The major recommendations in its second report were that:

- the use of donor gametes and donor embryos in IVF pro-grammes was acceptable;[29]
- hospitals should be specifically authorized to conduct IVF programmes using donor gametes or donor embryos;[30]
- donors of gametes should not receive payment (other than medical hospital and travelling expenses);[31]
- donations of gametes from children should be prohibited;[32]
- counselling should be mandatory for donors, as well as for infertile couples;[33]
- non-identifying information about donors should be offered to recipients of gametes or embryos, and to donors about recipients and successful pregnancies and live births;[34]
- comprehensive (that is, identifying) information about donors whose gametes were successfully used in an IVF programme should be stored in a Central Registry maintained by the Health Commission (now the Health Department of Victoria);[35]
- legislation should be enacted to establish clearly the relation-ship of father and child, or mother and child, or father and mother and child, where donor gametes or donor embryos were used to establish a pregnancy, provided it was with the consent of the spouse who made no genetic contribution to the child;[36]
- conscientious objection to participation by doctors and allied health professionals in approved IVF programmes should be recognized and protected.[37]

On the sensitive question of information about donors, and the established practice of complete anonymity for them, the Committee wrote:

> Whether or not a person pursues her or his origins, it should be possible for everyone to discover them . . .There is . . . a substantial and growing view that the values of honesty and integrity are crucial to the creation of a happy family . . . [T]he establishment and main-tenance of the Health Commission's registry will become a matter of common knowledge in the Victorian community. This will permit any person to request information about her or his own genetic background from the registry on such terms and in such circum-stances as the Commission from time to time shall determine.[38]

Its views and conclusions were influenced by the changes that had occurred in the counselling of adopting parents, and the moves for legislative change to reflect the value of honesty in that area of family development.[39]

While one member dissented from the central recommendation on the use of donor gametes,[40] and two from that on the use of donor embryos,[41] there was unanimous support for all the remaining recommendations.

The third report dealt with cryopreservation – freezing and storage – of embryos, with embryo experimentation, and with surrogate mother arrangements in IVF. On the first, the Committee recommended, albeit with one member dissenting[42] and another expressing a very specific qualification,[43] that freezing should be permitted.[44] It postulated a careful regime to avoid the establishment of embryo banks,[45] and to ensure that storage should be generally short-term,[46] in the context of a programme of reproductive technology support for the particular couple seeking to establish a family. Each couple agreeing to storage was to be obliged to decide what should happen in the event of an accident, or a death, or a break-up of the marriage occurring while the embryo or embryos derived from the gametes remained in storage.[47] The much publicized episode of the Rios embryos, the 'orphan embryos',[48] where no indications had been sought or given, led the Committee to recommend that in such a case (which it thought henceforth would very rarely occur) the embryos should be removed from storage and set aside.[49] 'The removal of the frozen embryo from storage is in some ways similar to the removal of life-support systems from a mortally ill person', we wrote. 'Life is allowed to end. This does seem to accord the embryo a measure of that respect which is so often spoken of in relation to it.'[50]

The issue of experimentation on embryos produced the widest division of opinion in the Committee. A majority of five members decided that embryo experimentation – of a destructive, non-therapeutic kind – might be conducted, but only on spare or excess embryos produced from the gametes of patients in an IVF programme.[51]

Recognizing the importance and potential benefits which could result from such research, those members went on to state 'that formation of embryos *solely* for research or experimentation is not acceptable in Victoria today'. Its reasons were these.

> From a moral perspective, it may be said that, regardless of the particular level of respect which different sections of the community would accord an embryo, this individual and genetically unique human entity may not be formed solely and from the outset to be used as a means for any other human purpose, however laudable. Where the formation occurs in the course of an IVF procedure for the treatment of infertility, the reasons which lead to the embryo's existence are not 'means to an end' ones.[52]

What was stressed was the intention or purpose of the scientists or clinicians working on human gametes in the laboratories of our hospitals and our institutions.[53] The understandings and intentions of the couple whose gametes are employed are also clearly at issue. Two members opposed all embryo research.[54] Two others, both highly distinguished professors of medicine, considered that it should not be restricted to spare or excess embryos.[55] They supported the recommendation promulgated by the National Health and Medical Research Council in 1982: embryos could ethically be created purely for research purposes.[56] (In 1986, a majority of the Senate Select Committee on Human Embryo Experimentation, established in the train of Senator Brian Harradine's Private Member's Bill on the subject, concluded that there should be no destructive, non-therapeutic experimentation on human embryos in any circumstances.)[57]

There was unanimous agreement that 'because of the very great public interest in and concern about research on human embryos all such research shall be regularly scrutinized by the Health Commission or the standing review and advisory body' which the Committee recommended should be established.[58]

The Committee, which had, in its second report, recommended that the sale of human gametes be prohibited (consonant with a general prohibition on the buying and selling of human tissue embodied in the uniform Australian transplantation legislation),[59] unequivocally condemned commercial surrogacy arrangements.[60] It said that the core of a surrogacy arrangement was the buying and selling of a baby: 'The buying and selling of children has been condemned and proscribed for generations. It should not be allowed to reappear, and no technological assistance, available to infertile couples, should be afforded to any such arrangements'.[61]

Nevertheless, the Committee considered that voluntary or altruistic surrogacy deserved different and more sympathetic consideration.[62] A particular instance, where sisters-in-law had offered to carry a child for an IVF patient who had been advised that treatment for a malignancy precluded pregnancy, was brought to its attention.[63] Even in such instances, however, it concluded that serious problems – which I have labelled as 'the agony of relinquishment' and 'the agony of rejection' – could arise.[64] There was also the contention, accepted by several members, that even in cases of 'surrogacy for love', with no element of commerce involved, 'there is still the deliberate manufacture of a child for others'. The Report stated: 'The Committee has grave doubts whether any such surrogacy arrangements are in the best interests of the child whose birth is so planned.'[65] Its recommendation was, accordingly, that surrogacy involving IVF should not be undertaken in Victoria *at present*.[66]

In its second and in its final report, the IVF Committee stated that there would be 'Developments in scientific research and in medical and surgical practice [which] may rapidly influence the future conduct of programmes to provide treatment for the infertile, and these may also be influenced by community attitudes'.[67] The Committee concluded that these matters could be best managed by an interdisciplinary group of people, drawn from, and representing, a wide range of interests in the community – a standing review and advisory body charged with the responsibility of advising the government, informing the Victorian community, and cooperating and collaborating with similar bodies throughout Australia.[68]

THE LEGISLATION

The foregoing account of the work of the Victorian IVF Committee between May 1982 and August 1984 is an important prelude to consideration of the legislation enacted in 1984, since the two pioneering statutes are based almost entirely on the recommendations in the Committee's Reports. The Victorian government had stated, in August 1983, that it would consider the Committee's recommendations on IVF and the use of donor gametes in IVF after allowing three months for community responses. By the year's end their acceptance had been announced, and in the New Year, the Attorney-General introduced the two measures in the Legislative Council.[69] While debate on the Infertility (Medical Procedures) Bill was still adjourned, the IVF Committee's third and final Report was published. The government immediately adopted its recommendations on commercial surrogacy, and introduced a second version of the Bill to incorporate what became section 30 of the Act. That prohibits both advertisements soliciting or offering surrogate mother services and the giving or the receiving of any payments or rewards for such services. It provides that all surrogacy contracts are void, and so unenforceable by legal action. The section does not prohibit altruistic or voluntary surrogacy.

Amendments dealing with embryo experimentation and the establishment of the Standing Review and Advisory Committee on Infertility were proposed by the opposition and accepted by the government in October 1984.[70] The Act was passed with that range of provisions included in it.[71] The new statutory Committee was charged with the responsibility, under the statute, of advising the Minister – and that Minister was to be the Minister for Health, to whom was assigned the administration of the Act – generally in relation to infertility and procedures for its alleviation, and on matters relating to that 'and any other associated matters referred to it by the Minister'.[72] It was also given the specific responsibility to consider, and, if it thinks fit, to approve requests for permission to conduct experimental procedures involving embryos.[73] The Act, although clearly contemplating approved embryo experimental work, is, however, subject to the significant restriction in s.6(5) of the Act of 1984, which states that ova removed from a woman may not be caused or permitted to be fertilized outside her body 'except for the purposes of the implantation of embryos derived from those ova in the womb of that woman or another woman in a relevant procedure in accordance with this Act'. It is my view that the clear intention of that provision was to give effect to the recommendation of the majority of the IVF Committee, that the intentional development of laboratory embryos for destructive experimentation should not be countenanced in Victoria but that spare or excess embryos could be used, in the development and improvement of programmes to circumvent infertility.[74]

The Act also prohibits cloning[75] (but does not define this procedure)[76] and the fertilization of human gametes by those of an animal.[77]

The sole provision introduced into this legislation which does not accord with a recommendation made by the IVF Committee is in s. 14 which states that where a laboratory embryo cannot be transferred to the woman from whose ovum it has been derived, because she has died, or been injured, or for any other reason, and she and her husband have not made any provision for such an event, or cannot be found, then 'the Minister shall direct the designated officer of the approved hospital where the embryo is stored to ensure that the embryo is made available for use in a relevant procedure'.[78] In other words, with the Rios embryos experience clearly in mind, it becomes available for donation.

THE STANDING REVIEW AND ADVISORY COMMITTEE ON INFERTILITY

The Standing Review and Advisory Committee on Infertility was constituted by the Minister for Health in 1985.[79] In consists of eight members, drawn from a range of disciplines — medicine, social work, law, philosophy, teaching — and a number of constituencies (religious bodies) in the Victorian community, spelled out in the Act.[80] Five of the members originally appointed had been members of the IVF Committee. I was appointed its Chairman. The Committee met first in October 1985, and since then has held more than 50 formal meetings, including consultations and extensive discussions with embryologists, clinicians, counsellors, and infertile couples. It has met with the Minister, with MPs of all parties, with Parliamentary

Counsel, and with officers from the Health Department, the Attorney-General's Department and Community Services, Victoria. It has provided advice to the Minister for Health on the implementation of the 1984 Act, including the making of regulations and the establishment of procedures and criteria for the approval of hospitals and of counsellors to conduct and participate in IVF programmes. It conducted, in 1986, a public twilight seminar on developments in IVF. In September 1987 it held a day-long symposium on embryo experimentation and possible future developments, including gene therapy, in the use of the new birth technologies. It is in regular communication with relevant committees, agencies and individuals in other states and overseas and its work has attracted local, national and international attention. In particular, its consideration − even before all the provisions of the 1984 Act were proclaimed − of several applications for approval of experimental procedures and of a remarkable voluntary surrogacy arrangement engendered great interest and considerable controversy.

The first application which the Committee examined, in late 1985, was for an experiment involving the chromosomal testing of embryos formed from ova which had been frozen and then thawed prior to fertilization. The purpose was to determine whether the freezing process and subsequent thawing − which had not been successfully developed, but which was being attempted when the IVF Committee considered the subject in 1984 − caused any damage to the chromosomes in the ovum. The IVF Committee had encouraged work on ovum freezing, since it was clear that, if it could be successfully employed, it would obviate the necessity for embryo cryopreservation in many cases, and so avoid problems of the Rios embryo kind, and others. Frozen sperm has been successfully used in donor insemination and in IVF programmes for a number of years. Section 6(8) of the 1984 Act specifically encourages research on, and development of, ova freezing techniques.

After extensive discussions with the scientists proposing the experiment, the Committee concluded that the provisions of s.6(5) prohibited it since it clearly involved the intentional formation of embryos which were to be damaged or destroyed in the process of chromosomal analysis. As Chairman, I advised the Committee that such experiments could only be conducted, with approval, on spare or excess embryos formed for transfer in an IVF programme, but not transferred.[81] The Committee's decision on this first application, however, was not unanimous. Three members[82] considered that the experiment could be approved because of the subject matter, and particularly because of the positive support for ova freezing research expressed in s. 6(8).

The Minister for Health, after receiving the Committee's advice, requested the Solicitor-General, the State's chief law officer, to provide an opinion on the matter. That opinion supported and reinforced the interpretation of s. 6(5) stated above.[83]

In pursuing its discussions on this most important subject, the Committee reviewed the work of Dr Christopher Chen, then of the Flinders Medical Centre in Adelaide. He had successfully achieved a pregnancy from freeze-thawed ova, without prior chromosomal testing, and a report had been published in a leading English medical journal.[84] As a result of the fertilization, live twins were born on 4 July 1986. Dr Chen subsequently informed the Committee that the twins showed no evidence of chromosomal deficiencies, nor did the foetus in a subsequent pregnancy which he had been able to establish.[85] The work had been undertaken with the approval of the institutional ethics committee of the hospital to which he was attached. On the other hand, in April 1986 the National Health and Medical Research Council advised the Fertility Society of Australia that embryos derived from freeze-thawed ova should not be transferred until appropriate chromosomal testing had been done.[86]

The second application concerned an experimental procedure involving the microinjection of a single sperm into an ovum. The researchers proposed to conduct analyses of the chromosomes released by the sperm, and those released by the ovum. They could thus confirm that the normal process of fertilization and cleavage[87] may be achieved with a single, introduced sperm both from fertile males and from infertile males with various forms of sperm dysfunction, such as, for example, oligospermia, (low sperm count). The ultimate objective was to ascertain whether certain forms of male infertility (resulting, sometimes, from illnesses such as mumps) could, accordingly, be alleviated by this novel procedure.

The applicants advised the Committee that after the entry of the spermatozoon[88] into the ovum there is a period when the two sets of chromosomes are found in two distinct nuclei – the male and the female pronuclei. These grow in size as the chromosomes decondense. After decondensation, the male and female chromosomes unite in what is termed 'syngamy' and which has been define as 'the alignment on the mitotic spindle of the chromosomes derived from the pronuclei'. It occurs approximately 22 or 23 hours after the spermatozoon penetrates the zona pellucida of the ovum. The first cleavage or cell division happens 26 to 36 hours after penetration, and two daughter cells result. The researchers proposed to block completely the movement together of the two pronuclei, by the introduction of a particular substance, and carry out karyotyping[89] of the unaligned, separate groups of chromosomes.

Was this, then, research on 'an embryo'? The Act did not, and does not, contain a definition or a description of that expression.[90]

Section 6(4) of the Act, which came into effect on 10 August 1986, defines an 'experimental procedure' as one 'that involves carrying out research on an embryo of a kind that would cause damage to the embryo . . .'. Section 6(5), which has already been discussed, was still unproclaimed when the Committee considered the microinjection proposal, but it was applied by all members as if it was. Its central place in the whole section dealing with embryo experimentation could not be ignored.

In March 1987 the Committee gave its answer. It was divided equally in opinion. Four of the members decided that, until syngamy, there is no 'individual and genetically unique human entity' – the expression used in the IVF Committee's final report to describe a human embryo.[91] There is no entity, those members concluded, separate and distinct from the two pronuclei, maternal and paternal. Since the Act made certain kinds of conduct criminal offences,[92] its terms should be interpreted in a restrictive fashion, in line with the well established approach to the construction of penal statutes. The langauge of s. 6(5) should be construed as referring to a *process* of fertilization, which begins with penetration but which is not complete until the kind of entity described in the IVF Committee's final report has developed.

The other four members of the Committee, while sympathetic to the general intent of the proposal in its search for a new treatment for a particular kind of infertility, concluded that it was prohibited by the terms of the statute. What was proposed *was* the formation of an embryo which was to be destroyed or irreparably damaged in the testing.[93] The IVF Committee's final report not only coined the description 'an individual and genetically human entity' for 'an embryo', it also earlier stated that an 'embryo is formed when a single sperm penetrates the ovum'.[94] They concluded that the terms in the Act should be understood in their common meaning, such that fertilization began and the embryo came into being with the entry of the sperm into the ovum. They also considered that if their colleagues' view of the legislation was accepted, 'then it would appear that the crucial initial stage of fertilization, i.e., the first 20 hours of development, *on which the whole subsequent development of the embryo depends* . . . [would be] left completely unprotected by the Act'.[95]

Some of the latter members favoured the amendment of the legislation to bring the kind of experiments proposed under the Committee's consideration, so that it could unequivocally consider them for the purpose of approval, or disapproval, on their merits, in the context of treatments for infertility. After discussions with the Minister, consideration of a further opinion from the Solicitor-General,[96] and much earnest debate, the Committee recommended that the Act should be amended.[97] The clear motive for that decision was to permit the encouragement of endeavours which might enable some infertile couples to establish their own families. Its recommendation was accepted by the Minister, and approved by the Cabinet. A Bill to amend the Act was introduced in the Legislative Council on 30 April 1987.[98] While Parliament was in recess, the Bill was discussed, examined and scrutinized in various fora, including the symposium attended by some 300 people which the Committee arranged in September 1987. It was debated on a number of occasions in the media. A redrafted version of the Bill was introduced in the Spring Session.[99] What is now s. 9A of the Act deals with experiments on fertilized eggs prior to syngamy, and spells out clearly the motive identified above. The Committee also advised the Minister in October 1987 that an amendment dealing with GIFT — gamete intra-fallopian transfer (a procedure related to but distinct from IVF) — and other new methods, such as PROST[100] and ZIFT[101] of seeking to alleviate infertility should be included in order to bring these clearly into the ambit of the legislative scheme of approval and regulation. What became s. 13A was speedily added,[102] and the Infertility (Medical Procedures) (Amendment) Act received the Royal Assent on 1 December 1987. Shortly after the amending provisions came into force, the Committee considered the resubmitted microinjection of sperm proposal and approved it as an experimental procedure under the terms of s. 9A.

The Standing Review and Advisory Committee has considered many questions not directly concerned with embryo experimentation. One was asked by a senior Melbourne infertility specialist, who sought its advice on a proposed voluntary surrogacy arrangement in June 1987. What was envisaged was the fertilization of an ovum from a woman who had no womb, and the transfer of the resultant embryo to her sister, who had several successful pregnancies. The latter would carry the baby to term and, after delivery, the genetic mother would take the child to rear it as hers, in every sense of that term. Before the Committee considered that matter it learned that the proposal had been submitted to the Ethics Committee of the Epworth Hospital, which had refused to approve it for ethical, not legislative, reasons. Since the Ethics Committee's conclusion was that the proposed arrangement was, at that time, unacceptable in the light of their understanding of moral values in the Victorian community, the Standing Committee decided not to consider the question further at that time.[103]

As is now well known, that particular fertilization and transfer was effected in another Melbourne hospital, and Alice Kirkman was safely born late in May 1988. When the surrogacy arrangement was made public, I said that the status legislation of 1984 affected the relationship of the baby and its genetic mother, and also the lawfulness of subsequent similar arrangements. It will be remembered that the 1984 Act does not proscribe voluntary surrogacy. The Status of Children (Amendment) Act 1984 provides, however, that where a woman becomes pregnant as a result of the transfer of a donor embryo, she — and not the woman whose ovum was employed — is to be denominated the mother of the child she carries, and to which she gives birth.[104] Her consenting husband is to be deemed its father.[105] If the relationship of mother and child — between Alice and Maggie Kirkman — was to be established firmly and unequivocally (and also that of father and child between her husband and the baby), there would have to be recourse to adoption. The provisions of Victoria's recently remodelled adoption legislation seem to discourage — but not altogether to foreclose — adoption within an existing family relationship.[106]

In addition, the provisions of s. 13 of the Infertility (Medical Procedures) Act 1984 preclude the transfer of an embryo formed from another woman's ovum unless the recipient is unlikely to become pregnant without IVF, or might transmit 'an undesirable hereditary disorder' if she became pregnant naturally. Those provisions were not in force when the Kirkman arrangements were put into effect, nor when the Perth triplets were conceived.[107]

The Standing Review and Advisory Committee decided that, as a result of the range of questions it posed in that case and the public interest it aroused, it should consider voluntary or altruistic surrogacy, with the object of providing advice to the Minister for Health — which might include advice that the legislation of 1984 should be amended to allow such arrangements to be undertaken in certain circumstances.

The birth of Alice Kirkman resulted in great public interest in surrogacy. Strong opinions in favour of and against voluntary or altruistic surrogacy were expressed. In December 1988, the New South Wales Law Reform Commission published its Report on Surrogate Motherhood, completing its examination of artificial conception begun in October 1983. The Commission recommended that the practice of surrogate motherhood should be discouraged, and that all forms of commercial surrogacy should be prohibited.

The National Bioethics Consultative Committee, established by the federal and state Ministers for Health, published a Report on Surrogacy in July 1990. It recommended that surrogacy should not be totally prohibited, nor should it be freely allowed. In March 1991, a Joint Meeting of Australian Social Welfare and Health Ministers decided not to accept those recommendations, but resolved instead to support uniform legislation in Australia to prohibit commercial surrogacy, the provision of technical or professional services for surrogacy, and advertising relating to surrogacy arrangements. As a result, the Ministers decided that there was no need for further work on the feasibility of regulating the practice of surrogacy.[108]

The Committee has recently reviewed its first three years of work, and submitted a report to the Minister which briefly records that initial period.[109] On the near horizon are several new applications for approval of experiments. One foreshadowed is on embryo biopsy — which could, if successful, lead to laboratory identification of some embryos unsuitable for transfer because of chromosomal abnormalities.

REVIEW AND CONCLUSIONS

Since the Victorian legislation was first enacted, it has attracted general and specific comment, commendation and criticism. The Infertility (Medical Procedures) Act 1984 uses the well known legislative techniques of prohibition and authorization: it employees the weapons of the criminal law; it creates offences and prescribes punishments. It is a far cry from the postulation of ethical guidelines devised, and declared by, a learned profession for its members, or by a specialist college or a particular society of practitioners. It is also a far cry from the technique of adding by regulation to the list of forms of behaviour that count as 'unprofessional conduct' or 'infamous behaviour in a professional respect', in the context of the disciplinary responsibilities of, say, a medical board. What justifies it?

The answer begins, I think, with a view expressed by a former Governor-General of Australia when he was a Justice of the High Court. Although he was contrasting the law made by courts with that by parliaments, his statement applies generally to statutes. He said:

> The passage of a measure through the legislature confers a unique stamp of democratic legitimacy, valuable in a country possessing democratic traditions. Moreover the legislative process is exposed to, and provides a safety valve for, those community pressures which, if not released in this way, may otherwise build up to levels dangerous to the system itself. An elected legislature as the identified and visible maker of laws can be seen to be responsive to legitimate pressures and to the strongly held views of the community.[110]

The creation of statutory offences means that those 'strongly held views of the community' are expressed in the most emphatic manner.

Both the 1984 and 1987 debates in the Parliament of Victoria saw the democratic process at work in relation to a subject where the Victorian IVF Committee had stated, in its first report, that it had found strong support for, and strong opposition to, the new birth technologies and their clinical applications.[111] Parliament finally agreed, in substantially bipartisan fashion, that the matter of new life in the laboratory should not be left to the ethical determinations of scientists or medical practitioners, nor to private conscience, nor to the chances of a forensic lottery in the superior courts. It was to be regulated by statute. The establishment of the Standing Review and Advisory Committee is an important part of that legislative arrangement. The Committee is obliged to submit Annual Reports to the Minister, covering the activities of hospitals approved to conduct IVF and related programmes,[112] and also to submit a report on each experimental proposal the Committee approves.[113] The Minister must table each such Report in the Parliament within 14 sitting days of its receipt.[114] This ensures that Parliament, and hence the community, knows of, and has the opportunity to consider and comment upon, developments in the challenging field of novel birth technologies.

When the legislation was enacted, it was criticized specifically on a number of counts. One was that legislation was altogether too cumbersome here and that it would fall rapidly behind new developments in the area to which it applied, where the frontiers of scientific knowledge and clinical practice were being pushed forward with an unprecedented vigour and urgency. It would be at best, as Mr Justice Windeyer once said of the courts' response to another controversial issue, '[L]aw, marching with medicine but in the rear and limping a little'.[115] Subsequently, one critic inferred that the delay in proclaiming the main regulatory provisions betokened, perhaps, a decision *sub silentio* by the government to leave the novel legislation in limbo – enacted but unenforceable.[116] It was also stated that Victoria was, and would remain, alone in embarking on legislation to regulate and control new birth technologies, and that would result in the departure of scientists and clinicians, and also 'border-hopping' by persons determined to employ relevant procedures, but apparently ineligible under the local statutory provisions.[117] That comment has been made in relation to the Perth IVF surrogacy,[118] but it may be that it is the nature and administration of the adoption legislation in various states which is of more weight in that case.

The process of amendment initiated and completed in 1987 should quieten some of those who claim that Victoria's infertility legislation is 'according to the law of the Persians and the Medes that it be not altered'.[119] The equal division within the Standing Review and Advisory Committee and its subsequent wholehearted recommendation that the law be changed attracted much public attention. That set the stage for the extensive debates in both Houses of Parliament on the amending Bill[120] – debates clearly informed by the expression to the members of all parties of the views and the values of many of their constituents. In a modern democratic society, where the Parliament sits regularly, statutes may be altered, and altered swiftly – if the will is there. The great advantages of that recent process are apparent. It was public – indeed carried out in the unremitting light of media scrutiny. It was reported by the media, so that the whole community could know what was happening. It was carried out by men and women who are elected and regularly accountable to the people, and who were solicited by groups and by persons advancing a range of interests which were, and are, considered highly in society. The legislators were informed through the statements prepared by the Standing Committee, and the opinion of the Solicitor-General, all of which were published and widely circulated.

The delays in proclaiming the balance of the legislation were occasioned by the need to prepare the regulations, guidelines and administrative procedures necessary to enable a new system of law to operate effectively. The Standing Committee provided advice on all these matters, and is represented on the Hospital Approval Advisory Panel and the Counsellor Approval Advisory Panel, both established by the Minister at its suggestion to give advice to him in relation to the exercise of his powers under the legislation.

The birth technology programmes have not stopped. There have been important developments since 1984, and indeed the institution of new procedures in both of the hospitals which initiated the first IVF programmes[121] and in at least one other Melbourne hospital.[122] Research in embryology has continued. The legislation is losing its air of novelty. Today the distinct issue of allocation of scarce resources has been finally added to the agenda of items of concern about the new birth technologies. What proportion of the federal health budget should be directed to IVF? A swingeing cut in funding could do more than any regulatory legislation to restrict existing programmes and implementation of new ones.

Victoria is no longer unique in the field of legislation in this area. In fact the first state to pass a relevant status statute was New South Wales in March 1984 – although it dealt only with children born as a result of artificial insemination or the use of donor sperm in IVF.[123] Every state in Australia, and the ACT and Northern Australia, now has legislation on the status of children born as the result of the use of donor gametes in the new technologies, or as a result of what is called today 'donor insemination' (DI) rather than 'artificial insemination by donor' (AID).[124] (The DI programmes in Victoria – and the rest of Australia – were suspended for some months in 1986 not because concerns about cessation of sperm donations due to the requirements of recording and preserving information were borne out, but because of justified fears of the transmission of HIV disease, or AIDS, through the use of untested stored sperm.) Queensland was last, enacting its status statute in October 1988. A number of these status measures, enacted between 1985 and 1988, are faithful copies of the Victorian, which was the first to deal with the position of children born from donor ova and donor embryos.

In March 1988 South Australia joined Victoria in the field of regulation, when it enacted the Reproductive Technology Act, 1988, which provides a system of licensing and control for that state's artificial fertilization procedures. This statute was preceded by the In Vitro Fertilization (Restriction) Act, 1987, which restricted IVF programmes to those established in three named Adelaide hospitals,[125] pending the enactment of the comprehensive legislation briefly described below. The Act of 1988 establishes the South Australian Council on Reproductive Technology, consisting of 11 members, of which five are nominated by the Minister for Health.[126] The Council's chief task is to formulate a comprehensive code of ethical practice to govern both the use of artificial fertilization procedures, and all research involving experimentation with human reproductive material.[127] The scheme of licensing incorporates submission to the code of practice, and careful oversight by the South Australian Health Commission, which is given wide-ranging powers of inspection.[128] The Council on Reproductive Technology may authorize experimentation with human reproductive material,[129] but s. (14) (2)(b) of the Act states that any such 'licence will be subject to . . . a condition prohibiting research that may be detrimental to an embryo . . .'.

A week earlier, the Governor of South Australia gave assent to the Family Relationships Act Amendment Act, 1988. That statute deals with surrogacy contracts and surrogacy procuration contracts; both varieties are declared to be void.[130] It also creates several new offences in connection with commercial surrogacy arrangements.[131] In 1988, the Queensland Parliament enacted the Surrogate Parenthood Act, which creates a range of offences in relation to both commercial and voluntary surrogacy[132] and also provides that surrogacy contracts are void.[133] It encompasses not only acts carried out in Queensland but also those where 'the offender is ordinarily resident in Queensland at that time, irrespective of where the act occurs'.[134] The Perth births, from a 'sister-surrogacy' arrangement employing IVF, must concentrate the attention of Ministers and civil servants – and others – in that State on the same subject.[134a]

Outside Australia, Denmark enacted legislation in 1987[135] which provides for a 17-member Advisory Council charged with the responsibility of proposing detailed statutory provisions to address all aspects of the new birth technologies. The Danish legislation prohibits a wide range of experiments involving human embryos. The

Federal German government has enacted comprehensive legislation on birth technology, based on the recommendations in the Benda Report of 1985.[136] The UK government published a White Paper late in 1987,[137] specifically canvassing several modes of legislation, and foreshadowing the introduction of a statute late in 1988. The enactment of regulatory legislation was clearly recommended in the Warnock Report on Human Fertilisation and Embryology in 1984.[138] The Surrogacy Arrangements Act 1985,[139] enacted after the notorious Baby Cotton case,[140] was designed to prohibit the operations of agencies procuring surrogate mother contracts. It has now been followed by the comprehensive Human Fertilization and Embryology Act 1990. This establishes a legislative framework for the regulation of the new reproductive technologies through the establishment of the Human Fertilization and Embryology Authority, empowered to control and licence centres undertaking embryo research, and centres providing IVF and donor insemination. The legislation also contains provisions dealing with the status of children born as a result of gamete or embryo donation, and for counselling of infertile couples seeking to avail themselves of novel reproductive technologies.[141]

In the United States, a variety of enactments affecting the use of new birth technologies, and surrogacy in general, have been introduced into state legislatures, and several have been passed. The protracted litigation between Ms Mary-Beth Whitehead and Dr and Mrs William Stern over the custody of the child born to Ms Whitehead after her insemination with Dr Stern's sperm – the case of Baby M[142] – which filled the front pages and the television screens of America and beyond in 1987 and the early part of 1988 has, unsurprisingly, resulted in a variety of proposed measures to deal with surrogacy, particularly where, to quote a Michigan judge in a 1981 surrogacy case, there are 'The evils attendant to the mix of lucre and the adoption process . . .'.[143] It is safe to predict that there will be a range of legislative measures enacted in that country in the near future. In 1988, indeed, Louisiana passed a statute which avoids commercial surrogacy contracts,[144] while Nevada exempted surrogacy contracts from its general prohibition on the sale of babies.[145]

Thus the development of a variety of statutory patterns of regulation and control of birth technologies, in Australia and in the common law world, is already under way. In Australia, the Senate Standing Committee on Constitutional and Legal Affairs, in 1985, pointed to significant differences in the several status enactments, decried the variety and the inconsistency and urged uniformity.[146] A similar call may be strongly voiced in terms of the regulatory legislation on the new birth technologies. It is discreditable, in a country such as ours, that there should be no uniform legislation on a subject where common considerations affect all Australians. The establishment, in April 1988, of the National Bioethics Consultative Committee, endorsed by the Australian Health Ministers' Conference, may result, in time, in proposals for uniformity. That Committee had surrogacy as the first issue in its list of priorities.[146a]

In the meantime, the Victorian legislation governs what happens in this state, and continues to provide a model for other jurisdictions. Its context, as its title clearly signals, is infertility and its treatment.

Infertility is not only a serious deprivation, as the IVF Committee had it in 1982, it is a scourge for many married couples. Can any person who is not a partner in an infertile union entirely share the range and the depth of those emotions which are experienced by those who want a child and find they cannot conceive one, or that they cannot sustain a pregnancy? The heritage we share, as members of Western society, includes many accounts in sacred literature where those feelings are poignantly described. While there has been − surprisingly, perhaps, in a secular society − a parade of Biblical examples to support the case for surrogacy, which the stories of Sarah's and Rachel's generosity to their husbands do not buttress, there is in those episodes, and in other scriptural narratives, the clearest expression of the pain of childlessness. One such is the account of Hannah, the infertile wife of Elkanah, whose passionate but silent prayer for a child was finally answered by the birth of Samuel, recorded in the prophetic book which bears his name. The Midrash − the Jewish homiletic commentary on the Bible − fills out that brief chronicle by ascribing the following text to Hannah's prayer:

> Sovereign of the Universe, among all the things that Thou hast created in a woman, Thou has not created one without a purpose. Our eyes to see, our ears to hear, our nose to smell, our mouth to speak, our hands for work, our legs to walk with, our breasts to give suck. Didst Thou not create these breasts that Thou hast put on my heart to give suck? Give me a son so that I may suckle with them. . . .[147]

An American rabbi, himself a partner in a childless marriage and an adoptive father, wrote: 'I am amazed by how well the rabbis of the Talmud captured the sense of injustice aroused by infertility. I have felt it personally.'[148]

That sense of injustice found strong recognition in the Victorian IVF Committee's first report,[149] and affected the rest of its work. It also finds recognition in the Infertility (Medical Procedures) Act 1984.

But the legislation also recognizes and imposes limits on what may be undertaken to redress it. It is structured only for married couples.[150] It mandates for them information and counselling, and thus constrains them in their autonomy.[151] It imposes controls of a specific sort on, and draws boundaries for, experiments involving damage to or destruction of human embryos.[152] It is a statutory system of checks and balances struck in our community, embedded in a carefully drawn rule-framework which gives force and effect to the principles it enunciates, providing, at the same time, clear legislative protection for all the persons involved in approved activities employing the new birth technologies. Nowhere is this concept of balancing competing considerations more clearly expressed than in the heart of the provision establishing the Standing Review and Advisory Committee on Infertility. Section 29(7) states that

In the exercise of its functions, the Committee —

(a) shall have regard to the principle that childless couples should be assisted in fulfilling their desire to have children;

(b) shall ensure that the highest regard is given to the principle that human life shall be preserved and protected at all times; and

(c) shall have regard to the spirit and intent of the several provisions of this Act.

The Committee has often reflected on those adjurations during its existence. It is work which has been done, and is being done, in what may be accurately described as the very first moments of new science and pioneering medicine, and it is not final and complete. I am reminded, again and again, of what is attributed to Alfonso X, King of Castile, an enthusiastic amateur natural philosopher, who was entitled 'The Wise'. 'Had I been present at the Creation', he is reported as saying, 'I would have given some useful hints for the better ordering of the universe.' That was comfortably spoken with the advantage of hindsight. We are, all of us, present at a creation. It is our special privilege to be here when, for the first time in the history of the world, the beginnings of new human lives are being formed in glass dishes in laboratories. The marvellous birth technologies are being undertaken in, and are being proposed for, institutions in our community today — affecting our fellow citizens and resulting in the birth, sometimes, of children who will live and hopefully flourish among us as we move towards the end of this awful, wonderful century.

How will posterity view our human ordering of this creation? Twenty-five years ago Dr Martin Luther King uttered this chilling commentary upon another of the greatest scientific discoveries and technological applications of our time:

The means by which we live have outdistanced the ends for which we live. Our scientific power has outrun our spiritual power. We have guided missiles and misguided men.[153]

It is my hope that, when judgement is passed on what has been done on the law and infertility in Victoria, in the years between the State's sesqui-centenary and Australia's Bicentenary, it will be this — that we did manage to strike a wise balance, where the best ends were pursued, but only by the best means.

NOTES

1   The Hon J. H. Kennan M.L.C., 20 March 1984 Parliamentary Debates 1983–4, vol.373, p. 1840 second reading: 21 March 1984; debate adjourned until 18 April 1984. See *Victorian Parliamentary Debates*, 1983–4, vol. 374, pp. 2316–38.
2   Idem.
3   Section 29(1) of the Infertility (Medical Procedures) Act 1984 provides that the committee shall consist of

   (a)   a person holding a qualification in the study of philosophy;
   (b)   two medical practitioners;
   (c)   two persons representing religious bodies;
   (d)   a person qualified in social work;
   (e)   a legal practitioner; and
   (f)   a person qualified as a teacher with an interest in community affairs

   to be appointed by the Minister [of Health], one of whom shall be appointed as chairman.
   Section 29(6) establishes the functions of the Committee:

   (a)   to advise the Minister in relation to infertility and procedures for alleviating infertility;
   (b)   to consider requests for approval of and, if it sees fit, to approve, experimental procedures for the purposes of s.6(3) [which are experimental procedures prohibited but for this approval by the Committee];
   (ba) to consider requests for the approval of, and if it sees fit, to approve a procedure to which s.9A applies [viz. an experimental procedure involving the fertilization of a human ovum from the point of sperm penetration prior to but not including the point of syngamy]; and
   (c)   to advise and report to the Minister on any matters relating to infertility and procedures for alleviating infertility and any other associated matters referred to it by the Minister.
4   See notes 68, 72, 74 and 75, below.
5   *Victoria Government Gazette*, No. 67, 6 August 1986, pp. 3011–12; sections 3, 6(1–4) and 6(6–8), 7, 8, 9, 24–8, 30–3.
6   The Infertility (Medical Procedures) (Amendment) Act 1987 was passed 'to make provision for the regulation of certain procedures involving human gametes' (s.1).

   S.4(1) amended s.6(5) of the Principal Act;

S.4(2) inserted s.9A into the Principal Act;

S.4(3) inserted s.13A into the Principal Act; and

S.4(4) inserted a definition of 'approved experimental procedure' in s.3(1) and slightly altered several other definitions within that section.

And see *Victorian Government Gazette*, no. G16, 4 May 1988, p. 1123.

7   On 11 March 1982 the then Attorney-General for Victoria, the Hon H. Storey, M.L.C. and the then Minister of Health, the Hon W. Borthwick, M.L.C. announced the government's intention to establish a committee to investigate the social, ethical and legal issues surrounding the procedure of *in vitro* fertilization in Victoria. Victoria, Committee to Consider the Social, Ethical and Legal Issues Arising from In Vitro Fertilization, *Interim Report*, September 1982, p.1, para.1.

8   The composition of the Committee was as follows: *Professor Louis Waller*, Sir Leo Cussen Professor of Law, Monash University, and Law Reform Commissioner (appointed chairman in March, 1982); *Reverend Dr Francis Harman*, Parish Priest of Clifton Hill and Presiding Judge of the National Tribunal of the Catholic Church; *Mrs Jasna Hay*, former teacher with interests in migrant welfare and education; *Reverend Dr John Henley*, Lecturer in Christian Ethics and Dean of Melbourne College of Divinity; *Professor Priscilla Kincaid-Smith*, Professor of Medicine, University of Melbourne; Director, Department of Nephrology, Royal Melbourne Hospital; *Ms Eva Learner*, social worker and Director of Human Resource Centre of La Trobe University and the Lincoln Institute of Health Sciences; *Dr James McDonald*, general practitioner with a substantial practice in obstetrics and gynaecology and Area Coordinator for the Family Medicine Programme; *Miss Lynette Opas*, barrister-at-law of the Victorian Bar in family law; *Professor Roger Pepperell*, Professor of Obstetrics and Gynaecology, University of Melbourne.

The remaining members of the Committee were appointed on 24 May, 1982, by the Cain government: Victoria, Committee to Consider the Social Ethical and Legal Issues Arising from In Vitro Fertilization (1982), *Interim Report*, September, p.1, para. 1.

9   The Committee's terms of reference were:

'To consider whether the process of in vitro fertilization (IVF) should be conducted in Victoria, and, if so, the procedures and guidelines that should be implemented in respect of such processes in legislative form or otherwise.'

Ibid.; more specific considerations are listed on pp. 2–3.

10   Examples, as follow, appear in *The Age* (Melbourne), in the latter half of November 1981:Barnard, M. (1981), 'Time for conscience to catch up', *The Age*, 24 November, p. 13, col. 5; 'Embryo test programme called grisly', *The Age*, 20 November, 1981, p. 16, col. 3; Kearney, B. (1981), 'Certainly, life does not begin at birth', *The Age*, 17 November, p. 12, col. 1; Little, Archbishop T.F. (1981), 'Grant for research on human embryos must cause gravest concern', *The Age*, 19 November, p. 16, col. 1; McIntosh, P. (1981), 'Test tube baby ban urged', *The Age*, 23 November, p. 5, col. 3; Miles, Mrs. L. (1981), 'Research helps childless couples', *The Age*, 27 November, p. 12, col. 2; Santamaria, Dr J.N., (1981), 'In vitro fertilization is morally wrong', *The Age*, 27 November, p. 12, col. 1; Singer, Professor P. and Kuhse, H. (1981), 'Personal view on bioethics', *The Age*, 25 November, p. 12, col. 4; Uren, J. W. (1981), 'To initiate human life for experiments defies medical ethics', *The Age*, 30 November, p. 12.

11   See 'The first test tube baby', *Time*, 31 July 1978, p. 46 at p. 49.
12   Ibid., p. 52.
13   Ibid. See *Newsweek*, 7 August 1978, p. 47: Leo Abse, British MP, stated that 'the issue is how far we play God, how far we are going to treat mankind as we would animal husbandry'.

   British geneticist Robert J. Berry, consultant to the board set up by the Church of England to consider issues like the Brown baby, said, 'Western society is built around the family; once you divorce sex from procreation, what happens to the family?'

   Dr Malcolm Potts, executive director of the International Fertility Research Program in North Carolina, USA, suggested that 'it's a human and useful thing, but it's a cookbook thing . . . [Fertilization outside the body] is something frogs do in a dirty stream'.

   And from the Reverend William B. Smith, spokesperson for the Archdiocese of New York: 'I call it switching the marital bed into a chemistry set', *Time*, 31 July 1978.
14   Some examples are: Louise Brown, *Time*, 31 July 1978; *Newsweek*, 7 August, 1978, p. 44; *International Herald Tribune* Sat.–Sun. 29–30 July 1978; also Candice Reed: McIntosh, P.(1980), 'Test tube baby Candice enters a silent world', *The Age*, 24 June, p. 3, col. 1.
15   Metherell, M. (1981), 'Test tube team increases pregnancy success rate', *The Age*, 27 October, p. 5, col. 3.
16   Metherell, M. (1981), 'Grant for study of embryos', *The Age*, 19 November, p. 3, col. 5.
17   Carbines, L. (1981), 'Archbishop urges rethink on embryo experimentation', *The Age*,. 10 December, p. 20, col. 3.
18   O'Callaghan, M.-L. (1985), 'Halt test-tube baby work: two churches', *The Age*, 25 January, p. 3, col. 1.
19   Oke, K. and Aitken, J. (1982), 'The implications of IVF for the individual', in M. Brumby (ed.), *Proceedings of the Conference — In Vitro Fertilization: Problems and Possibilities*, Clayton: Monash Centre for Human Bioethics, p. 7 at p. 70.
20   Metherell, M. (1982), 'Test-tube ethics: doctor calls for study', *The Age*, 9 January, p. 3, col. 1.
21   Victoria, Committee to Consider the Social, Ethical and Legal Issues Arising From In Vitro Fertilization (1982), *Interim Report*, September, p. 4, para. 2.
22   Ibid., p. 20, para. 5.5.
23   Ibid., p. 20, para. 5.6.
24   Ibid., pp. 21–2, para. 5.8.1.
25   Ibid., pp. 22–3, para. 5.8.2.
26   Ibid., p. 23, para. 5.8.3.
27   Ibid., p. 27, para. 5.10.2.
28   See Victoria, Committee to Consider the Social, Ethical and Legal Issues Arising from In Vitro Fertilization (1983), *Report on Donor Gametes in IVF*, August, Appendices C, D and E, pp. 62–7; also Victoria, Committee to Consider the Social, Ethical and Legal Issues Arising from In Vitro Fertilization (1984), *Report on the Disposition of Embryos Produced by IVF*, August, Appendices D, E, F and G, pp. 79–88.
29   Victoria Committee, *Report on Donor Gametes*, op. cit., pp. 10–12, paras 2.6, 2.7 and 2.8 (donor gametes) and p. 40, para 5.5 (donor embryos).
30   Ibid., p. 30, para. 3.40.
31   Ibid., p. 18, para. 3.10.
32   Ibid., p. 18, para. 3.12.

33 Ibid., p. 19, para. 3.14 (donors) and p. 15, para. 3.4 (couples).
34 Ibid., pp. 24–5, paras 3.26–8.
35 Ibid., p. 27, para. 3.32.
36 Ibid., p. 36, paras 4.9–11, with reference to pp. 33–5, paras 4.5–6.
37 Ibid., p. 31, para. 3.42.
38 Ibid., pp. 26–7, paras 3.29–30, and 3.33.
39 Ibid., p. 26, para. 3.30.
40 Ibid., p. 11, para. 2.6 (Rev. Dr Frank Harman) and Appendix A, p. 49, especially pp. 50–1.
41 Ibid., Rev. Dr Frank Harman, Appendix A, pp. 52–6; Mrs Jasna Hay, Appendix B, pp. 59–61.
42 Victoria Committee, *Report on Disposition of Embryos*, op. cit., Rev. Dr Frank Harman, pp. 17–18, paras 1.27–29, and Appendix A, pp. 62–71, paras A1.1–A5.
43 Ibid., Mrs Jasna Hay, pp. 21–2, para. 1.38, and Appendix B, pp. 72–4, paras B.1.1–B.3.2.
44 Ibid., p. 22, para. 1.41.
45 Ibid., pp. 24–5, paras 2.1–3.
46 Ibid., p. 19, para. 1.30.
47 Ibid., p. 32, para. 2.17.
48 Ibid., p. 17, para 1.25, and p. 30, para. 2.14.
49 Ibid., p. 32, para. 2.18.
50 Ibid., p. 29, para. 2.12.
51 Ibid., p. 46, para. 3.26.
52 Ibid., p. 46, para. 3.27.
53 Ibid., p. 47, para. 3.28.
54 Ibid., p. 45, para. 3.24 (Rev. Dr Harman and Mrs Hay) and Appendix A, p. 70, para. A4.2.
55 Ibid., pp. 47–8, paras 3.30–31, and Appendix C, pp. 75–8, paras C1.1–C.2.5 (Professor Kincaid-Smith and Professor Pepperell).
56 Ibid., pp. 40–2, paras 3.18–19.
57 Commonwealth, Senate Select Committee on the Human Embryo Experimentation Bill 1985 (1986), *Human Embryo Experimentation in Australia*, Canberra: AGPS, p. 25.
58 Victoria Committee, *Report on Disposition of Embryos*, op. cit., p. 48, para. 3.32.
59 Victoria Committee, *Report on Donor Gametes*, op. cit., p. 18, para. 3.10.
60 Victoria Committee, *Report on Disposition of Embryos*, p. 50, para. 4.6, and p. 52, para. 4.11.
61 Ibid., pp. 52–3, para. 4.11.
62 Ibid., p. 53, paras 4.12–13.
63 Ibid., pp. 51–2, para. 4.9.
64 Ibid., p. 53, para. 4.14.
65 Ibid., p. 54, para. 4.16.
66 Ibid., p. 54, para. 4.17.
67 Victoria Committee, *Report on Donor Gametes*, op. cit., p. 8, para. 1.8; also *Report on Disposition of Embryos*, op. cit., p. 55, para. 5.2.
68 Ibid., pp. 56–7, paras 5.4–7.
69 See note 1. And see Victoria, *Parliamentary Debates*, 1984, vol. 374, p. 2316. When this debate recommenced, the opposition called for the debate to be adjourned again until the publication of the Committee's *Final Report*, so that its recommendations could be incorporated into the Bill, thus creating a broader Act. The government wished to accelerate the passage of the Bill in its then form, arguing that the Bill should be made law as the

issue had been left unlegislated for too long already. The government also suggested that if the Bill was not passed at that particular time, but instead, debate was adjourned, there was a distinct possibility that the Bill would never become law. Nonetheless, debate on the Bill was adjourned until 4 October 1984.

70   Ibid., vol. 375, pp. 556–7; vol. 376, p. 738.
71   Ibid., vol. 376, pp. 805–37, and pp. 1313–15.
72   Infertility (Medical Procedures) Act 1984 (Vic.) s.29(6)(a) and (c).
73   Infertility (Medical Procedures) Act 1984 (Vic.) s.29(6)(b).
74   Victoria Committee, *Report on Disposition of Embryos*, op. cit. pp. 45–6, paras 3.26–27.
75   Infertility (Medical Procedures) Act 1984 (Vic.) s.6(1) and (2)(a).
76   See Brumby, M. and Kasimba, P. (1987), 'When is cloning lawful?', *Journal of In Vitro Fertilization and Embryo Transfer*, **4(4)**, pp. 198–204, esp. at p. 199, where the authors state that a basic criterion for a definition of cloning requires that 'the members of a clone are identical in character one with another' (relying on *Dorland's Illustrated Medical Dictionary*, (26th edn), Philadelphia: W.B. Saunders, 1981.
77   Infertility (Medical Procedures) Act 1984 (Vic.) s.6(1) and (2)(b).
78   Infertility (Medical Procedures) Act 1984 (Vic.) s.14(1)(b).
79   Victoria, Standing Review and Advisory Committee on Infertility (1988), *First Report to the Minister for Health in Terms of Section 29 of the Infertility (Medical Procedures) Act 1984*, September, p. 1. The Committee was appointed in June 1985.
80   Ibid., p. 7. The eight members, and their categories, are: *Miss Jan Aitken*, s.29(d); *Dr Christine Bayly* (who replaced *Professor Roger Pepperell* in June 1988), s.29(b); *Professor Max Charlesworth*, s.29(a); *Rev. Dr Frank Harman*, s.29(c); *Mrs Jasna Hay*, s.29(f); *Rev. Dr John Henley*, s.29(c); *Mr Peter Paterson*, s.29(b); *Professor Louis Waller* (Chairman) s.29(e).
81   Ibid., p. 14, para. 3.4.3.5.
82   Ibid., p. 14, para. 3.4.3.6.
83   Ibid., p. 14, para. 3.4.3.7.
84   Chen, C. (1986), 'Pregnancy after human oocyte cryopreservation'. *The Lancet*, 19 April, p. 884.
85   Victoria, Standing Review and Advisory Committee, *First Report*, op. cit., p. 15, para. 3.4.3.9.
86   National Health and Medical Research Council (1987), *Consideration by Institutional Ethics Committees of Research Protocols Involving Frozen-Thawed Human Ova: Statement by the NHMRC Medical Research Ethics Committee*, Canberra: AGPS, p. 1. Also noted in Victoria Standing Review and Advisory Committee, *First Report*, op. cit., p. 14, para. 3.4.3.8.
87   *Dorland's Illustrated Medical Dictionary* (1988), Philadelphia: W.B. Saunders, p. 344, 'Cleavage' is defined as 'the mitotic segmentation of the fertilized ovum, the size of the structure remaining unchanged, as the cleavage cells . . . become smaller and smaller with each division'.
88   Ibid., p. 1556. 'Spermatozoon' is defined as 'a mature male germ cell . . ., the generative element of the semen which serves to fertilize the ovum'.
89   Ibid., p. 871. 'Karyotype' is defined as 'the full chromosome set of the nucleus of a cell'.
90   The *Dorland* definition is as follows: 'Embryo' is defined as being '. . . those derivatives of the fertilized ovum that eventually become their offspring . . . in man, the developing organism is an embryo from about two weeks after fertilization to the end of the seventh or eighth week'. Two definitions are quoted by Members of the Legislative Council of Victoria during the

drafting of the Infertility (Medical Procedures) (Amendment) Bill 1987: Victoria, *Parliamentary Debates*, Council, Spring Session 1987, vol. 388. At p. 784, the Hon G.P. Connard quotes and approves the definition of 'embryo' as stated in a letter from the Standing Review and Advisory Committee on Infertility to the Minister for Health, signed by Professor Waller. That definition stated that an embryo is 'the developing organism formed directly or indirectly as a result of any penetration by human sperm of the cytoplasmic membrane of a human ovum or any parthenogenetic activation of a human ovum'. The Hon B.A. Chamberlain (at p. 793) repeats this definition. attributing it to the Rev. Dr Frank Harman. The Hon M.T. Tehan (at 790) submits that an embryo is 'The organism formed by the sperm penetration of the membrane of the human ovum'.

91   Victoria Standing Review and Advisory Committee, *First Report*, op. cit., Appendix 8A, p. 135.

92   See Infertility (Medical Procedures) Act 1984 (Vic.) ss.5(1), 6(1),(3),(5), (6),9A(2)(b),(3), 11(2),(3),(4),(5),(6), 12(5),(6), 13(5),(6),(7),(9), 13A(5),(6), 17, 18, 19, 23(1), 25, 27, 28, 30, 33.

93   Victoria Standing Review and Advisory Committee, *First Report*, Appendix 8A, pp. 137–8.

94   Ibid., p. 139.

95   Ibid.

96   Ibid., Appendix 8B, p. 142.

97   Ibid., Appendix 8D, p. 150.

98   See Victoria, *Parliamentary Debates*, Council, Autumn Session, 1987, vol. 387, pp. 1304–6.

99   See ibid., Spring Session 1987, vol. 388, pp. 775–94; vol. 389, pp. 1695–7.

100   Pronuclear surgical transfer.

101   Zygote intrafallopian transfer.

102   Victoria, *Parliamentary Debates*, Council, Spring Session, 1987, vol. 389, pp. 1695–7.

103   Victoria Standing Review and Advisory Committee, *First Report*, op. cit., p. 40, paras 5.4.2.1 and 5.4.2.2.

104   Status of Children (Amendment) Act 1984 (Vic.) s.10E(2)(a) and (b).

105   Status of Children (Amendment) Act 1984 (Vic.) s.10C(2)(a); s10D(2)(a).

106   Adoption (Amendment) Act 1987 (Vic.) s.13(3)(d).

107   Section 13 of the Infertility (Medical Procedures) Act 1984 (Vic.) came into force on 1 July 1988: *Victorian Government Gazette*, no. G16, Wednesday 4 May 1988, p. 1123.

108   See now New South Wales Law Reform Commission (1988), *Artificial Conception Surrogate Motherhood*, December and Australian Health Ministers Conference and the Council of Social Welfare Ministers: *Communique*, Adelaide, 26 March 1991.

109   Victoria Standing Review and Advisory Committee, *First Report*, op cit.

110   Stephen, Sir N. Southey, Memorial Lecture 1981: 'Judicial Independence – A Fragile Bastion', *MULR*, **13**, 334 at 342.

111   Victoria Committee, *Interim Report*, op. cit., p. 19, para. 5.1.

112   Infertility (Medical Procedures) Act 1984 (Vic.) s.29(8).

113   Infertility (Medical Procedures) Act 1984 (Vic.) s.29(8).

114   Infertility (Medical Procedures) Act 1984 (Vic.) s.29(12)(a).

115   In *Mt Isa Mines* v. *Pusey* (1970) 125, CLR, 383 at 395.

116   Corns, C. (1987), 'In vitro fertilisation: the problem of regulation', *LIJ*, p. 791 at 792–3.

117   See Jansen, R. (1987), *Med. J. Aust*, **146**, p. 338, and also p. 362.

118   Terry, P. (1988), 'Surrogate mother to be "Special aunt"', *The Australian*,

20 October, p. 1, col. 3.
119 Esther 1.19.
120 See notes 99 and 102.
121 The Queen Victoria Medical Centre (now the Monash Medical Centre) and the Royal Women's Hospital.
122 Mercy Maternity Hospital (now the Mercy Hospital for Women) initiated a GIFT programme in 1986.
123 Artificial Conception Act 1984 (NSW).
124 Status of Children (Amendment) Act 1985 (Tas.); Artificial Conception Act 1985 (WA); Status of Children (Amendment) Act 1985 (NT); Family Relationships (Amendment) Act 1984 (S.A.); Artificial Conception Ordinance 1985 (ACT); Status of Children Act (Amendment) Act 1988 (Qld).
125 In Vitro Fertilization (Restriction) Act 1987 (SA). Section 4(2) limits IVF procedures to:

    (a) the University of Adelaide and The Queen Elizabeth Hospital;
    (b) the Flinders University of South Australia and the Flinders Medical Centre;
    (c) the IVF programme conducted by Repromed Pty Limited at the Wakefield Memorial Hospital.

126 Reproductive Technology Act 1988 (SA), s.5(1) and (2).
127 Reproductive Technology Act 1988 (SA), s.10.
128 Reproductive Technology Act 1988 (SA), s.13.
129 Reproductive Technology Act 1988 (SA), s.14.
130 Family Relationships Act Amendment Act 1988 (SA). Section 6, which inserts (amongst other provisions) s.10g(1) and (2) into the Family Relationships Act 1975 (SA).
131 Family Relationships Act Amendment Act 1988 (SA), s.6, amending s.10h of the Principal Act.
132 Surrogate Parenthood Act 1988 (Qld), s.3(1).
133 Surrogate Parenthood Act 1988 (Qld), s.4(2).
134 Surrogate Parenthood Act 1988 (Qld), s.3(2).
134a Western Australia enacted its Human Reproductive Technology Act in November 1991.
135 See *IME Bulletin*, August 1987, and *Bioethics News*, **7**(2), 1988, pp. 4–5.
136 *Nature*, **331**, 18 February 1988, p. 555, and see *The Times*, 25 October 1990.
137 United Kingdom, Department of Health and Social Security (1987), *Human Fertilisation and Embryology: A Framework for Legislation*, Cmnd 259, London: HMSO.
138 United Kingdom, Department of Health and Social Security (1984), *Report of the Committee of Inquiry into Human Fertilisation and Embryology* (The 'Warnock Committee'), Cmnd 9314, London: HMSO, pp. 80–6.
139 Surrogacy Arrangements Act 1985 (UK), s.2(1).
140 See Rozenberg, J. (1985), 'Commercial surrogates', *The Listener*, 17 January, p. 9.
141 See Human Fertilisation and Embryology Act 1990: on status, ss. 27 ('mother'), 28 ('father'), 30 ('commissioning' parents in altruistic surrogacy); on counselling see s. 13(6), conditions of licence for treatment.
142 *Stern* v. *Whitehead*, 1988, 56, USLW, 3442. For further discussion see Chapter 9 of this volume.
143 In *Doe* v. *Kelly*, 1980, 6, FLR, 3011.
144 See OTA (1988), *Infertility – Medical and Social Choices*, Washington DC: OTA, May, pp. 285 and 288.

145   Ibid.
146   The Parliament of the Commonwealth of Australia (1985), *IVF and the Status of Children: Report by the Senate Standing Committee on Constitutional and Legal Affairs on National Uniformity of law Relating to the Status of Children Born through the use of In Vitro Fertilisation*, Canberra: AGPS.
146a See pp. 26–7, above.
147   *TB. Berakhot*, 31 b.
148   Gold, M. (1985), *And Hannah Wept*, Philadelphia: JPSA, p. 5.
149   Victoria Committee, *Interim Report*, op. cit., p. 4, para. 2.
150   Infertility (Medical Procedures) Act 1984 (Vic.) s.10(3)(a), s.11(3)(a), s.12(3)(a), s.13(3)(a), s.13A(3)(a).
151   Infertility (Medical Procedures) Act 1984 (Vic.) s.18.
152   Infertility (Medical Procedures) Act 1984 (Vic.) s.6(3) and (4).
153   King, Martin Luther (1963), *Strength to Love*, New York: Harper and Row, p. 57.

3 Canada: The Ontario Law Reform Commission Project on Human Artificial Reproduction

BERNARD DICKENS

INTRODUCTION

The Ontario Law Reform Commission (OLRC) received its terms of reference for the Project on Human Artificial Reproduction and Related Matters in November 1982, and initiated its research at the beginning of 1983. The Commissioners concluded their substantive deliberations before the September of 1984. The Report of the United Kingdom Committee of Inquiry into Human Fertilisation and Embryology,[1] known as the Warnock Committee, was released in July of that year, after the Commissioners had decided on almost all of their recommendations. The OLRC Report was ready for release by January 1985, but, because the Project was initiated by the Ontario Attorney-General's reference, the Report could not be released until its presentation to the Attorney-General and tabling before the Ontario provincial legislature, which was prorogued early in 1985 pending a provincial election. Following the election, the Report was tabled and released to the public.

The delayed publication of the Report, following the release of the Warnock Committee Report by some months, caused several commentators to conclude that, to the extent that the OLRC recommendations were congruent with those of the Warnock Report, the Commissioners had simply adopted the Warnock approach.[2] In fact, however, the Commissioners independently arrived at many recommendations that were also favoured by the Warnock Committee in the areas of gamete (sperm and ovum) and embryo donation, *in vitro* fertilization and related techniques. The OLRC departed fundamentally from Warnock, however, and indeed all other pre-existing and most other subsequent governmentally-related reports on reproductive technologies, in their recommendations on surrogate motherhood.

This chapter reviews the factual and political history leading to the OLRC Project's terms of reference, the method of approach adopted by the Commissioners, the main reasoning behind the Commission's principal recommendations, and some responses to the recommendations.

HISTORY OF THE PROJECT'S TERMS OF REFERENCE

The population and government of Ontario were aware of the potential for surrogate motherhood agreements to be reached from the time when they gained general publicity in North America in the late 1970s, but felt no need to respond legally or otherwise to the prospect of such arrangements involving Ontario couples until such a case came to light early in 1982. It appeared that a couple resident in the Toronto suburb of Scarborough had engaged the services of the Dearborn, Michigan lawyer, Noel Keane, to arrange and negotiate an agreement for surrogate motherhood. The couple were infertile, and Noel Keane had attracted considerable attention in North America for identifying and recruiting women who were willing to serve infertile couples as surrogate mothers, usually for payment. The Scarborough couple, through Noel Keane, agreed with a woman from Florida that she would be artificially inseminated with the husband's sperm, conceive and give birth to a child and surrender it to the couple. The agreement was successfully concluded when the woman gave birth in a Scarborough hospital, where she left the baby on her return to the United States. The biological father, the husband of the commissioning couple, went to the hospital to take custody of his child. The hospital declined to surrender the child to him, however, since it considered the child to have been abandoned by its mother, and was not prepared to hand it to a stranger who claimed to be a relative. In the province of Ontario, responsibility for an abandoned child falls on a Children's Aid Society, a quasi-public agency mandated by statute to protect children who are abandoned or otherwise in need of protection. In Toronto, Hamilton and Windsor in the province of Ontario, in addition to secular societies, religious denominational Children's Aid Societies exist, largely because of the sizeable Roman Catholic communities in those cities. Public hospital regulations require that, on admission, patients' religions should usually be noted, and that if a child is suspected to be in need of protection and its parent is known to be Roman Catholic (or, in Toronto, Jewish), the Children's Aid Society to be notified shall be that of the parent's religious affiliation. On her admission to the Scarborough hospital the woman from Florida had stated that she was Roman Catholic. Accordingly, when the hospital found itself in custody of her abandoned baby, it notified the Toronto Catholic Children's Aid Society.

The father meanwhile took legal advice, and went to the Ontario Supreme Court to obtain a declaration of paternity, giving evidence that established his biological link to the child. The Society declined to surrender the child to him without a judicial order to this effect, but it had a major secondary concern. The infertile couple were also Roman Catholic, and had earlier applied to the Society to be considered to receive a child for adoption. They had been assessed as unsuitable to be adoptive parents, however, on the grounds both of advanced paternal age (the husband was aged over 40 years) and his physical disability, although this appeared to be relatively minor.

Staff of the Society were particularly exercised by this experience not simply because it offended their sense of religious precepts but because it demonstrated how social workers' professional role as gatekeepers against those whom they assess as unsuitable to become parents can be evaded and rendered futile by surrogate motherhood agreements. Agency staff showed considerable hostility to the Scarborough couple gaining custody of the child, but were compelled to surrender it to them when the Supreme Court granted the husband a declaration of his paternity. The Society presented no evidence that the child in his custody would have been in need of legal protection, or that he or his wife were unfit parents according to any legally set standard. The fact that standards of suitability to adopt a child were much higher than legal standards set for parents to retain custody of their existing children reflected the scarcity of adoptable children and the artificially high standards that Children's Aid Societies had come to apply regarding their placement.

The provincial minister responsible for child welfare and for the operation of Children's Aid Societies was the Minister of Community and Social Services, who at the time was Frank Drea. As a Roman Catholic, he was particularly responsive to complaints from the Toronto Catholic Children's Aid Society that the Scarborough couple had prevailed to obtain custody of the husband's child. He asked the Ministry's legal department to initiate whatever proceedings they could against the couple. It was anticipated, correctly as it happened, that the wife of the couple would soon initiate adoption proceedings in order to regularize her legal relationship to the child she intended to rear as her own, and it was speculated that, although the father did not have to undertake such proceedings, he might do so in order to give the child a birth certificate revealing its surname as his.

The father's adoption proceeding was almost impossible to oppose on legal grounds, and such proceedings by the wife, as a step-parent, would be approved almost as automatically, both because step-parent adoption would serve the child's best interests and because refusal would be of little effect since the wife would continue to rear the child of which her husband had lawful custody, in their joint home. Legal consideration was given to whether the payment to the woman who bore the child and who would consent to any adoption proceedings was a violation of the provincial statute that made it an offence to offer, and to receive, money in exchange for consent to adoption. It was legally concluded, however, that adoption consent was, if at all, only a minor part of the surrogate motherhood agreement, and that, in any event, adoption could proceed without the birth mother's consent, so that any promise she made to give consent for the purpose of adoption proceedings was largely inconsequential. Although news media at the time carried rather frenzied discussions of baby-selling, prostitution and even slavery analogies, the Ministry's legal department advised that there were no legal proceedings that could be taken in good faith against the Scarborough couple. Reinforcing the conclusion that no proceedings should be brought was the realization that to bring unsuccessful proceedings would show that the Ministry had acted ineptly and perhaps oppressively, and that surrogate motherhood agreements were lawful. It was considered inappropriate to initiate legal proceedings that were unlikely to succeed, would compromise the child's privacy and advertise to the watching public that surrogate motherhood agreements were beyond legal regulation.

Questions and statements in the Legislative Assembly of Ontario showed concern that the legalities surrounding surrogate motherhood appeared uncertain, the Minister of Community and Social Services being particularly indignant that such a transaction could be completed without restriction or liability to any form of prior scrutiny. He rejected arguments that the same is true of natural procreation of children by pointing to the presence of commercial brokerage and payments. The Minister went further by observing that he would ensure that the matter would be considered by the OLRC. In fact he lacked legal authority to do this, since by law only the provincial Attorney-General was able to refer issues to the OLRC for deliberation and report. The Attorney-General, R. Roy McMurtry, QC, recognized the political pressure on the government to take some action, and was sympathetic to the OLRC preparing a study of the area and proposing to the government any reform of the law it considered appropriate.

Officers in the Policy and Planning Division of the Attorney-General's Department consulted informally with the OLRC staff and others about how the project could best be defined, and in particular about what its scope should be. It was quickly accepted that concentration simply on surrogate motherhood would be too narrow. The process could be undertaken by such crude means as insemination in private through use of such instruments as turkey-basters or through natural intercourse, but could also be related to such reproductive technology as is used in *in vitro* fertilization (IVF), which would involve the services of health professionals and hospital or related facilities. Clinics might be run on a private basis, but the overwhelming majority of health services in Ontario are delivered through public hospitals and related facilities over which the provincial Ministry of Health has influence and for the quality and nature of whose services the Minister of Health is responsible. It was therefore decided that the occasion should be taken to review legal aspects of the general medical practice of assisted or artificial human reproduction.

Awareness had arisen that sperm donation was being arranged in order to overcome some forms of infertility, and that ovum donation was an immediate prospect. Donation of pre-embryos was not addressed in the drafting of the OLRC Project's terms of reference, but the rate of development of reproductive technologies was such that between the first meeting the Commissioners held on the project in mid-November 1982 and the second meeting early in January 1983 it was announced in California that a healthy baby had been born by pre-embryo transplantation. The intention of the terms of reference was to permit a comprehensive examination of the practice of artificial reproduction. The OLRC described the Project in its earliest stages as involving human artificial insemination, because this was employed in the surrogate motherhood instance in which the Project originated, but it was quickly recognized that much more was involved. The Project was accordingly renamed to address human artificial reproduction and related matters. The title of neither the project nor the Report it was designed to produce referred to surrogate motherhood, because the Commissioners did not want the Project or Report to be known, as they feared it might be because of news media preoccupation with surrogacy, as the Surrogate Motherhood Project and Report.

The Project's terms of reference were defined in the Letter of Reference of 5 November 1982 sent by the Attorney-General of Ontario to the then Chairman of the OLRC, Dr Derek Mendes da Costa, QC,[3] which read:

I wish to request that the Ontario Law Reform Commission inquire into and consider the legal issues relating to the practice of human artificial insemination, including 'surrogate mothering' and transplantation of fertilized ova to a third party. I would be pleased to have the Commission report on the range of alternatives for resolution of any legal issues that may be identified.

In conducting your study, I would be grateful if you would include the following considerations within the scope of the review:

1. The legal status and legal rights of the child and the safeguards for protecting the best interests of the child.
2. The legal rights and legal duties of each biological parent.
3. The legal rights and legal duties of the spouse, if any, of each biological parent.
4. The nature and enforceability of agreements relating to artificial insemination and related practices.
5. The nature and enforceability of agreements respecting custody of the child.
6. The legal rights and liabilities of medical and other personnel involved in performing artificial insemination and other related practices.
7. The legal procedures for establishing and recognizing the biological parentage of children born as a result of these practices.
8. The applicability of present custody and adoption laws in such cases.
9. The availability of information to identify the child and the parties involved.
10. Such medical and related evidence as may have a bearing on the legal issues raised in these cases.

I am certain that the Commission will appreciate the deep importance of these issues for the persons involved, particularly the children, and accordingly in the interests of these children, make the report available as soon as possible.

COMMENTARY ON THE TERMS OF REFERENCE

Both favourable and unfavourable responses to the OLRC Report failed in many cases to observe the essential conditioning of the project implicit in its being sought from and produced by a Law Reform Commission, and made explicit in the terms of reference. The Report requested by the Attorney-General, the senior Law Officer of the province, prepared in collaboration with legal consultants, by staff lawyers employed by the Commission was only concerned with matters of law. The terms of reference defined the Project to inquire into and consider 'the legal issues', including the 'legal status' and 'legal rights' of children produced by artificial reproduction, the 'legal rights' and 'legal duties' of biological parents and their spouses and of medical practitioners and other personnel involved, the 'legal procedures' for establishing and recognizing parentage of children, the applicability of custody and adoption laws and the bearing of medical and related evidence on legal issues. The Commissioners were 'acutely aware that these technologies pose ... profound philosophical, moral, ethical, social, and psychological questions that form the context within which the legal issues ultimately will have to be decided',[4] but undertook the Project as an exercise in potential law reform.

The Commissioners themselves – all distinguished lawyers – initially approached the project with some ambivalence. They were gratified that, when the goverment sensed public pressure to take effective action to resolve social perplexities presented by the new reproductive technologies, the Cabinet entrusted the task of resolution to the Commission. One Commissioner believed the issue of surrogacy to be so far outside the type of work to which the Commission was accustomed and that it was appropriate for it to tackle, however, that he considered resigning his commission in protest against the Attorney-General's reference. Public commentary on surrogate motherhood had been largely from religious doctrinal, philosophical, sociological and related orientations which were not of inherent legal interest, and it appeared that a legal response would be received in an emotionally charged and critical atmosphere in which legal principles were little appreciated. As the legal issues raised became evident, however, he recognized how suitable they were to be addressed by the Commission, and indeed at the conclusion of the Project observed that it had been one of the most rewarding and creative exercises of prospective law reform in which he had been engaged because of the important legal issues which the Project had disclosed. This satisfaction underscores the point, however, that the OLRC Project was undertaken and executed as an exercise in lawmaking. It was informed of ethical and related concerns, but accomplished its purpose by proposing legal reforms that were compatible with the surrounding jurisprudence – particularly recent legislation protecting the human rights and civil liberties perceived to contribute to the prevailing secular and pluralistic environment of the province and the country.[5]

Another key feature of the terms of reference is that they make no mention of infertility or of the concerns of those who suffer impaired fertility, but emphasize the protection of children who may be born through their parents' resort to artificial means of reproduction. The first enumerated consideration of the Attorney-General's reference concerns 'safeguards for protecting the best interests of the child', and the closing request for expedition is made 'in the interests of these children'. This emphasis controlled many of the Commissioners' approaches. A different emphasis might have produced differently directed recommendations. For instance, an emphasis on the best interests of couples who want to have children, or on individuals, or specifying that a goal such as the protection of women's interests be promoted, would probably have led to different recommendations on a number of issues, and indeed on which issues warrant consideration. The recommendations the OLRC made may be compatible with different priorities or agendas, but the prioritization of issues in the project was set not by the Commissioners, but through the terms of reference.

A point of context, rather than of commentary, should be made concerning the OLRC Project's terms of reference. In Canada, the Constitution Act 1867 allocates exercise of Criminal Law powers to the federal government. Provincial legislatures have jurisdiction over most family law matters, health care services, regulation of professions, and, for instance, commercial and contractual transactions. Provinces can, by legislation, create quasi-criminal offences provided that they are auxiliary to the pursuit of a legitimate provincial goal, but cannot criminalize acts because they are considered inherently wrong or immoral. The terms of reference of the Project must accordingly be read to preclude consideration and recommendation of truly criminal sanctions for misconduct on grounds of its wrongfulness or social harm. A goal related to control of medical practice or, for instance, pursuit of individuals' domestic well-being, might be reinforced through introduction of a summary offence of violating a newly enacted provincial statute that deals primarily with medical practice or family law or welfare.

While Canadian provincial legislation cannot create nor directly relieve criminal liability because this power is constitutionally given to the federal government of Canada, the federally promulgated Canadian Charter of Rights and Freedoms governs provincial legislation. The Charter, which is applicable to governmental activities including payment for health services, came into general effect in 1982. Its provision on rights to equal protection of the law and to non-discrimination came into effect in 1985, however, after a three-year period during which provinces were intended to adjust their laws to remove offensive terms. The prevailing atmosphere of accommodation to the Charter, including its provision opposing discrimination, notably on grounds of physical disability, influenced the Commissioners' selection of options available to meet the terms of reference. Further, the provincial Human Rights Code had been re-enacted in 1981, and it was presumed that the Project was intended to comply with its terms. The Code, which is applicable to all who offer services to the public, proscribes discrimination on grounds not only of physical disability, but also of marital status. An amendment made more recently prohibits discrimination on grounds of sexual orientation.

CONDUCT OF THE PROJECT

Shortly after the Project's terms of reference were settled and the Attorney-General's formal Letter of Reference was received by the Chairman of the OLRC, the Commission initiated its work by appointing the present writer as Project Consultant. A scheme of approach was developed with the Commission's legal staff and agreed in principle with the Commissioners, outlining major components of the study, indicating how they might be addressed, and proposing to invite particular people to join an Advisory Board to the project. The Board was designed to bring in relevant perspectives from outside and also within the discipline and profession of law, and to consider drafts of papers before their presentation to the Commissioners and offer their thoughts on the issues and proposals set out.

The Project was particularly fortunate in the calibre and dedication of members of the Advisory Board, which was a working board in every sense. Members brought in necessary information, sometimes after extensive individual research, professional perceptions and personal sensitivities of extraordinary richness and value. Members included Dr Michael D Bayles, a renowned Professor of Philosophy who was at the time Director of the Westminster Institute for Ethics and Human Values in London, Ontario. His book, *Reproductive Ethics*,[6] was being written at that time, reflecting a philosophically Utilitarian orientation. Reinforcement of the ethical contribution to the Advisory Board came from Dr Abbyann Lynch, another Professor of Philosophy, then at St Michael's College, a Roman Catholic college of the University of Toronto. Invaluable medical information was offered by Dr John Jarrell, then Director of the Infertility Centre at McMaster University Medical Centre in Hamilton, Ontario. Dr Jarrell introduced the perceptions not only of an active clinician leading patients through the most advanced reproductive techniques, but also of a scholar; he initiated a questionnaire survey of Ontario practitioners of donor insemination for the project, and maintained continuous vigilance of the contemporaneous medical literature for those working on the project. Also of immense benefit to the Project, on the latest biological techniques in use around the world and in foreseeable prospect, was the contribution of Dr David Armstrong, a professor at the University of Western Ontario's medical school department of physiology and obstetrics and gynaecology. Although not a member of the Advisory Board, Dr Murray Kroach of the Toronto East General and Orthopaedic Hospital's artificial insemination and *in vitro* fertilization services made himself available for discussions regarding patient management and clinical techniques.

A social work and sociological perspective was introduced by Dr Ruth Parry, a senior Professor of Social Work at the University of Toronto's graduate Faculty of Social Work and then Director of the Family Court Clinic in Toronto. She explained that surrogate motherhood was not new to the province or country, and that members of some ethnically distinctive communities where infertility was a stigma would accept privately conducted artificial insemination of a barren wife's consenting sister or, for instance, cousin, and the rearing of the resulting child in the immediate family of the wife and husband/father as the child of them both. Dr Parry was the only participant in the Project to have had direct experience of surrogate motherhood, which she found had proven unexceptional in practice. She provided a stabilizing influence when more wild and scandalous scenarios were imagined. Dr Paul Steinhauer, a leading authority in child psychiatry from the Hospital for Sick Children in Toronto, professor in the University of Toronto Medical School's department of psychiatry, where he was Director of Training in the Division of Child Psychiatry, introduced what was known about the effect on children's mental health and personalities of birth and growth in an unstable or unorthodox domestic environment. He was most influential in shaping some key recommendations on surrogate motherhood intended to serve the Project's terms of reference concerning promotion of the best interest of children so conceived.

Judge J. Wilma Scott, a Family Court judge from St Catherines, brought in her experience as a family law practitioner and jurist, particularly concerning the practicalities of different legal options and the role the courts might play, and David Aston, a lawyer from London, Ontario, perceived the prospective legal impact of proposals from a more generalized viewpoint including, for instance, their likely effect on inheritance and succession. Harry Nixon, a Toronto chartered accountant, addressed a variety of taxation questions raised by births of children and their arrival in families other than those of their birth mothers, but served mainly as the voice of an intelligent layperson in a world of medico-legal perplexities and introverted options.

The Advisory Board functioned collectively to review draft papers prepared by the Project Consultant based on research conducted in large part through the OLRC legal staff, particularly Larry Fox and Mel Springman, and then Commission Counsel M. Patricia Richardson. Following Advisory Board consideration, papers were then presented to the Commissioners, sometimes as amended and always accompanied by commentary on the Advisory Board's responses. The Commissioners considered the analysis of issues, presentation of legal options and the Project Consultant's and Advisory Board's recommendations, and arrived at their decisions. The OLRC Vice Chairman, H. Allan Leal, QC, dissented regarding most of the surrogate motherhood proposals made by the Commissioners,[7] and their preferences, while generally consistent with prevailing views in the Advisory Board, were not necessarily approved by every Board member.

When the Project was initiated following receipt of the Attorney-General's Letter of Reference, the OLRC announced the terms of reference through advertisements in each daily newspaper published in Ontario and sought written submissions from any person or organization wishing to make representations. In addition, the Chairman wrote to leading medical and related health professional associations, representatives of religious organizations, hospitals and medical schools, Children's Aid Societies and to the Ontario Branch of the Canadian Bar Association. In response, 35 briefs were submitted, all of which were made available to the Commissioners and members of the Advisory Board. The Project also convened meetings of the majority of medical practitioners of artificial insemination in Ontario, and of all actual and imminent IVF practitioners in Canada in 1983.

A particular challenge which the OLRC recognized was the introduction of women's or feminist perspectives. Women were present on the Advisory Board because of their potential to make specialized contributions to the Project and not simply because of their gender or experience of gestation and motherhood. Research was undertaken into feminist, women-oriented and women-derived literature in law, sociology, psychology and related areas, but the literature that has arisen in recent years was not available at the time the Report was in preparation; in Ontario, indeed, much feminist writing has been undertaken in response to the OLRC Report. The research that was possible disclosed no distinct feminist approach to surrogate motherhood and the new reproductive technologies. Fears had been expressed that surrogate motherhood and its means were exploitive particularly of poor women, and that the physical and emotional burden on women of chemical treatments for infertility had been understated. Countering this, however, was a policy emphasis, influenced by feminist writing on abortion, on legislation not being applied to control or direct women's medical choices, and more radical suspicion of institutions (notably some Churches) not generally accommodating of women's advancement or independence and seeming to direct women's behaviour by invoking women's need of protection. In the result, it appeared that feminist literature that expanded sensitivities gave no clear guidance and that women, as such, held as many varied opinions on artificial reproduction and surrogate motherhood as did men.

THE GENERAL APPROACH

Before addressing specific details of the reproductive technologies and surrogate motherhood, the Commissioners developed their general philosophy or orientation in the setting of which the details would be resolved. A full analysis of prevailing legislation and case law relevant to the reproductive technologies and surrogate motherhood had shown that considerable uncertainty and risk of dysfunctional effects had resulted from recourse to laws that were applicable only inadvertently or by reference to inexact analogies. This conclusion is of some historical interest, because the Commissioners' recommendations of 1985 remain unacted upon, but the practice of artificial reproduction in Ontario appears to have been neither obstructed nor facilitated by the unsatisfactory state of the law, and no discernible problems have arisen in the province from resort to surrogate motherhood. Discussion of these issues has been ideological and speculative, triggered at times by events elsewhere, notably the 1987 New Jersey *Baby M* case,[8] and not resting on any demonstrated local experience of harm or accommodation of outrageous or generally unacceptable practices.

It appeared that three general orientations might be applied in developing legal responses to artificial reproduction and surrogate motherhood, namely the approach of maximally accommodating individuals' private ordering of their reproductive behaviour, whether giving, acquiring, selling or purchasing reproductive services; the approach of establishing one of several levels of regulation of the ways in which individuals may act to achieve their own and other people's reproductive preferences; and the approach of legally prohibiting, denying or frustrating any pursuit of a reproductive deviation from procreation within marriage or a conservatively defined alternative stable domestic union.

The Private Ordering Approach

This approach predicates basically facilitating, non-judgemental laws through which individuals may plan, negotiate and complete their consensual reproductive activities according to their own goals, confident that the legal consequences that they intend will actually follow from their conduct, such as legitimacy of children in the families in which they will be reared, and non-recognition of mere gamete donors. Liberal or accommodating though this approach may be, it simply applies to artificially assisted reproduction the expectation of the state's accommodation of – or, at worst, non-involvement in – married couples' reproduction that prevails concerning natural reproduction, and recognizes what is already customary in many jurisdictions when full confidentiality is maintained of pregnancy through sperm donation – namely that all participants achieve what they intend. The approach respects the principle of not placing persons at disadvantage or visiting discrimination upon them when they suffer disability, which in this case will include reproductive disability.

The limit of this approach is implicit in the model on which it draws, namely marriage. The law sets conditions for marriage, such as minimum age and prohibition of consanguinity, and has traditionally not been accommodating of a spouse's reproduction that is achieved through the biological contribution of a third party. Further, at separation and divorce, spouses are not free to enforce any agreement they may reach on custody of children of the marriage; courts tend to recognize such agreements when they serve, or do not violate, the best interests of the children in question, but will disregard custody agreements that are inconsistent with children's best interests. The emphasis that the Project's terms of reference gave to pursuit of children's best interests has been noted above.

Nevertheless, the state's respect for the autonomy of married persons to initiate pregnancy, and their general freedom to agree to gamete donation for the purpose of reproduction, furnishes a model generally sympathetic to private ordering. Laws requiring prior screening of prospective gamete donors do not really limit reproductive freedom but may be seen to encourage responsible choice and reasonably to balance reproductive freedom with protection of prospective children's best interests. Similarly, the marital model is not harmed by legislation that bars the sale and purchase of sperm, as in principle do the Human Tissue Gift Acts of Ontario and other Canadian provinces, although such legislation that is restrictive of commerce may offend political principles favouring deregulation that have been developed in recent years. Influential legal writers have come to urge minimal public paternalism and greater respect for individual parental choices.[9]

The Regulatory Approach

In contrast to the *laissez-faire* philosophy underpinning the private ordering approach, the regulatory approach postulates a legal regime in which normative standards are set on the basis of *a priori* principles that rest on values transcending the preferences of those the law immediately affects. Such values may originate in ethical or moral precepts, or, for instance, rest on empirical data or perceptions regarding the public interest or the best interests of children. Ideally, regulatory principles will be rational and congruent with associated principles and practices, but they may also rest primarily on intuition, experience or the conditioning effects of culture. Public statement of the basis of regulation exposes it to scrutiny, criticism, debate and, if appropriate, correction from time to time.

Regulation may be undertaken at different levels of intensity or penetration, on a scale from the minimal to the almost prohibitive. The law on adoption illustrates not simply an area of operative regulation but an area relevant to artificial reproduction and applicable to surrogate motherhood; indeed, the approach the Commissioners took to surrogate motherhood has been conveniently described as 'surrogate adoption'. The goals of adoption regulation are to facilitate adoption of easily adoptable children and to encourage the adoption of so-called 'hard to place' children, but also to ensure, as far as possible, that children go to suitable homes and are likely to become happily settled where they are placed. Commerce is discouraged, in that public agencies are presumed to be most suitable to match children in need of adoption with applicants to adopt, but a margin of privately arranged adoptions is accommodated and private agencies may be licensed to operate.

A regulatory approach allows selection of particular elements of a scheme for special scrutiny. For instance, commercial aspects, profiteering tendencies or unwelcome potentials can attract high levels of control, and proven or trusted practices can receive almost automatic approval. Different agencies can be appointed or created to discharge regulatory functions, such as governmental department, ad hoc authorities or the courts. Where the scope for discretionary decisionmaking is sizeable and the interests affected are particularly significant or profound in their impact on personal happiness (as opposed, for instance, to their impact on material matters), the courts may be more suitable to exercise regulatory functions than governmental bureaucracies. Courts, in principle, function in public, although sensitive family matters in which children's well-being may be jeopardized by publicity can be conducted *in camera*; the legal principles applied in trial decisions are usually appealable; and the sense of procedural regularity or of due process is commonly more developed in courts of law than within administrative agencies.

The Prohibitory Approach

Practices that it is considered should be not just discouraged but actively prevented can be subjected to legislated prohibitions. It has been seen that a Canadian provincial law reform agency cannot recommend provincial legislation to render conduct a crime, although it can send its own recommendations on criminalization to the federal government of Canada, perhaps in particular to the federal Minister of Justice. Because provinces have constitutional authority to act regarding such matters as child welfare, personal and public health and the protection of the public against the unqualified and the unethical practice of medicine and law, however, disapproved conduct regarding artificial reproduction can be prohibited through the creation of appropriately directed provincial offences. At present, for instance, it is an offence to offer and receive money in exchange for consent for adoption of a child, and in exchange for the donation of body materials except blood or blood constituents. Leaving dependent children in need of protection and abusing children are provincial offences, even though incidents of assault of children or recklessly endangering them are concurrently punishable under the federal Criminal Code of Canada. Conducting an unlicensed private adoption agency may be provincially prohibited, and by analogy conducting a surrogate motherhood agency could be similarly prevented.

At the time of their deliberations, the Commissioners were unaware of the direction the Warnock Committee would take, but had become familiar with legal developments in other jurisdictions, notably the United States and Australia.[10] Gamete donation and IVF were seen to present acutely sensitive social issues but relatively few major problems of legal policy, the main legal tasks appearing to be to maintain standards of conscientious practice and to regularize relationships among different actors and resulting children in a reasonable and protective manner. The central prohibitory issue concerned surrogate motherhood. The Australian State of Victoria had pioneered prohibitive legislation that was somewhat more comprehensive than that which followed the Warnock Report in the UK, but similarly concentrated on the elimination of financial incentives to participation, operation of agencies designed to arrange transactions, and advertisements of, or for, surrogate motherhood services.[11]

The legal conclusion was reached that, in Ontario, surrogate motherhood agreements would be held unenforceable by the courts and probably void as being against public policy. While agreements would not be enforced *per se*, however, courts might be prepared to attach legal significance to the consequences of voluntary compliance with them, so that they would achieve their substantive goals on a consensual basis. The Commissioners therefore had to address whether and, if so, how they should be prohibited. Prevention of human organ and other tissue sales had been achieved with adequate success through the combination of human tissue gift legislation and control of the practice of medicine, but surrogate motherhood was not dependent on medical technology nor resort to health professional services. Establishment that artificial insemination and its equivalent of ovum transfer was 'the practice of medicine' would bring it under existing legislation regarding the unqualified and unethical practice of medicine, and so subject it to the regime of provincial offences, but natural intercourse for the purposes of surrogacy would remain unaffected and unsanctioned.

The Commissioners seriously considered the appropriateness of more strongly and directly prohibitive legislation, but finally accepted that such an approach would be dysfunctional, inadequate and a disservice to the terms of reference remitted by the Attorney-General. The penalization of some forms of voluntary parenthood seemed excessive and unduly stigmatizing of children who were born following a breach of the law, as well as creating a constitutionally suspect distinction between the fertile and the reproductively disabled. Further, strong prohibitions would compromise the development of legislation regularizing the domestic relations of children born despite the prohibitions, minimizing the legal uncertainty and potential for friction of integrating them into the homes in which they would be reared. The obligation to give priority to the best interests of the children militated against the establishment of rigorous and consistent prohibitions against their births. Prohibitive laws were considered likely not to serve the interests of such children, but rather to sacrifice them to abstract moralistic or ideological commitments.

The OLRC Approach

At the conclusion of their deliberations on fully analysed legal issues raised by artificial reproduction and surrogacy (the OLRC Report is in two volumes and contains 390 pages), the Commissioners rejected both extremes of the private ordering and the prohibitory approaches in favour of a hybrid approach. Different techniques of assisted reproduction were found to warrant different legal approaches, the governing factors being not the techniques *per se* but, rather, related to the wider settings in which the techniques are to be applied. It was noted, for instance, that legal regulation of adoption is quite intense regarding both the conduct of agencies and the procedures that result in completion of lawful adoption, but that, in contrast, recourse to therapeutic donor insemination is analogous to unregulated recourse to such therapies as microsurgical repair of damaged fallopian tubes that may result in natural fertilization. The area found to warrant a high level of regulation, namely surrogate motherhood, presented the issues discussed in the previous section, and also the possibility of the evasion of prohibitory laws by the execution of banned agreements in other easily accessible jurisdictions. Such agreements might be lawfully concluded there, perhaps resulting in judicially approved adoption that Ontario courts would recognize, if only on the humanitarian grounds of not leaving infants parentless out of the jurisdiction and separated from the only adult guardians willing to care for them.

The first principles of the OLRC approach were conditioned by the Common law tradition, which may differ from the Civil law's codified tradition, that individuals are free to act according to their wishes without first having to demonstrate a legal right of action. Those who oppose their activities bear the burden of showing that they violate a prohibitory provision of the law. In contrast, however, public officers cannot act without first being satisfied that they enjoy legal authorization to intervene in others' pursuit of their intentions. In the context of prospective lawmaking, the Commissioners observed that:

> When considering the legal regime that ought to apply in the case of artificial conception, we start with the basic governing proposition that there should be no intervention, in any form, unless the public interest is likely to be threatened or frustrated by the absence of some form or degree of regulation. Indeed, this formulation of the role of the state and its many organs applies generally to all facets of human endeavour: our traditions require that a reasonable justification must be found for legislative or other intervention.[12]

Accordingly, the OLRC recommendations reflect a pragmatic, functional approach, resisting intervention on slight grounds or grounds of ideology not supported by clearly demonstrated experience or risk of personal or compelling social harm. In an area where tendencies to overreaction and moral panic had been seen, the recommendations aimed at moderation. They were most directive concerning surrogate motherhood, where, as an exercise in damage control, a process of judicial screening was proposed. They also considered, however, that the non-interventionist position taken by the state regarding natural reproduction was inappropriate for artificial reproduction, in part because some regulation of services was justified and in part because legal accommodation of the former was often lacking or uncertain regarding the latter. That is, legal regulation was justified in order to afford some forms of artificial reproduction the recognition that natural reproduction enjoyed.

The Commission considered whether, where regulation was felt to be appropriate, it should be by direct and specific legislation, or by general parent or enabling legislation that authorized detailed subordinate regulations to be made by, or in consultation with, bodies capable of interpreting medical and scientific information. The latter was found to hold many attractions, because knowledge about means and effects of human reproductive technology appeared to be developing at a rapid pace. The parliamentary process might prove too cumbersome to respond quickly to, for instance, newly found safer techniques, or newly disclosed perils in practices that had received legislative approval. Further, the provincial College of Physicians and Surgeons already had the legislated mandate to protect the public against the unqualified practice of medicine, and against incompetent and unethical behaviour by licensed physicians, and had access to means to understand what practices were lawful and medically appropriate, or otherwise. It was felt that many matters in artificial reproduction were already subject to regulation through the College of Physicians and Surgeons of Ontario, or could be brought under regulation through existing legislation affecting public hospitals, child welfare and, for instance, registration of births. Accordingly, it was felt that comprehensive new legislation was unnecessary, since many recommendations could be implemented under prevailing legislative structures. Surrogate motherhood was the main exception, where new legislation appeared desirable.

THE OLRC RECOMMENDATIONS

The Commission made the following recommendations:

A. THE PROPRIETY OF ARTIFICIAL CONCEPTION TECHNOLOGIES

1. Artificial conception technologies, that is, artificial insemination, *in vitro* fertilization, and *in vivo* fertilization followed by lavage, should continue to be available and accepted as legitimate techniques to be used (except where a fertile and genetically healthy single woman receives treatment: see Recommendation 5) where medically necessary to circumvent the effects of infertility and genetic impairment.

2. (1) The use of the new artificial conception technologies should be subject to the recommendations proposed below.

    (2) Unless otherwise stated, the recommendations proposed below should not apply to artificial insemination where the sperm used is that of the recipient woman's husband or partner (A.I.H.)

B.   GENERAL RECOMMENDATIONS FOR REFORM

3.   Legislation should expressly provide that artificial conception procedures, that is, artificial insemination (including A.I.H.), *in vivo* fertilization followed by lavage, constitute the 'practice of medicine' under the Health Disciplines Act.

4.   Physicians should not be required to obtain a special licence or to practise in a specially licensed health facility in order to perform artificial conception procedures.

5.   Eligibility to participate in an artificial conception programme should be limited to stable single women and to stable men and stable women in stable marital or nonmarital unions.

6.   The proposed criteria for participation in an artificial conception programme (see Recommendation 5) should be set out in regulations made under the Health Disciplines Act.

7.   Given the present variety of means by which grievances may be redressed, no additional or different means of challenge or appeal should be made available to a person who is denied access to artificial conception services.

8.   Subject to Recommendation 9, legislation should remain silent on criteria for the selection of gamete donors. Questions of reproductive history, marital status, and genetic and other medical status should be left to professional standards to be set by the medical profession.

9.   Having regard to recent federal initiatives respecting the setting of standards for donor selection, at least in the context of licensed sperm banks, and in the belief that such standards should be uniform across Canada, there should be consultation between the provincial governments and the federal government so that such uniformity may be furthered.

10.   The issue of sperm donation by minors should be left to the general law, which now permits such donation.

11.   (1)   Minors should be prohibited from undergoing any procedure undertaken deliberately to donate ova.

   (2)   However, so long as they have given their free and adequately informed consent (see Recommendation 12), minors should not be prohibited from donating ova acquired indirectly as a result of therapeutic surgery, such as a hysterectomy.

12.   Legislation should expressly require a donor's free and adequately informed consent as a precondition to the donation or use of his or her gametes.

13.   At the time of donation, a donor should be entitled to restrict the use of the donated gamete to a specified purpose. Such a restriction should continue in effect even after the gamete has been used in a fertilization procedure, unless, prior to fertilization, the donor has altered the specified purpose or has indicated that the restriction is no longer to apply.

14.   (1)   After donation, but prior to the use of their gametes in a fertilization procedure, donors should be entitled either to

require their donation to be wasted or returned to them, so that the gametes may not be used for artificial conception, research, or any other purpose.

(2) A donor's consent to the donation of his or her gametes, given at the time of donation, should remain of legal effect until withdrawn or otherwise altered (see paragraph (1) and Recommendation 13), so that a fresh consent should not be required at each time the gametes are used.

15. (1) Donors of sperm should be allowed to be paid their reasonable expenses. Such payment should be based roughly upon the time and inconvenience involved in the initial screening with a view to recruitment into donor programmes, and the periodic follow-up checking while remaining active donors. However, payment for 'discomfort' should not be available. The sum paid should not be so great as to be an incentive to deceive, nor so great as unduly to burden a clinic having to pay for the time of applicants it rejects. In Ontario, existing payments tend to fall within the $25–50 range, which is acceptable.

(2) The same principles as those proposed in paragraph (1) should be applied to ovum donors, although payments may prove to be greater where ovum recovery involves invasive procedures, such as laparoscopy, or where a woman's naturally released ovum is recovered nonsurgically, by means of *in vivo* fertilization and lavage.

16. The frequency of employment of individual gamete donors should be left to the professional judgement and ethics of medical practitioners and to the preference of participants in artificial conception programmes.

17. (1) Gamete banks, that is, banks that buy and sell sperm, ova, and embryos, should be permitted to operate on a commercial basis. However, they should be allowed to operate only under licence and under stringent regulations setting standards of operation, with respect, for example, to payment by users to defray reasonable costs and, perhaps, to provide a reasonable profit. They should be operated subject to public accountability or under the auspices of a public organization, preferably on the model of the Canadian Red Cross Society blood donor clinics.

(2) Having regard to the recent federal initiatives respecting the licensing of sperm banks, there should be consultation between the provincial governments and the federal government so that the goal of uniformity of standards across Canada may be furthered. (See, also, Recommendation 9.)

(3) Licensed gamete banks should be prohibited from supplying gametes or embryos to any person or agency other than a licensed physician, a hospital or other approved health care facility, or another licensed gamete bank.

18. (1) The use of gametes and embryos imported from outside Ontario should be permitted but should conform to the

standards governing gamete banks in the Province. (See Recommendation 17.)

(2)   Having regard to recent federal initiatives in this general area, there should be consultation between the provincial governments and the federal government to ensure that uniform standards in regard to importation of gametes and embryos are established for the whole of Canada. (See, also, Recommendations 9 and 17(2).)

19.   (1)   For all purposes, a woman bearing a child through artificial conception in order to rear it should be conclusively deemed to be the child's legal mother, and the woman's husband or male partner who consents to the initiation of the artificial conception procedure or procedures (having regard to paragraph (3)) should be conclusively deemed to be the child's legal father.

(2)   A donor of sperm or an ovum should have no legal relationship to the child arising from the fact of donation; in other words, a donor should have no parental rights or duties regarding the artificially conceived child.

(3)   The consent of the husband or partner (referred to in paragraph (1)) should be presumed as a matter of law. However, this presumption should be rebuttable at his instance or at the instance of another person with a legitimate interest.

(4)   The proposed legislation respecting the status and legal parentage of artificially conceived children should be retroactive in effect.

20.   With respect to registration of the birth of an artificially conceived child,

(a)   in the case of artificial conception with donor gametes, the woman who bears and intends to rear the child should be registered as the child's mother, and the mother's spouse or partner who, under Recommendation 19(1), is deemed to be the natural father, should be registered as the child's father.

(b)   the gamete donor should not be named in the register of births, nor should the fact of artificial conception appear in such register.

(c)   where a woman gives birth to a child conceived posthumously by means of her deceased husband's or partner's preserved sperm, the woman should be entitled to register the birth showing the deceased as the father of the child.

21.   (1)   A child conceived artificially with donor gametes

(a)   should acquire inheritance rights to the estates of those persons who are legally recognized as his or her parents (see Recommendation 19), and to the estates of others as if the child was the natural child of such parents, unless the contrary is expressed by the testator, and

(b)   should have no inheritance rights through the gamete donor, unless the donor expressly provides for the child in his or her will.

(2)   A child conceived posthumously with the sperm of the mother's husband or partner

    (a)   should be entitled to inheritance rights in respect of any undistributed estate once the child is born or is *en ventre sa mère*, as if the child were conceived while the husband or partner was alive, and

    (b)   should be entitled to inheritance rights where the child is born or is *en ventre sa mère* when the time for the ascertainment of possible beneficiaries arrives.

22. (1)   Subject to the recommendations that follow, no specific legislation or rules dealing with medical records relating to the provision of artificial conception services should be enacted or established.

    (2)   In order to ensure that the legislation and other guidelines respecting medical records are as comprehensive as possible, particularly in light of the proposal to be made in paragraph (3) concerning a system of linkage between donors and recipients, the relevant statutes, regulations, and professional rules should be amended to make it clear that gamete donors are patients for the purposes of record keeping.

    (3)   Pursuant to the power given to the Council of the College of Physicians and Surgeons of Ontario under section 50 of the Health Disciplines Act, and subject to the approval of the Lieutenant Governor in Council and the prior review of the Minister of Health, the Council should make regulations that would establish a system of record keeping permitting doctors to link gamete donors with recipients, subject, however, to paragraph (4).

    (4)   Anonymity concerning the identity of all parties involved in artificial conception — the donor, the recipient, her spouse or partner (if any), and the child — should be preserved in the medical records.

    (5)   (a)   Where a genetic or transmissible defect or disease in a donor or a donor's child becomes known to a doctor, the doctor should be under a duty, imposed by regulations governing the medical profession, to make all reasonable efforts to report all relevant information to any person whose health and welfare the doctor reasonably believes may be affected by it.

        (b)   Sanctions for the failure to abide by such a regulation should lie in potential civil liability in negligence and in the 'professional misconduct' regulations under the Health Disciplines Act, rather than in a specific new penalty.

    (6)   There should be no positive duty on artificial conception practitioners to take steps to ascertain whether conception and birth have taken place or to ascertain the medical status of any child. However, should it be thought necessary or desirable to deal more formally with this matter, any legal obligation to follow up the outcome of artificial conception treatment should be

incorporated in the regulations governing the medical profession under the Health Disciplines Act.

(7) (a) The decision to disclose to the child the nature of its biological origins or parentage should not be regulated or dealt with by legislation or other formal rules.

(b) The decision concerning access to medical records by the parties involved – the woman, her husband or partner (if any), the child, and the donor – should be left to individual members of the medical profession. However, under no circumstances should any doctor or other person disclose information that could in any way identify the parties.

23. It should be made a provincial offence knowingly to conceal or misrepresent information in offering or agreeing to donate gametes for artificial conception purposes.

24. Legislation should provide that principles of strict liability, and particularly the implied warranties of merchantable quality and fitness for purpose, should not be applied to the direct or indirect donation or supply of gametes or embryos; rather, recovery in such a transaction should be dependent upon general principles of the law of negligence.

25. The claims by a parent known as wrongful conception and wrongful birth claims, and the claims by a child known as wrongful life and dissatisfied life claims, should not be resolved in a study on human artificial reproduction. Rather, these claims should be the subject of a separate study, in the context of tort law generally, so that an integrated jurisprudence in the area may be adequately developed.

C. PROPOSALS RELATING TO THE FERTILIZED OVUM OUTSIDE THE BODY

26. There should be no prohibition of the practice of transferring multiple fertilized ova to a woman, regardless of whether the ova are her own or are donated, and, where the ova are donated, regardless of whether a single donor or different donors are used.

27. (1) (a) A fertilized ovum outside the body, produced with the gametes of the intended recipient and her husband or partner, should be under the joint legal control of the man and woman.

(b) Where one of the couple dies, legal control of the fertilized ovum should pass to the survivor. If both should die, control should pass to the physician, clinic, gamete bank, or other authority that has actual possession of the ovum.

(c) Where the couple cannot agree concerning the use or disposition of the fertilized ovum, legal control should pass to the physician, clinic, gamete bank, or other authority that has actual possession of the ovum.

(2) Subject to Recommendation 13, concerning the case where a

gamete donor has imposed a restriction on the use of his or her gamete,

(a)   a gamete donor should have no right in law to control the use or disposition of a fertilized ovum to which he or she has contributed genetic material;

(b)   where a fertilized ovum has been produced from donated sperm and a donated ovum, and is not to be transferred to the woman for whom it was originally intended, legal control over the fertilized ovum should reside in the physician, clinic, gamete bank, or other authority that has actual possession of the ovum; and

(c)   where a fertilized ovum has been produced by a donor gamete and a gamete from one spouse or partner of a couple for whom the ovum was originally intended, and is not to be transferred to the woman for whom it was originally intended, legal control over the fertilized ovum should reside in that spouse or partner alone.

28.   Legislation should not be enacted to deal with whether a woman or couple should be entitled to obtain information concerning the sex of a fertilized ovum intended to be transferred to the woman.

29.   (1)   Research and experimentation on a fertilized ovum outside the body should be permitted, subject to the recommendations that follow.

(2)   Research and experimentation involving a fertilized ovum outside the body should be restricted to research centres approved by the Ministry of Health.

(3)   A research centre should be entitled to be approved only where it has established an ethical review committee for the internal screening of research projects. The Ministry of Health should develop minimum requirements respecting the composition and operation of ethical review committees in research institutions.

30.   A fertilized ovum that has been the subject of experimentation that has no direct therapeutic purpose in relation to the ovum should not be transferred to a woman.

31.   Having regard to the information now available to medical science respecting embryonic development, regulations should provide that no fertilized ovum outside the body should be allowed to develop beyond fourteen days after fertilization. Should the state of medical knowledge at some future date indicate that the fourteen day period is not appropriate, by being either too short or too long, the regulations should be amended.

32.   There should be a maximum of ten years for the cryopreservation or similar storage of a fertilized ovum, after which time the storage authority should be under a duty to have the ovum wasted.

33.   The question whether, having regard to the rule against perpetuities, a testator should be able to bind property by relation to the birth of a child from a fertilized ovum in cryopreservation at the time of the testator's death (and, therefore, whether such an ovum is a 'life in

being' under the rule) should be left to judicial, not legislative, resolution.

D. SURROGATE MOTHERHOOD

34.   Legislation should be enacted to establish a regulatory scheme governing surrogate motherhood arrangements.

35.   Before an artificial conception procedure may be employed in furtherance of a surrogate motherhood arrangement, the approval of the Provincial Court (Family Division) or the Unified Family Court should be obtained in accordance with the proposals made below.

36.   All surrogate motherhood agreements should be in writing. The court should be required to approve the terms of the agreement and to ensure that they adequately protect the child and the parties and are not inequitable or unconscionable.

37.   On the hearing of the application for approval of a surrogate motherhood arrangement, the court should be required to assess the suitability of the prospective parents for participation in such an arrangement.

38.   Before the court approves a surrogate motherhood arrangement, the prospective parents should be required to satisfy the court that there is a medical need that is not amenable to alleviation by other available means, including the artificial conception technologies.

39.   The availability of surrogate motherhood to prospective parents should not be restricted on an *a priori* basis, but should depend on an assessment of the prospective parents by the court according to legislated standards. The court should be required to be satisfied that the intended child will be provided with an adequate upbringing; in making this determination, the court should be required to consider all relevant factors, including the marital status of the prospective parents, the stability of their union, and their individual stability.

40.   Where a donated gamete is to be used in a surrogate motherhood arrangement from a donor who is neither the prospective surrogate mother nor a prospective social parent of the intended child, the treatment of the donor should be governed by the previously recommended provisions concerning gamete donors.

41.   There should be no restriction on the eligibility of women to serve as surrogate mothers, so long as they have reached the age of majority at the date of the application for court approval of their participation in a surrogate motherhood arrangement.

42.   On the hearing of the application for approval of a surrogate motherhood arrangement, the court should be required to assess the suitability of the prospective surrogate mother.

43.   In assessing the suitability of a prospective surrogate mother, the court should consider, among other factors, her physical and mental health, her marital and domestic circumstances, the opinion of her spouse or partner, if any, and the likely effects of her participation in

a surrogate motherhood arrangement upon existing children under her care.

44. The question of the standard of proof for approval of surrogate motherhood arrangements should be left to the courts responsible for determining the matter.

45. The surrogate mother should be a co-applicant in proceedings to approve a surrogate motherhood arrangement, but should not be required to be in attendance at the hearing of the application in every case. The surrogate mother should receive separate legal representation.

46. In order to minimize uncertainty concerning a child's parentage upon birth, the court should require that information relating to the blood type and other relevant biological characteristics of the surrogate mother, her husband or partner, if any, and the persons who produced the gametes involved should be placed before it prior to approval of the surrogate motherhood arrangement.

47. Notice of an application to the court for approval of a surrogate motherhood arrangement should be served upon the appropriate children's aid society, and the society should have standing to attend at the hearing of the application. However, a children's aid society should intervene only where its records disclose information demonstrating the unsuitability of either the surrogate mother or the prospective social parents for participaton in the surrogate motherhood arrangement.

48. The anonymity of the prospective social parents and the surrogate mother and the confidentiality of court records pertaining to surrogate motherhood proceedings should be preserved. The application should be heard and determined *in camera*, the court records should be sealed, and access to the records should be granted only upon judicial approval for good reason.

49. A child born pursuant to an approved surrogate motherhood arrangement should be surrendered immediately upon birth to the social parents. Where a surrogate mother refuses to transfer the child, the court should order that the child be delivered to the social parents. In addition, where the court is satisfied that the surrogate mother intends to refuse to surrender the child upon birth, it should be empowered, prior to the birth of the child, to make an order for transfer of custody upon birth.

50. Where, following approval of a surrogate motherhood arrangement, there has been a change in circumstances, or new information has become available, indicating that the approved social parents are unsuitable to receive the child, the surrogate mother or the children's aid society should be permitted to apply, at any time prior to the date of the birth of the child, for a review of the approval of the surrogate motherhood arrangement, and the judge should be empowered to rescind the agreement.

51. Legislation should provide that no payment may be made in relation to a surrogate motherhood arrangement without the prior approval of the court.

52.   In light of Recommendation 56, to the effect that, upon the birth of a child pursuant to an approved surrogated motherhood arrangement, the social parents will be the parents of the child for all legal purposes, legislation should not require that surrogate motherhood agreements contain special provisions dealing with legal responsibility for a handicapped child that is born pursuant to a surrogate motherhood agreement.

53.   The court should be required to ensure that a surrogate motherhood agreement contains adequate provision dealing with the allocation of the power of decision relating to the medical care of a newborn handicapped child, and with the nature of that decision.

54.   The matter of spontaneous abortion during a surrogate pregnancy should be left to agreement between the parties, as should the possibility that conditions may arise that justify a therapeutic abortion in accordance with the Criminal Code.

55.   (1)   The parties to a surrogate motherhood agreement should be free to include in the agreement terms of their choosing; however, they should be required to consider, and to agree upon a resolution of, the following issues:

        (a)   health and life insurance protection for the prospective surrogate mother;

        (b)   arrangements for the child should the intended social father or mother, or both, die before the birth of the child;

        (c)   arrangements for the child should the intended social parents cease to live together as a couple;

        (d)   circumstances regarding the particular manner in which immediate surrender of the child to the social parents is to be effected;

        (e)   the right, if any, of the surrogate mother to obtain information respecting, or to have contact with, the child after surrender;

        (f)   prenatal restrictions upon the surrogate mother's activities before and after conception, including dietary obligations; and

        (g)   conditions under which prenatal screening of the child may be justified or required, for example, by ultrasound, fetoscopy or amniocentesis.

56.   Upon the birth of a child pursuant to an approved surrogate motherhood arrangement, the social parents should be recognized as the parents of the child for all legal purposes, and the surrogate mother should have no legal relationship to the child.

57.   Where a child is born prematurely, after an application by the surrogate mother or the children's aid society to review the surrogate motherhood arrangement (see Recommendation 50), but before the court has determined the matter, the court should have the power to make an order that the social parents are not to be recognized in law as the parents of the child.

58.   The birth of a child pursuant to an approved surrogate motherhood arrangement should be registered under the Vital Statistics Act,

showing the social parents as the mother and father. The surrogate mother should not be named in the register of births; nor should the fact that the child has been born to a surrogate mother appear in the register.

59.   Children born pursuant to an approved surrogate motherhood arrangement should acquire inheritance rights through the approved parents. The child should have no inheritance rights against the estate of the surrogate mother simply by virtue of the biological relationship.

60.   The Ministry of Community and Social Services should be required to regulate any agencies that arrange surrogate motherhood agreements.

61.   Where a woman undergoes *in vivo* fertilization of an ovum intended for donation and becomes pregnant, she and the intended social parents should be able to apply to the court for approval of a surrogate motherhood arrangement in accordance with our previous recommendations. In approving the arrangement, the court should be empowered to determine unresolved terms of the agreement where all parties have approved the terms in principle, but have been unable to settle the details thereof by the time that the application for approval is presented.

62.   Where an approved surrogate mother who is the intended recipient of a fertilized ovum becomes unavailable, there should be a summary procedure for the approval of a replacement surrogate mother where this is necessary to secure transfer of the fertilized ovum in order to avoid its wastage.

63.   For the initial period during which surrogate motherhood agreements are regulated by statute, no specific provision should be enacted to address the question of such agreements made outside Ontario and intended for implementation in the Province.

64.   No legislation need be enacted concerning the maintenance of medical records specifically in the context of surrogate motherhood. Rather, the previous recommendations dealing with medical records relating to the provision of artificial conception services should apply (see Recommendation 22).

65.   A penalty of a fine should be provided for participation in a surrogate motherhood arrangement where it is known or believed that the arrangement is intended to evade the proposed regulatory scheme. However, where a professional whose assistance is sought is confronted with a *fait accompli* — for example, where an obstetrician is asked to deliver a pregnant surrogate mother's baby — he or she should not be subject to the proposed penalty for giving such assistance.

66.   (1)   Social parents who acquire custody of children born pursuant to unapproved surrogate motherhood arrangements should be allowed to utilize existing procedures, as modified by paragraph (2), to establish their parentage in law after the fact.

       (2)   Where social parents seek an adoption order in relation to a child who is born pursuant to an unapproved surrogate mother-

hood arrangement and transferred to them, notice of the application should be served upon the appropriate children's aid society. Upon receipt of the notice, the children's aid society should be required to conduct a homestudy and submit to the court a report in relation thereto.

E.   FURTHER REVIEW

67.   Five years after the recommended regulatory regime has been implemented in whole or in part, a review of all aspects of the regime should be undertaken by an appropriate governmental body.

GENERAL COMMENTARY ON RECOMMENDATIONS

The OLRC did not break new ground in Canada in proposing legislation to regularize the practice and consequences of artificial insemination. Quebec and the Yukon Territory already had legislation that aimed to integrate children born by such means into their social environments with a minimum of difficulty.[13] Indeed, the Yukon Children's Act adopted, almost verbatim, the provision of the Uniform Child Status Act proposed by the Uniform Law Conference that dealt with human artificial conception.[14] The Uniform Law Conference is composed of representatives of provincial law reform agencies who agree on drafts of model legislation that may be proposed for adoption by provincial legislatures. The OLRC recommendations were considerably more detailed than such legislation, but followed a sympathetic direction. The recommendations projected the thrust of earlier laws and proposals onto ovum and embryo donation, and IVF and its analogies.

The results of artificial insemination through use of the sperm of a woman's husband or male partner were equated as far as possible with the results of natural insemination. The perception at the time was that care had to be taken expressly to distinguish laws on artificial insemination by donor from those on artificial insemination by a woman's chosen partner, but the perception may have been incorrect. Courts might consider legislation on donor insemination inapplicable, because they might find that such a partner is not a 'donor' as understood in the expression 'artificial insemination by donor'. A latter donor tends not to be selected by the recipient woman but to be selected by health professionals, and to be anonymous to her. Further, the donor intends not to have maintenance responsibilities to a resulting child, and is expected not to seek access to the child. Similarly, the child is denied claims of succession to the estates of the donor and his family, and on the child's premature death the donor will not succeed to any assets or rights of legal action possessed by the child. In contrast, a husband or chosen partner will intend to rear the child in his home as his own, discharge financial and related responsibilities regarding the child, serve as custodian and, in the event of legal separation from the mother, have a right at least to access to the child. As an heir of the husband or partner, the child would enjoy family succession rights, and, if suffering early death, would be succeeded by him. Accordingly, the man would probably not be held in law to be a 'donor' as understood in laws on artificial insemination by donor, and the results the OLRC recommended should be legislated would probably be secured in any event by ordinary functioning of the courts interpreting legislation on donor insemination.

The recommendation that therapeutic donor insemination (TDI)[15] be taken to constitute the 'practice of medicine' was directed by the opinion that the private, non-medical practice of artificial insemination created dangers that inadequate screening of donors is risked by private practices, that appropriate counselling of all actors may be lacking, and indeed that the unskilled insertion of objects such as turkey basters into women's bodies, even when the women freely agree, is not to be encouraged. As the 'practice of medicine', such activities fall under the provincial Health Disciplines Act, which reserves the practice of medicine to those approved by the College of Physicians and Surgeons of Ontario, such as physicians and appropriately trained nurses. It may be countered, of course, that artificial insemination has been successfully and safely undertaken by unqualified personnel for many years, and that artificial insemination is no more the practice of medicine than natural insemination. The OLRC was conscious that its recommendation reinforced the medicalization of human reproduction, and would be offensive to such activists as members of lesbian organizations, which had already publicized their private performance of artificial insemination. It was considered, however, that such activities would be judicially found to violate the provincial Health Disciplines Act, and that the recommendation simply declared prevailing law. The presence of health professional involvement was also believed to underwrite standards of safety for all participants.

It was also believed that the practice of artificial reproduction is not so special or sensitive that it warrants special licensure of practitioners or facilities. Guidance from health professional licensing authorities and, for instance, from professional specialty organizations such as the American Fertility Society and the Canadian Society of Fertility and Andrology was considered appropriate for initial reliance. A case for special licensing might be made in the future if professional standards were found to prove inadequate in substance or enforcement, but the health professions were found to apply a more balanced approach to assisted reproduction than was offered the public by, for instance, sensation-seeking news media and public activists who viewed practices from sometimes unstated ideological bases.

All but one of the Commissioners[16] considered it unlawful to limit access to reproductive technology to married persons because the Ontario Human Rights Code 1981 proscribes discrimination based on marital status. It was questioned whether there truly would be such discrimination, since couples are admitted to treatment not simply on proof of marriage but after satisfying some minimal criteria of personal stability of a nature that would reduce risk to children under their care. It was concluded that only criteria of personal stability were appropriate for admission to programmes. It was noted that if, for instance, the condition of a woman's fallopian tubes prevented her from conceiving but that surgery or microsurgery could remove the disability, her marital status, prospective capacity to parent or, indeed, criteria of her personal stability would not bar her from access to treatment.

Standards of screening for gamete donation were considered of major significance, but better addressed through professional regulation than legislation or subordinate provisions. Some legislated exclusions might prove unnecessary or too rigid regarding some populations among whose members certain genetic conditions are common. The recent need to screen for acquired immunodeficiency syndrome (AIDS) or the human immunodeficiency virus (HIV) has shown how professional perceptions can be protectively applied in advance of governmental or legislative action, and render it of secondary effect. Professional self-regulation may be reinforced by judicially set standards, although these may be determined only *ex post facto*. Because of Human Rights Code provisions on marital status, the status of gamete donors was similarly considered better addressed on a clinical than a normative basis.

When the OLRC was developing its project in 1983–84, the Supreme Court of Canada's decision on informed consent to medical treatment, *Reibl* v. *Hughes*,[17] was still relatively recent, and not well acknowledged by the medical profession.[18] Because the thrust of the decision was to move Canadian jurisprudence from its English-derived principles in favour of the approach gaining strength in the United States, the Commissioners found it appropriate that legislation should direct health professionals to observe the prevailing standard of disclosure of information. Recent evidence indicates that professional practice is now considerably closer to the legal requirement of disclosure,[19] so that legislation may no longer be required to effect change.

Payment is prohibited under the Human Tissue Gift Act of Ontario for 'any tissue for a transplant, or any body or part or parts thereof other than blood or a blood constituent, for therapeutic purposes, medical education or scientific research'.[20] 'Tissue' as defined 'includes an organ, but does not include any skin, bone, blood, blood constituent or other tissue that is replaceable by natural processes of repair'.[21] It thus appears that sperm are not tissue, although ova are, but that in any event neither may be sold, unless it is claimed that their use is not for a therapeutic purpose, medical education or scientific research but is, for instance, for cosmetic use. Payment for sale of materials is distinguishable, however, from payment for a service,[22] and sperm donation has long been paid in Ontario because of its service character. The OLRC saw no need to limit this practice regarding sperm or ova, but was anxious to keep payment modest in order to emphasize that it is for inconvenience and real out-of-pocket expenses, and should not be allowed to become a source of individual enrichment. Because at the time the Report was being prepared ovum or ova recovery was a surgically invasive procedure, it was supposed that any such donation offered in its own right (as opposed to arising, for instance, from treatment of infertility or when surplus ova remained from participation as a patient in IVF) would warrant higher payment than for sperm donation.

Limitations on the frequency of use of gamete donors was considered an important issue, but better left to professional scrutiny and practice. Many uses, perhaps up to 30, may be made from a single donation of sperm, so limiting the number of donations to, say, five, would not really reduce to a comparably small number the children that may result. A donor who exhausts donations that may be made at one centre may go to another in the same city, so again limits may be difficult to enforce, except if time- and resource-consuming services were used. Because epidemiological evidence indicates that most reasonable employment of sperm donors will not increase the chance of male and female children of the same man later meeting and marrying beyond the general level of community risk from natural reproduction outside marriage, the matter was considered better not placed under legislated control.

The risk of inadvertent inbreeding would be reduced if gametes from one donor could be distributed in a widely based region. The prohibition of commercial payments reduces the chance of this happening, however, because non-profit agencies will be hospital-based and serve their local communities. Neither commercial nor cost-recovery gamete banks exist in Canada, because of the prohibition on payments other than for modestly assessed services. The OLRC found this dysfunctional, however, and accordingly recommended that commercial sperm and ova banks be allowed to make charges for their reasonable costs, and perhaps charge a minor related service fee. A licensing system was urged, however, and it was hoped that non-profit agencies might be created modelled on Canadian Red Cross Society blood donor clinics, whose motives are altruistic rather than profiteering and whose donors are preponderantly, if not exclusively, unpaid, or modestly repaid their necessary costs of donation. It was noted, however, that some not-for-profit clinics providing various medical services in the United States are owned and operated by professionals who are also exceptionally highly paid staff members, and that clinic costs reflect their elevated salaries in high charges for services. Accordingly, the operation of not-for-profit facilities may still be a source of personal enrichment, unless payments can be limited to only publicly regulated fees.

Consistent with the aim of regularizing family relationships in which gamete donation was involved, a central recommendation was that women who gestate children with the intention of rearing them should be conclusively and exclusively deemed to be their mothers for all purposes, and be registered as such in the birth register, and that their male partners who consent prior to initiation of pregnancy similarly be deemed their fathers. A rebuttable presumption was favoured that partners consented to assisted reproduction. No status was given to female partners of such mothers. True donors of gametes were reciprocally to have no legal relationship to children born of their donation. It was also proposed that regularizing legislation be retrospective in effect, notwithstanding the consequences this might cause in theory to legal provisions such as court orders requiring sperm donors to support children born of their donation. The Commission had received no evidence that families created through gamete donation functioned in practice other than in the way the Commission considered that they should be able to function in law – that is, according to the intentions of all adult participants in the artificial reproduction. Sperm donors had apparently never become liable under paternity findings.

Regarding children conceived posthumously through stored sperm of the mother's deceased partner, the Commissioners responded favourably to the outcome of the French *Parpalaix* case permitting a woman's choice to conceive by this means,[23] and did not follow the unsympathetic approach the Warnock Committee took to a genetic offspring who was not *in utero* at the time of its father's death. It was preferred that the mother be entitled to have the partner registered and otherwise recognized as father, and the child have inheritance rights to any of the father's estate undistributed when the child is born or is diagnosed as *en ventre sa mère*, as if conceived during the partner's life. This would not disturb rights to inherited property that had vested in successors at the time of birth or diagnosis of pregnancy, and might create some problems for judicial resolution in unusual circumstances. Under their mandate to serve the best interests of children of reproductive technologies, the Commissioners felt obliged to seek to protect children's status as the children of their mothers' partners as far as legally possible, although they may have risked such children's material interests in recommending that they should have no inheritance claims through gamete donors, except by a testator's clearly expressed intention.

The Commissioners concluded that no specific legislation or regulations were required regarding confidentiality of medical records where gamete donation for assisted reproduction was concerned. Existing legal means were found to preserve the personal confidentiality that was considered necessary for successful management of assisted reproduction, provided that such existing means were reviewed in light of gamete donation and amended accordingly. In particular, it was considered that prevailing means should be applied to link gamete donors with recipients and their resulting offspring, with preservation of personal anonymity. A condition of such linkage was that existing practice be amended in order to consider and treat a gamete donor as a patient, whereupon obligations of record-keeping and confidentiality would arise.

Patient status was not a precondition to physicians' and clinics' fiduciary responsibilities being created in law to donors, recipients and consequent children, however, since such responsibilities were considered to be legally inherent in the relationships that gamete donation created. Donors were entitled to be informed of any dysgenic risks they were found to face, dysgenic and otherwise harmful donations had to be traceable in order to warn recipients and discontinue use of affected donations, and resulting children's medical records would have to include information on their genetic origins that was apparently relevant to their health care. Accordingly, means of record linkage appeared legally required, and the medical record system was expected to be amended to achieve linkage of anonymous information. The subsequent HIV-inspired abandonment of fresh sperm application has reinforced the practice of record-keeping of gamete donors.

Attention was given to the perception emerging in adoption experience that anonymity of genetic origins was not necessarily an essential or desirable feature of sound practice, and that, by mutual agreement of gamete donors and their genetic offspring who had reached maturity, disclosures or exchanges of personal identifications might be accommodated. In the absence of reliable data, neither the Project's Advisory Board nor the Commissioners knew how best to respond to this perception. They therefore decided that correct policy was to preserve data under customary anonymity, but to provide that the review of effects of implementation of their recommendations that was proposed after five years (see the final recommendation) should include reconsideration of anonymity.

A limit on potential disclosure, and indeed on record linkage, was that practitioners might be unaware whether a gamete recipient had conceived through the donation. Many recipients conceive naturally, particularly when admitted to treatment programmes after a relatively brief period of infertility such as twelve months' inability to conceive with a partner, and others who conceive through donation do not inform the assisting practitioners. They leave those practitioners' care and present themselves to their regular physicians as women pregnant through their partners, either to preserve their and their children's anonymity from donors, or because they do not want to pay such practitioners' additional expenses. The Commissioners considered that obligations to yield confidentiality should not be a condition of receiving care, and accordingly recommended that practitioners should not fall under a positive duty to ascertain whether conception or birth had resulted from treatment. The duty of record-keeping was to achieve linkage of what was known, but not necessarily to know more than recipients of care chose to disclose. The provincial Ministry of Health could take initiatives to compel more rigorous duties of tracing and disclosing treatment outcomes.

The Project became involved in some depth in consideration of the place that would be occupied in the legal management of artificial reproduction by legal principles raised in the actions known as wrongful conception, wrongful birth, wrongful life and dissatisfied life actions.[24] Much study and discussion were given to these issues because of their inherent legal interest. The Commissioners' general approach was that neither patients' nor parents' claims for wrongful conception or birth, nor children's claims for wrongful or dissatisfied life, required legislation, because the courts were currently disposed to accommodate the former claims and to reject the latter, which the Commissioners considered at first view was the desirable response to such claims. In any event, however, it was found that the contribution to development of jurisprudence and legislation on these matters that would be made by artificial reproduction was at its highest quite secondary, and that the issues should not first be addressed by the Commission in this context, lest the tail of reproduction may wag the dog of transcending legal policy. It was accordingly proposed that claims of this nature should be the subject of more general study that could develop law more integrated with the affected jurisprudence. It cannot be stated to date, however, that the Commission's subsequent members have shown an appetite to promote such a study.

The Commissioners' general approach to pre-implanted embryos (now increasingly described as 'pre-embryos') when outside a woman's body was to require that they be treated with special respect, but not that they be treated as being the same as born children or foetuses. They had to be preserved from being the subject of research beyond development of the primitive streak, taken to occur at 14 days' gestation, unless compelling medical knowledge indicated that another limit was appropriate, but even before such limit they warranted protection against inappropriate research, such as in high school laboratories. Although the Project made residual proposals on control, it was anticipated that assisted reproduction practitioners and clinics would appreciate the wisdom, based on the Australian experience with the misleadingly described 'orphan embryos' of the Rios family,[25] of determining legal control of pre-embryos when they were outside a woman's body in advance of any uncertainties arising. They might require participants in their programmes to say in anticipation of events such as separation, death or disagreement, in whom control was to rest, with the practitioners or clinics themselves filling any gap in certainty. Wasting pre-embryos was considered regrettable because of their intended role in the achievement of pregnancy, but the Commissioners observed that more advanced pre-embryos than were involved in IVF loss were intended to be wasted by fitting women with intrauterine devices, and that such treatment was considered generally acceptable and was funded by the provincial health plan.

Expert evidence showed that pre-embryonic sex could be determined, and fears were raised that potential parents with information would be inclined to select to have male offspring in preference to female, reflecting and reinforcing the lower value of female children and women in society. The Commissioners appreciated the fear and the proposal that sex not be disclosed, but felt unable to recommend punishment for persons who gave true information of pre-embryonic sex to those to whom it was material to ask and to be influenced by the answer, in light of legal principles on free and informed consent to medical treatment.[26] It was accordingly preferred that no legislation be enacted and the issue be left to the general law.

The Commissioners were aware of the concerns that arise on the prospect of research being undertaken on pre-embryos, and of the elaborated limits on such research that had been enacted in Australia and urged elsewhere.[27] The matter could have been left to the guidelines developed by the Medical Research Council of Canada,[28] whose standards for funding research are frequently adopted by

Canadian institutions that regulate research without regard to sources of funds. It was considered appropriate to indicate procedures and limits according to which pre-embryonic research might be conducted, including the approval of institutions where such research would be permitted and institutional operation of an ethical review committee to screen research proposals.

It was proposed that the maximum term for which a pre-embryo should be preserved should be 10 years. This duration was somewhat arbitrary, but was based on estimates of the greatest time for which the patients for whom they were developed were likely to require their preservation and the need in time for cryopreservation facilities to clear their deposits. An esoteric legal issue concerning whether the Rule Against Perpetuities, a rule that prevents estates from being legally tied up for too long, could be related to cryopreserved pre-embryos, was considered best left to the courts. Estates can be tied only for the duration of a 'life in being' at a testator's death plus 21 years. The Commissioners had reservations about whether a court would consider a preserved pre-embryo to be a 'life in being', but felt no need for legislation to resolve the issue.

RECOMMENDATIONS ON SURROGATE MOTHERHOOD

The most innovative, contentious and misunderstood OLRC recommendations concerned surrogate motherhood. The Commissioners were aware that surrogate motherhood might be either partial, in which the gestating mother is also genetic mother, or full (or total), in which IVF produces a pre-embryo for implantation in a woman other than the one who supplied the ovum, the born child that results being intended for surrender to the ovum-supplying woman. At the time of deliberation, experience was almost entirely confined to partial surrogate motherhood, although instances of full surrogate motherhood had been publicized by the conclusion of the study. It was not anticipated that publicity concerning the New Jersey *Baby M* case[29] would both intensify ideological opposition to legal accommodation of surrogate motherhood, and increase interest in and apparently the incidence of full surrogacy, where the maternal-bonding features that led to the *Baby M* circumstances might be less likely to occur.

Full surrogate motherhood is dependent on medical aid for either IVF or natural fertilization and the recovery of the pre-embryo by lavage for transplantation. Partial surrogate motherhood is dependent on little medical aid, however, and may be accomplished by natural insemination, such as in condoned adultery. The legal freedom with which participants in partial surrogate motherhood may achieve their reproductive goals presented many obstacles to pursuit of the aim to prohibit and punish surrogacy. The scope for legitimate evasion of controls is so vast as to render effective control unfeasible. Draconian measures, violative of privacy, that discriminated against those for whom surrogacy presented the only real opportunity for parenthood, such as infertile couples and women who ovulated but could not complete gestation, and that punished parenthood and altruism and jeopardized the welfare of surrendered children, appeared objectionable to the Commissioners, although measures that would have such effects were strongly urged in a small number of the briefs and representations that the Commissioners received.

The control not of commissioning parents and gestating mothers *per se* but of commercially inspired intermediaries or brokers appeared more feasible and attractive, but not necessarily to call for new legislation. Such professionals as lawyers and physicians were already amenable to regulation on account of professional misconduct by their provincial licensing authorities, and commercial initiatives in private adoption were already controlled through provincial laws. The Commissioners were impressed that their obligation to serve the best interests of children of surrogate motherhood might not be discharged by confining prospective gestating mothers to women the commissioning couples knew as friends or relatives. Women coming under strong pressure to act as gestating mothers for relatives or friends because strangers could not be found might accept but be resentful of the burden, and disposed to intervene in the rearing of children they had not willingly surrendered and with whom they retained family or other close links. More significantly, the Commissioners were advised that children might experience confusion if their parents' friends or their aunts, second cousins or other relatives, including, as a South African case illustrated, their grandmothers, were also their genetic or gestating mothers. Children of surrogate motherhood might be favoured by having gestating mothers who would be unlikely to retain a close interaction with their parents, and an intermediary's role in finding such strangers is not necessarily offensive where such children's interests are concerned.

The Commissioners approached their task regarding surrogate motherhood in no sense as supporters of the practice, but as undertaking an exercise in damage control. Surrogate motherhood was seen as an option that could not be eliminated or suppressed, but that might perhaps inadvertently be directed either into adjacent or more remote jurisdictions where it is lawful, or into the most undesirable of pathways and practices. The risk that particularly poor women or vulnerable relatives might be overinduced, manipulated and abused to serve in surrogacy agreements seemed to be aggravated rather than prevented by rendering surrogate motherhood illegal and driving its practice underground or into the hands of unscrupulous operators. Critics of surrogate motherhood likened it to, among other practices, prostitution. The analogy may be apt in that the illegality of public soliciting has proven dysfunctional in controlling the practice because it has led to exploitive pimping, a woman's feeling of need to conceal her occupation and relationships, and practices of well advised higher-priced call-girls that may not constitute illegal soliciting. Prostitution *per se* is not illegal in Canada, the United Kingdom or many other countries that have inherited English criminal law.

The approach to surrogate motherhood that the Commissioners favoured reflected proposals that had been made in such US jurisdictions as South Carolina and Minnesota,[30] to adapt adoption practice to surrogate motherhood through a judicial procedure described as surrogate adoption. The general model was that participants in surrogacy agreements, with separate legal representation of commissioning couples and prospective gestating mothers, would agree terms and, before initiation of procedures, present them for approval to a Family Court judge. The judge would be mandated to address a number of key issues and empowered to raise any others that appeared to the judge appropriate to consider before any agreement could be judicially endorsed. When the judge was satisfied that the parties had acted freely, with due information and counselling, and that the terms were conscionable and mutually understood in sufficient detail, the judge would approve the agreement and legal effect would be given to its terms.

The agreement, like others for personal services, would not be specifically enforceable before birth of the child. That is, a gestating mother's agreement not to take teratogenic substances, not to undertake risky behaviour or positively to receive prenatal care, would not be enforceable by judicial order violation of which could be punished as contempt of court. Non-compliance with the surrogate motherhood agreement could be pursued as breach of contract, for which financial payments or adjustment might be made — for instance by withholding a portion of payments due on completion of the agreement. Enforced surrender of the born child is physically achievable, and the Commissioners favoured this both in order to deter women who were considering acting as gestating mothers by removing any sentimental idea that they might retain the children, and also because it was consistent with the advice they received from paediatric psychiatrists regarding the best interests of such children.

This was by far the most contentious of the OLRC recommendations, and in hindsight has probably proved to be the greatest obstacle to adoption of its approach, although it is operationally severable from the surrogate adoption proposal itself. Experience in other jurisdictions, notably Michigan,[31] has indicated that a procedure is workable in which a gestating mother is financially supported during pregnancy but retains a discretion on birth to surrender or retain and rear the child. The instances of retention have always apparently been few even with partial surrogate motherhood, and are likely to be reduced with skilful screening of applicants and with full surrogate motherhood agreements. Commissioning couples may therefore consider the possibility of a gestating mother deciding to retain the child a social, psychological and financial risk that is worth taking. The financial risk might, indeed, be an insurable interest against which they might seek protection by payment of an insurance premium.

The recommendation for obligatory surrender of a child born of a judicially approved surrogate motherhood agreement rested on the evidence and arguments presented by paediatric and general psychiatrists that it was not in the interest of gestating mothers that they should undertake pregnancies with any ambivalence about whether they would rear the children, and that it was not in the interests of the children themselves, with whom the Commissioners were most concerned, that the commissioning couples to whom they would be surrendered in all but a few cases should be ambivalent about whether they would have children for whom they were morally and otherwise responsible. In particular, it was shown to be potentially harmful that commissioning couples should suspend their emotional commitment and bonding to a child, for fear of aggravating their grief if it were not to be surrendered. Ambivalent commissioning couples might feel able to change their minds and cancel the moral and legal commitments they had made, abandoning children before or at birth to settings in which neither their gestating, genetic nor potential social parents would want to rear them. It was proposed to the Commissioners that children were best served by commissioning couples considering themselves irrevocably committed on judicial approval of the surrogate motherhood agreement, and assuming responsibilities to children comparable to those that would arise on their natural gestation.

A reason reinforcing the OLRC approach emerged from one or two anecdotal experiences related by highly informed sources in the United States, which were not at that time documented and which the Commissioners did not discuss in the Report. One or two gestating mothers were reported to have declined surrender of the children on grounds not of emotional bonding to them but that they considered their agreed fees inadequate and wanted increased or additional payments. The anecdotes indicated that commissioning parents had met these demands. It was perceived that, if gestating mothers were legally entitled to retain custody of children, subject perhaps to court-ordered rights of visitation by their natural parent(s), they might make the grant of exclusive custody depend on payments that, even if made illegally, commissioning parents would have a strong incentive to conceal and deny. The children might thereby become the object of commerce, commodification and ransom. An irony of this realization is that those opposed to surrogate motherhood often claim that baby-buying and commodification would follow were agreements to be enforceable. The Commissioners saw that the same was at least as likely to occur if agreements were not enforceable, and perhaps worse would result from legal attempts at prohibition.

In judicial proceedings for approval of surrogate motherhood agreements there was no legal need to advert to the role of the provincial Attorney-General as guardian of the public interest, because the Law Officer has ubiquitous standing (*locus standi*) to intervene. It was provided, however, that notice of proceedings be served on the appropriate Children's Aid Society, which is legally mandated to guard children's interests in its area of the province, and which might appear and present evidence relevant to the hearing. It has been observed that Roman Catholic participants are found in surrogate motherhood relationships in overproportion to their numbers in the community. Notice would accordingly be served on Roman Catholic Children's Aid Societies where they exist, namely in the Ontario cities of Hamilton, Toronto and Windsor. The Commissioners recommended that any Children's Aid Society could present specific evidence to support or oppose an applicant's prospective role in the surrogacy agreement, but not argue against approval of such agreements on general philosophical, religious or public policy grounds, since the issue would have been resolved by a legislature that enacted the OLRC proposal.

The Commissioners had formulated their damage-control approach, designed to mitigate potential harm, before arguments appeared indicating surrogate motherhood might, in some circumstances, positively promote the best interests of children. Instances were raised however, of women with phenylketonuria (PKU) and uncontrollable diabetes who would almost invariably cause their foetuses immense neurological and physical damage in the course of gestating them. Later experience added women with AIDS or HIV positivity, which might be vertically transmitted to their foetuses either *in utero* through exposure to amniotic fluid or blood, or by passage through the birth canal. In such cases, it would be in the best interests of the foetuses themselves that, on early detection as pre-embryos or embryos, they be recovered by lavage and be transplanted for gestation in the uterus of an unaffected woman. The case for surrogate motherhood might be more compelling when a woman suffered from chronic spontaneous abortion, and had a sad history of repeatedly aborting embryos or more developed foetuses. Embryo transplantation might alone permit embryonic and foetal survival, and surrogate motherhood for this purpose might be tolerable to Roman Catholic and comparable 'Pro-Life' opinion which considers any measures designed to preserve human embryonic and foetal life to be legitimate.

RESPONSES

By the time they were released, the main body of the OLRC recommendations had been so discussed as a result of the proposals of the Warnock Committee Report that, except with regard to surrogate motherhood, they appeared orthodox and relatively non-contentious, except among opponents basing their rejection on general ideological or moralistic grounds. Feminist sensitivities were beginning to arise at that time, and in some discernible measure these were fuelled locally by the OLRC Report, which was conditioned, as had been seen, by the perceived best interests of resulting children rather than by a perception of the best interests of women partici-pants in assisted reproduction.[32] Although it was hoped that the Report was not anti-feminist it was clearly non-feminist in its deve-lopment,[33] and was therefore not accepted by those seeking feminist laws.[34] Several recommendations regarding gamete donation, such as on donor screening and non-parenthood of donors, particularly non-paternity of sperm donors, caused some surprise in that they revealed that the existing situation, in practice or law, was not as many had supposed it to be. The recommendations for reform therefore appeared to them only to urge the obvious, and to require the law to become what many thought it already was.

Religious groups' responses to the Report were predictably mixed, those who generally accepted the new reproductive techno-logies tending to approve the Report and opponents disfavouring it. Hostile responses appeared to urge restrictive approaches that the Report explained would violate the provincial Human Rights Code — for instance concerning discrimination on the basis of sex, marital status or sexual orientation. The Canadian Charter of Rights and Freedoms would probably be similarly violated, as the Supreme Court of Canada indicated when it struck down the prohibitive abortion provisions of the Criminal Code in 1988.[35] In the years following the 1985 release of the Report, some feminist opinions were formed that shared the direction of conservative religious views, although for different reasons. Other feminist views, not necessarily supporting the Report's recommendations, were more cautious about urging alternative proposals to limit choice of reproductive technologies because of their implications for women's general reproductive choice and access to abortion services. They were reluctant to support other feminist demands for governmental regulation of access to reproductive technologies for fear that it would lead to wider controls than they favoured, and reluctant to react to men's influence over reproduction and demand their disempowerment because this might run counter to the emerging empowerment of women reinforced by the assertion that 'biology is not destiny'. That is, those urging that women should not face legal or other limitations due to their gender did not want to urge that men should be subject to legal constraints on grounds of their gender.

No provincial action was taken immediately on the Report, or is currently pending, largely because the Project served the government's political goal in 1982 and for some time thereafter, of taking Ministers off the firing line on use of the reproductive technologies. By the time the Report was issued the matter was less politically volatile. The recommendations other than those on surrogate motherhood were not contentious among the general public nor in obvious need of legal enactment, and the surrogate motherhood recommendations were too far-reaching to be embraced without political costs. However, women's groups, sensitive to a women's perspective that might lead to different conclusions on some issues from those reached by the OLRC in attempting to pursue the best interests of children, took political initiatives to press for the issues and recommendations to be further reviewed in accordance with their agenda.

An irony of some women's groups' responses, in light of general provincial disinterest and inactivity, was fear that the province of Ontario might rush headlong into legislation and become a Mecca for those seeking to use reproductive procedures that such groups had not yet assessed to their own satisfaction. They have accordingly urged that a Canada-wide study be undertaken. The pressure that was applied at the federal level of government, although at times inducing an ambivalent response, was finally successful in persuading the federal government of Canada to appoint a Royal Commission on New Reproductive Technologies, chaired by Professor Patricia Baird, a highly respected geneticist at the University of British Columbia. The Commission, appointed late in 1989, is scheduled to report by the end of 1992. This counteracts any provincial dispositions to take legislative initiatives. The Royal Commission's final report will have to be studied, of course, and will almost invariably address many issues that can be legislated only at the provincial level of government, so that the question of provincial disparity is likely to recur at that time.

Academic commentators on the OLRC Report have compared the depth of its consideration favourably to that of, in particular, the Warnock Report, the discussion in which was generally superficial and the legal perceptions in which were confusing and poorly structured. Commentators strongly opposed to surrogate mother-hood, for instance, have nevertheless observed that the Report 'argues persuasively' in favour of its recommendations.[36] Some mis-understanding, misrepresentation and distortion of the Report and its recommendations was inevitable. Some commentators from disci-plines other than law – such as philosophy, for instance – have not understood that courts do not enforce personal service agreements through orders of specific performance, and have incorrectly sup-posed that surrogate motherhood agreements would be enforceable under the OLRC scheme by courts compelling gestating mothers to receive prenatal care and to refrain from conduct endangering a foetus. Others have so misrepresented this issue, claiming, for instance, that a gestating mother would 'be subject to coercion specifically enforcing the use of her body by third parties',[37] that it appears[38] that they have not actually read the Report. A special irony of the criticism quoted is that it appears in defence of the Roman Catholic viewpoint, but employs the same criticism that has been made of the Roman Catholic approach to induced abortion.[39]

Although not legislated, the Report has been influential in condi-tioning or reinforcing legal reforms to such enactments as the Vital Statistics Act on birth registration, which no longer requires infor-mation on paternity of a child, and in giving IVF and related clinics the legal confidence to proceed to treat patients. They can manage the legal aspects and implications of their practices, and reasonably assure participants in their procedures that many of their goals can be legally achieved, and advise on the areas of uncertainty. Such clinics also now appreciate the need and means to minimize legal concerns by anticipating them and avoiding them or resolving them as far as possible in advance. Even regarding surrogate motherhood, the atmosphere in the province has been affected so much as to persuade a High Court judge late in 1988 to order, on the application of all parties to an agreement for full surrogate motherhood, that on birth of the twin children, the commissioning genetic mother (who had earlier had a hysterectomy) be named as mother in the provincial birth registry, rather than the gestating mother. This followed a decision of a Michigan Court[40] and a recommendation[41] of the OLRC Report. This shows, in a specific setting, the more general point that the Report has had the effects, which are not necessarily incompatible, of indicating what the prevailing law is and might develop to become through legislative and judicial initiatives, and also the targets at which opponents may aim in order to pursue alternative goals to those the OLRC considered should be sought.

NOTES

1   Cmnd 9314, 1984.
2   See, for example, Elias, S. and Annas, G.J. (1987), *Reproductive Genetics and the Law*, Chicago: Year Book Medical Publishers, Inc., p. 236, incorrectly claiming that the OLRC Report 'was prepared following Warnock' and relies heavily on it.
3   Now a judge in the Unified Family Court, Hamilton, Ontario.
4   OLRC Report, p. 2.
5   See the Ontario Human Rights Code, 1981 and the Canadian Charter of Rights and Freedoms, 1982.
6   Bayles, M.D. (1984), *Reproductive Ethics*, Englewood Cliffs, NJ: Prentice-Hall, Inc.
7   OLRC Report, pp. 287–91.
8   See *In re Baby M.*, 537 A.2d 1227 (NJ Sup.Ct., 1988). For further discussion see Chapter 9 below.
9   See, for example, Goldstein, J., Freud, A., and Solnit, A.J. (1979), *Before the Best Interests of the Child*, New York: The Free Press, 1979.
10 The Appendix to the OLRC Report, pp. 295–390, summarizes Reform and Proposals for Reform in Other Jurisdictions available by the conclusion of the OLRC study.
11 For further discussion, see Chapter 2, above.
12 OLRC Report, p. 119.
13 OLRC Report, p. 374.
14 OLRC Report, p. 373, n. 589.
15 This expression has superseded the former expression Artificial Insemination by Donor, because the acronym AID may be confused with that of Acquired Immune Deficiency Syndrome, AIDS.
16 See note 7, above.
17 (1980), 114 DLR (3d) 1 (S.C.C.).
18 See Robertson, G. (1984), 'Informed consent in Canada: an empirical study', *Osgoode Hall LJ.*, **22**, p. 139.
19 See Dickens, B. M. (1991), 'The effects of legal liability on physicians' services', *University of Toronto LJ*, **41**, p. 168.
20 Section 10.
21 Section 1(c).
22 This common distinction appears, for instance, in the UK legislation prohibiting human organ sales, where expenses incurred in altruistic donation may be repaid; see the Human Organ Transplants Act 1989, s. 1(3).
23 See Jones, D. (1988), 'Artificial procreation, societal reconceptions: legal insight from France', *American J. Comparative Law*, **36**, p. 525.
24 See Dickens, B. M. (1989), 'Wrongful birth and life, wrongful death before birth, and wrongful law', in S. McLean, (ed.), *Legal Issues in Human Reproduction*, Aldershot: Dartmouth, 1989, ch. 4, pp. 80–112.
25 OLRC Report, pp. 352–5.
26 See *Reibl* v. *Hughes*, note 17 above.
27 OLRC Report, pp. 343–69.

28   See now Guidelines on Research Involving Human Subjects, 1987.

29   See note 8, above.

30   See Dickens, B. M. (1985), 'Surrogate motherhood: legal and legislative issues', in A. Milunsky and G. J. Annas (eds), *Genetics and the Law III*, New York: Plenum Press, pp. 183–214.

31   *Doe v. Attorney-General of Michigan State*, 19 September 1988, discussed in *Bio Law*, II,U: 1149, and Lewin, T. (1988), 'Surrogacy: a consensus', *New York Times*, 22 September, p. A25.

32   Contrast Brodribb, S. (1986), 'Off the pedestal and onto the block? Motherhood, reproductive technologies, and the Canadian state', *Canadian Journal of Women and the Law*, **1**, p. 407.

33   See Overall, C. (1986), 'Reproductive ethics: feminist and non-feminist approaches', ibid., p. 271.

34   For example, see Coffey, M. A. (1986), 'Of father born: a lesbian feminist critique of the Ontario Law Reform Commission Recommendations On Artificial Insemination', ibid., p. 424.

35   *R. v. Morgentaler* (1988), 44 DLR (4th) 385 (SCC).

36   See, for example, Elias and Annas, op. cit., p. 229.

37   Wagner, W. J. (1988), 'The new reproductive technologies and the law: a Roman Catholic perspective', *J. Contemporary Health Law and Policy*, **4**, p. 37 at p. 46.

38   The author refers not to the OLRC Report itself but to an interpretation derived from Elias and Annas, op. cit., p. 237.

39   See, for example, Rubenfeld, S. (1989), 'The right to privacy', *Harvard LR*, **102**, p. 737.

40   *John Smith and Mary Smith v. Mike Jones and Jane Jones*, Wayne County Circuit Court, 1986; see (1986) *Bio Law*, **II**, U:65.

41   OLRC Report, recommendation 58.

4 Czechoslovakia: Legal Regulation of Human Reproduction

JIŘÍ HADERKA

INTRODUCTION

In his famous work, *Les grands systèmes de droit contemporains*,[1] René David classifies the European countries into three groups: the Romance–Germanic law group, the socialist law group and the common-law group. If we observe this division, then Czechoslovakia would belong to the second group, often also called 'the East European group'. No objection can be made against such a method of categorization although we must also bear in mind the remark of the above-mentioned author that Czechoslovakia – as well as Poland, Hungary and western parts of Yugoslavia – belongs to areas in which, for many centuries, the development of law took a parallel course with the development of law in Germany, Austria and France. Events and conditions influencing its evolution were the same as in the countries of the Romance–Germanic law group. Czechoslovakia was always under a noticeable influence from legal tradition: the rule of law was considered one of the principal cornerstones of society and lawyers enjoyed considerable esteem.

Since the enactment of the Common Civil Code in 1811, an uninterrupted advancement of legal thinking found propitious conditions at the universities and in the courts. Legal techniques have attained a high level; judicial decisions have been published periodically and have enjoyed deserved esteem; editions of commentaries and analytical monographs have been an indispensable constituent part of the national life. All of this has been too deeply imbued in the national character to be changed by temporary pressures from the outside.

At the same time, Czechoslovakia is a country where medical

science is well developed: Czechoslovak medical specialists have played an important role in the development of many branches of medicine, and the standards of medical care have always been very high.

Both of these characteristics were favourable prerequisites for the gradual introduction of necessary law reform coinciding with the changes in human sexual attitudes – on one hand, efforts to regulate the birth rate and, on the other, the desire to apply assisted fertilization methods.

THE ROLE OF LAW IN REGULATING HUMAN REPRODUCTION IN GENERAL

From the medical point of view, contraception, induced abortion and voluntary sterilization are relatively old problems, the questions connected with their legal admissibility and mass application emerging approximately in the middle of this century – although they were concerned with only partial dilemmas, and did not relate to the admissibility of techniques as a whole.

In Czechoslovakia there was no major public discussion of such problems, probably because the first Abortion Act was enacted in 1957 and was relatively moderate and also because the social climate was not particularly propitious for dealing with such topics. Nor did the recognition of the legal admissibility of voluntary sterilization arouse much attention: it was never widely used, the principle conceding its legality being hidden in one of the numerous sections of the Public Health Care Act 1966, and the detailed arrangements being left to a rather obscure instruction of the Ministry of Health in the same year. The problems of the legality of contraception have always been dealt with in connection with abortion in statute law. Especially after the Second World War the limitation of the birth rate found little favour in Czechoslovakia; public policy always preferred higher birthrates, and this was stimulated by various social means. Contraception and induced abortion were stressed as being methods to avoid unwanted pregnancy and to facilitate planned parenthood.

Moreover, there was never public media interest in such matters, as there was in Great Britain in the *Gillick* case,[2] or a series of important judicial decisions, as in the United States.[3] The Churches, especially the Roman Catholic Church, showed only a token resistance. Broadly the public seemed prepared to accept the legal admissibility of all these methods.

In contrast to the relatively slow and gradual advance of birth limiting or delaying methods, the arrival of assisted human fertilization methods was rather hasty – as it was in the whole industrialized world.[4] The problems of artificial insemination, particularly in its heterologous form, began to be acute at the end of the 1960s and early 1970s. In Czechoslovakia the first child from *in vitro* fertilization and embryonic transfer/reimplantation (IVF + ET/ER) was born only four years after Louise Brown on 4 November 1982 – a boy born to a 32-year-old mother. The second IVF baby followed on 7 January 1984, the third on 8 September and the fourth one on 24 October of the same year and so on. Thus, when the first test-tube twins were born on 4 January 1988, the event was accepted without surprise or undue comment.

Up to now no case of surrogate motherhood has been reported. Indeed, in a newspaper interview, a member of the medical staff carrying out IVF and ET in Brno said that he could not imagine that a woman in Czechoslovakia could be found to fulfil such a mercenary role.[5] To date, no experiments in respect of flushing embryos and implanting them have been carried out in Czechoslovakia.[6] The technique of freezing human sperm is available but no cryopreservation of ovocytes or embryos has been reported.[7] Nevertheless, nobody can know what tomorrow will bring. . . .

However, it seems that some stereotypical lawyers' approaches to assisted fertilization methods have evolved. They are typical, and are repeated, with some variations, in all the countries where such problems are topical. One significant feature of the lawyers' approach to assisted fertilization and connected problems is their apparent aversion to legislative intervention.[8]

In a previous paper[9] I quoted a series of opinions of high judicial and legislative authorities from the common-law countries that were united in urging for caution and against any rush into legislating on assisted human fertilization or genetic engineering. The situation in Europe is no different. The dictum of Dean J. Carbonnier seems the most symptomatic and clear. He said, at the Paris colloquium in 1985:

> La législation nécessite toujours une certaine expérience, c'est à dire un certain nombre de cas et une certaine durée pendant laquelle ces cas ont été mis à l'épreuve. Pour la plupart des questions soulevées aujourd'hui, cette expérience fait encore défaut.[10]

In general, then, we can observe our inclination to delay legislation – if possible – and permit other mechanisms to control activity in this area. This may happen in a number of ways.

First, there is a tendency to use existing statutes or judicial decisions to solve new problems by old means, reinforcing the view that there are no *lacunae iuris*. There is always the possibility of a broad interpretation or *praeter legem* interpretation, or even judicial creation of law based on the famous model of s. 4 of the French Civil

Code 1804, or s.7 of Allgemeines bürgerliches Gesetzbuch /ABGB/ 1811. Bear in mind, for example, the answer to the question 'Who is the mother?' in the case of heterologous IVF + ET with donated ova according to the French Civil Code 1804,[11] or the response of British courts to the question of surrogacy contracts between commissioning couples and womb-leasing women.[12]

Second, there is a common trend to give way to the self-regulating mechanisms of bodies of medical professionals such as ethical committees. Such bodies may also be created on a broader level.[13]

The third possibility is to form committees of inquiry to study the acute problems and make recommendations for legislation. This phenomenon frequently occurred in the first half of the 1980s in a worldwide movement, resulting in a flood of reports, recommendations, guidelines and so on from Western Europe, North America and Australia.[14]

Leaving aside the Australian example,[15] it is generally only a real shock to public opinion that results in rapid legislation, as in the British *Baby Cotton* case, which led to the passing of the Surrogacy Arrangement Act 1985; otherwise evolution remains relatively slow.[16]

In Czechoslovakia in particular, and in East European countries in general, similar trends have been operating, although with some variations. It has been clear from the outset that the legal problems arising from the use of assisted fertilization techniques cannot be solved legally without changes in the legal order. There has, therefore, been hesitation and some doubt about how to proceed. In Czechoslovakia, the Czechoslovak Medical Society has played a very important role in preparing the basis for clarification of the substance of legal problems and for legislation.

The first, most pressing, problems became those concerning the status of children born as a result of artificial insemination and the prerequisites for use of this method. These complex issues were discussed in public for the first time at the third Medico-Juridica Conference in Bratislava in 1972.[17] Nevertheless, years passed without any result until the enactment of the Family Code Amendment Act 1982 at least gave an explicit answer to the question 'Who is and remains the father of a child born after the use of assisted reproduction?' – although it failed to provide an explicit answer to the question of maternity in such cases. Almost simultaneously, the 'binding instructions' of the Czech and the Slovak Ministries of Health on artificial insemination prerequisites appeared in late 1982 and 1983.

A further significant step was made at the sixth Medico-Juridica Conference in Olomouc in 1984 where legal problems connected with protection of unborn life, IVF in general and surrogacy were considered for the first time. Since then, increasing numbers of articles have been published on those topics, resulting in the dissemination of knowledge of developments worldwide and the acquisition of experience from abroad, reflected by Czechoslovakian participation in the World Congresses on Medical Law. The zenith of this evolution was represented in the Eighth World Congress on Medical Law held in Prague in 1988, where a number of Czechoslovak scientists and lawyers participated in the discussion of further problems which are topical, not only for Czechoslovakia, but also for nearly all the countries of the industrialized world. In my view, the Congress discussion will soon result in new legislative steps in Czechoslovakia.

The scope of legal reactions to assisted human reproduction problems can be seen in the excellent paper by Stepan in the Actes de Lausanne, 1986,[18] and also in one of my own papers.[19] To sum up, it can be said that the fundamental problems of the status of children, as well as the conditions for artificial insemination including AID, are expressly solved in the family codes of some 'socialist' countries — the former in all the Yugoslav Republic's codes originating from 1973–84, Hungary (1986), Bulgaria (1985), the latter in some Yugoslav Republics, Hungary and, since 1987, also the Soviet Union. Poland is an atypical case; there is no statute dealing with these topics, but the main issue of status is solved by a Supreme Court decision in 1985[20] and considerable academic writing on connected problems is now going on.[21]

Until now, East European countries have not attempted, as a group, to prepare a common recommendation or declaration on the main principles in respect of assisted human reproduction and genetic engineering, as the West European countries have done in part[22] and with only partial success. Although it is impossible to predict when the time might be right for such an undertaking, it could accelerate part-European harmonization of law which I believe to be absolutely necessary.

ORIGINAL LEGAL BACKGROUND

In the preceding section it was said that before any attempt is made to legislate, there is a strong tendency to attempt to cover the new situation by existing legal provisions using extensive interpretation, analogies and so on. This has been also the case in Czechoslovak legal development. To explain it, it is necessary to sketch the possibilities hidden in the principal legal codes, which may form the basis for regulating those problems arising from human assisted fertilization and related matters.

It is appropriate to begin with the consideration of the Czechoslovak Civil Code, 1964. In s.7 para. 1 the main content of the former s.22 of the Common Civil Code (ABGB) 1811, is preserved, concerning the *infans conceptus pro iam nato habetur quotiens de eius iure quaeritur*, (which comes from the old Roman law). This provision states: 'The capacity of an individual to have rights and obligations shall be established by birth. This capacity shall also belong to a conceived child if born live.' But there is no explicit provision on the possibility of instituting a *curator ventris*. Until now there has been no attempt, similar to that made in Austria (which also inherited the Common Civil Code 1811) to build up, on this ground, legal protection against annihilation or research for embryos created *in vitro*.[23]

Moving on to consider the Czechoslovak Family Code 1963, in this respect we should begin with the regulation of affiliation. Neither in this code, nor in any other act, is there any provision on 'who is the mother of the child'. It can be only deduced that, until it became possible to combine IVF and ET in a heterologous way (using a donated ovocyte or embryo), there was no doubt that the woman who gave birth to the child was considered the mother of the child as *mater gestatrix*. What is more surprising is that nowhere can be found any provision in respect of the denial or determination of maternity. But there are – albeit rarely – such cases in practice, and the doctrine recognizes the possibility of motions founded on those grounds.[24] It should be emphasized that an 'accouchement dans l'anonymat', as in French law, does not exist in Czechoslovakia, and recognition of maternity is not possible (unlike in the French Civil Code 1804).

Paternal affiliation rests on an unchangeable sequence of three paternity presumptions and, in this regard, the Czechoslovak system is very similar to other European legal orders. The first presumption results from the old Roman maxim that *pater est quem nuptiae demonstrant* and, in a dispute between a former and a subsequent husband, prefers the latter. In this regard s. 51 of the Family Code states:

S.51
(1) If a child is born within the period between the day the marriage was contracted and the expiration of the 300th day following the termination of the marriage or its invalidation, the husband of the mother shall be deemed to be the child's father.
(2) If a child is born to a remarried woman, her later husband shall be deemed to be the child's father, even if the child was born prior to the expiration of the 300th day following the termination or invalidation of the woman's previous marriage.
(3) When counting the time decisive for the determination of paternity, it is assumed that the marriage of a person declared dead became extinct on the day of death indicated in the decision declaring such a person dead.

The second legal presumption of paternity is formulated in ss. 52 and 53 of the Family Code as follows:

S.52
(1)   In general, the man whose paternity was determined by the concurrent declaration of the parents is deemed to be the child's father.
(2)   The concurrent declaration of the parents must be made before the national committee charged with keeping vital registers, or before a court.
(3)   The declaration of the mother is not required if she is unable to assess the significance of her action or if a serious obstacle is encountered in procuring her declaration.

S.53
The concurrent declaration of the parents may determine paternity of a child as yet unborn provided it has already been conceived.

In judicial practice and doctrine the content of the sections referred to above is very controversial in respect of the problem which might arise if a man who is not, and cannot be, the biological father declares his paternity in the prescribed way. It would appear that in this case the declaration can be regarded as valid if the declaring man makes his declaration of will in harmony with s. 37 of the Civil Code – that is, freely and seriously, definitely and understandably. The result of this approach is that what prevails is the optional, volitional element, not the biological truth.

The third presumption indicates that the man who has had sexual intercourse with the mother of the child in the so-called critical period is the father if a court so decides. The Family Code states:

S.54
(1)   If paternity has not been determined by the concurrent declaration of the child's parents, both the child and the mother may move that paternity be determined by the court.
(2)   The man who had sexual intercourse with the child's mother within the period of not less than 180 and not more than 300 days prior to the birth of the child shall be deemed to be the child's father, unless his paternity is precluded by serious circumstances.

In the second paragraph the use of the expression 'sexual intercourse' as an equivalent of coitus causes a problem – does this term permit of such a broad interpretation that the motion could be successful against the donor of the sperm? The passage at the end of para. 2 raises the possibility of preclusion of affiliation by a test proving that the child cannot originate from the defendant although his coitus with the child's mother in the critical period is evident. *Onus probandi* is on the defendant and can be fulfilled by the evidence of expert witnesses (in haematology, gynaecology, andrology, anthropogenetics and so on).

It is also possible to file the motion after the death of the presumed father.

Paternity can be denied by the husband (or the man who has declared his paternity), or by the child's mother, but not by the child. Such a right can be exercised only in a very short period of six months after the birth or the time at which the situation becomes known. Exceptionally this right may also be exercised by the Prosecutor General without regard to the lapse of time (s.62 of the Family Code).

In the case of the first presumption, the prerequisites for denial were originally based on paras 1 and 2 of s.58. If the child could have been conceived in wedlock, the husband's (or generally the plaintiff's) *onus probandi* would have been that he absolutely could not be the biological father of the child (s.1). In other cases the plaintiff's position is not so difficult: according to para. 2 it is sufficient to deny paternity, with the exception of situations in which the husband had sexual intercoure with the mother of the child in the critical period or knew that she was pregnant. On this point law does not concentrate on the way in which the pregnancy started.

As to the man who has declared himself the father of the child, he can deny his paternity according to s.61 of the Family Code only if he is precluded from the possibility of being the biological father of the child and he — as well as other plaintiffs (the mother, the curator) — has only the six months' preclusive term at his disposal.

It seems clear, therefore, that the quoted text offers considerable possibilities for the reinterpretation of affiliation matters by taking into consideration the changed situation arising from the availability of artificial insemination (AI) or IVF + ET/ER. These matters will be considered below.

A brief comment is now appropriate on vital registers. The principles for the operation of the book of births, the book of marriages and the book of deaths are based on the Vital Registers Act 1949, and on the Realizing Notice 1977. It is supposed that the person indicated as the mother of the child should be the woman who gave birth to the child, and that the man who is indicated as the father is her husband or, in relation to the child born out of wedlock, the man who has engendered the child, but the possibility of verifying his voluntary declaration is modest.

Another Act that must be mentioned is the Public Health Care Act 1966. The following provisions are the most important for our purposes.

S.11
(1) The state provides health services in its institutions in conformity with contemporary medical knowledge.
(2) Health services are provided to all citizens of the CSSR (now CSFR) free of charge to the extent, under the conditions and in the health institutions specified in the present Act and in the regulations issued for its implementation.
(3) The Ministry of Health [now the Ministries of Health and Social Welfare of the National Republics] may specify that in exceptional cases payment may be demanded for the provision of certain health services which are not indispensable.

S.12
(1) Health services are provided by health institutions which are integrated in a uniform system based on team work and an expedient division of work, while maintaining the unity of specialized care for human health and personal responsibility for the care provided. In these institutions, examinations and treatment may be provided only by authorized health workers.
(2) Specialized care is based on services provided in health communities. The health communities are based on territorial or factory level. . . .

S.26
(1) Health institutions may organize and carry out the collection of blood, tissues and organs for the needs of preventive and therapeutic care and scientific research.
(2) The above may be taken from live persons only with their consent and must not involve any danger to their health; donors shall receive special health care.

S.27
Sterilization may be carried out only with the consent or at the request of the person concerned and under conditions specified by the Ministries of Health and Social Welfare of the National Republics.

This provision was realized by a binding instruction in the same year, later replaced by another instruction. The aim of voluntary sterilization remained, even after this change, above all the preservation of the health of the woman or the man involved. The sterilization of minors or other persons without full legal capacity is allowed only at the request of their legal representative or with his consent (see s. 7 of the Binding Instruction on Realization of Sterilization 1972).

According to s.31, para. 1, the tasks of the health services are implemented by health institutions and other health organizations formed as a uniform system of health services.

Section 35 para. 1 states that the basic unit of the facilities for therapeutic and preventive care, which provides out- and inpatient care to the population of a particular area, is a hospital with a polyclinic.

As to the tasks of science and research, the provisions are as follows:

S.64
The bodies which control and coordinate the development of science and technology and their application in practice, as well as workers from all the fields of scientific research, shall fulfil their tasks in harmony with the findings of medical science and thus ensure that the development of science and technology contributes to the promotion of public health.

S.66
(1) In order to fulfil the tasks of the Ministries of Health and Social Welfare concerning the care for development of medical science and research activities in the health services, the Scientific Council of the Ministries has been established. The Members of the Scientific Council shall be appointed by the Minister. . . .
(3) The statute of the Scientific Council of the Ministries shall be approved by the National Government.

S.70
(1) In order to ensure uniform professional guidance in public health care and health services and in order to settle problems which call for uniform nationwide regulation, the Ministries of Health and Social Welfare shall, in particular
   c)   control the health services in a uniform manner and to this aim issue binding principles and instructions for the organization and operation of these services, and supervise their standards. . . .

The following provision is the basis for the problems of civil liability:

S.78, para. 2
Payment for damage caused during the provision of health services shall be governed by the provisions of the Civil Code; even if no obligation to pay damages has arisen, the state may, in extraordinary cases deserving special attention, pay a contribution to the injured person.

This provision leads us back to the Civil Code 1964 where two sections should be considered. The first one is of a general character:
S.421
(1) An organization shall be liable for damage caused to an individual through having broken a legal obligation.
(2) The damage shall be considered as having been caused by the organization if it was caused within the scope of the fulfilment of its duties by persons who are fulfilling their duties. These persons shall not be liable themselves, under the present Civil Code, for the damage thus caused; their liability under the labour law regulations shall not be affected.

(3) The organization shall relieve itself of its liability if it proves that it could not have prevented the damage even if it had made all the efforts that could be expected of it. However, it may not relieve itself by stating that it was implementing orders of superior authorities.

This general liability based on fault does not exclude a special liability that is objective under the following conditions:

S.238
The organization shall be liable for damage caused by circumstances originating in the nature of an instrument or other object used in performing the service; it may not be relieved of this liability.

Legitimate abortions were originally regulated by the Abortion Act 1957, as was noted above, and complementary notices from the Ministries of Health. These have been changed several times. At one time, the consent of a special commission was among the prerequisites for legitimate abortion. Besides medical, eugenic and ethical reasons, there was a group of social reasons for abortions which were only enumerated as examples. This regulation was an object of criticism, especially from gynaecologists.

Finally, this was abolished and has been replaced by two parallel new Abortion Acts of 1986 for the National Republics. They are implemented by realizing notices. The new Acts distinguish medical indications from the simple desire of a pregnant woman to have her pregnancy terminated as reasons for legal abortion. If there are no contraindications, the interruption of unwanted pregnancy is admissible provided that the pregnancy has not exceeded 12 weeks. The commissions were abolished and the plain request of the woman is now sufficient. Special prerequisites exist for minors and incapacitated women. The fee for abortions on non-health grounds is 500 koruna.[25]

The current Penal Code 1961 does not apply any punishment or penal sanctions against a pregnant woman who has terminated her own pregnancy, or asked another person to do so, or has permitted such a person to do it (s. 229). Under s. 228, however, any person who interrupts a woman's pregnancy, even with her consent, otherwise than in a way admissible according to the Abortion Act is punishable, as is also the assistant or instigator under s. 227. The aggravating circumstances resulting in heavier punishment (up to 12 years' imprisonment) are performance of abortion for gain or grave harm to the health of the woman, or performance against her objections, especially causing her death.

THE SEARCH FOR NEW LEGAL APPROACHES AND ACTUAL LEGISLATIVE STEPS

Administration of Artificial Insemination

Resolving the problems posed by the administration of artificial insemination (AI), which has been occurring to a certain extent in both forms – that is, artificial insemination by husband (AIH) and AID, without any regulation, has perhaps been the most urgent task for lawyers. It was estimated that at the end of the 1970s there had been approximately yearly 500 requests for AI in the Czech Republic alone. There was doubt as to the legal consequences of such proceedings and it was necessary to take a position on this. I was invited to analyse the problem and this resulted in the presentation of a paper to Medico-Juridica III, 1972, which met with the general approval of the assembly, and was subsequently published in a completed form afterwards.[26] This paper attempted to adopt a positive approach to AI in both forms and argued for their use only in cases of married women and only for medical treatment. In addition, it sought to show that there are not inevitably dangers for the legal status of the child if all the possibilities of interpretation of the Family Code in connection with the Civil Code are used.

However, years passed and no legal regulation appeared. The main reason probably was expectation of the promulgation of the Family Code Amendment Act which appeared only in 1982. Then, after long preparations, the Binding Instruction on Prerequisites for Artificial Insemination 1982 was published by the Czech Ministry of Health, and followed by the Slovak instruction in 1983 which is virtually identical. Those interested can find their shortened English translation in the Actes de Lausanne.[27] The instruction accepted the main postulates I fought for 10 years previously. I would have preferred the guidance to take the form of a parliamentary Act, but the legislator gave priority to a more elastic procedure, which was possible on the basis of s. 70 of the Public Health Care Act, as quoted above. It must be added that the binding Instructions were announced in the Czechoslovak *Digest of Laws* and this fact gives them the character of generally binding regulations which must be observed by all citizens and organizations.

Currently there are several articles analysing or explaining the Instructions.[28] Since, with only a few exceptions, they are written in Czech and therefore not directly accessible to foreign specialists, the following paragraphs describe not only the content of the Instructions but also basic comments on them.

Section 1, para. 1 states that AI may be administered only at the request of both the husband and wife and that the request is to be addressed to the gynaecologist treating the woman. That means that the administration of AI to unmarried couples, lesbian couples and other unmarried women is excluded. It can be also deduced that AI *post mortem mariti* is outlawed and, in the areas of Czechoslovak jurisdiction, such an attempt would be unsuccessful – in contrast to the French *Parpalaix* v. *CECOS*.[29]

Section 1, para. 2 states: 'AI is a medical act through which a woman is fertilized by the semen of either her husband or another man (a donor).' From this formulation it follows that AI can be legally administered only by a medical professional; autoinsemination is not admissible, and sale or other transmission of human sperm to patients is forbidden. Only AIH or AID are permitted, not AIC (with the use of a mixed sperm); AIH is preferred to AID, which can be used only if AIH cannot lead to the desired result.

The next sections state:

S. 2
(1)   Artificial insemination may be performed only if health reasons exist for such an intervention.
(2)   Health reasons for artificial insemination include, in particular, lack of fertility of the husband, anatomical or other defects of the female genital organs, risk of hereditary disease, or evolutionary defects.

The consequence of this section is that AI for the convenience of the woman, without medical indications – for example, if a woman wished to have a child by a donor with special endowments, especially high IQ and so on – is not permitted. The scope of health reasons for AIH or AID is indicated in para. 2.

S. 3
(1)   Spouses who apply for AI shall undergo a medical examination from the point of view of their general state of health, including fertility and genetic risks.
(2)   AI may be undertaken only by a woman who has reached majority and who, as a rule, is not over 35 years, provided her state of health or that of her husband does not preclude it.
(3)   AI may not be administered if both spouses are not legally fully competent.

There is nothing to add to para. 1; however, regarding para. 2, it must be said that the age of 35 years can also be exceeded if no contraindications exist. Para. 3 states nothing in relation to the age of the husband of the woman patient. By analogy to s. 5, para. 2, it can, however, be deduced that as a rule he should not be over 40. The minimum age of the woman is not indicated clearly in the Instruction. On this point we must respect s. 8, para. 2 of the Civil

Code in relation to s. 13 of the Family Code. That is, majority is generally acquired at the age of 18, but is also attained after conclusion of marriage, which is possible after the sixteenth year with the court's permission. What is meant in the Instruction, however, is the completion of 18 years for the woman, and it should be deduced that the same age is the minimum age for the husband. Nevertheless, in practice, the age level will be substantially higher because very careful treatment must take place before the physician takes AI into consideration.

As to the full legal competence mentioned in para. 3, which both husband and wife must satisfy, the Instruction is in harmony with ss. 10 and 38 of the Civil Code and with ss. 186 and following of the Civil Procedure Code 1963, on legal capacity proceedings.

S. 4

(1)   The spouses must file the application for artificial insemination in person and jointly. They must prove their identity and, if they apply for AID, they must state in writing that they were instructed on the legal consequences of AI and on the possible complications that may arise from the pregnancy. . . .

(2)   Before each fertilizing act the applicant spouses shall pay a fee of 200 koruna.

To the first paragraph it can be added that the formula for the declaration of spouses is contained in the annexe to the Instruction. This formula should be assessed in connection with ss. 37, 38 and 40 of the Civil Code and s. 20 of the Family Code. This means that it is a declaration of will of each of the spouses which must be made freely, seriously, definitely and understandably, in full sanity of mind and in the prescribed written form. It cannot be replaced by a declaration of another person (for example, the party's lawyer) and both the declarations must be in concordance. A discordant declaration cannot be substituted by a court's decision as in other cases according to s. 20, sentence 2 of the Family Code. It is an exclusively personal manifestation of will. It cannot be restricted by any condition but can be time-limited and loses validity as a result of dissolution of marriage. In this regard there is a newly published court decision containing this principle – D 49/1990. The spouses must make their decision after receiving sufficient information on civil and family law consequences. The consent of the husband must exist at the moment of the performance of AI by the physician; dissent has legal consequences from the moment at which it is communicated to the physician, not before.

If the fertilizing act is repeated the fee must be paid anew for each repetition according to para. 2.

S. 5

(1) If the husband's semen cannot be used, AI may, with the consent of the spouses, be performed with the semen of a donor chosen by the physician who performs the act (s. 6, para. 2). The donor must undergo a medical examination.

(2) The donor must be healthy, without a demonstrable medical defect and not older than 40 years. He must not be a relative of the woman in the direct line or be her brother. The spouses and the donor must not learn each other's identity. The sperm may be used for AI only with the express consent of the donor.

Para. 1 confirms the principle of the priority of AIH over AID, as has been noted in connection with s. 1. I believe that there is a difference between a request for AIH and for AID, and that the manifestation of will of the spouses must not be ambiguous in this regard. The spouses cannot influence the choice of donor — that is entirely the responsibility of the performing physician. But he/she must observe certain rules in order to ensure that the child is appropriate to the couple: for example, he has to consider their principal physical and psychical features. The physician should also observe the requirements to avoid the transmission of HIV/AIDS in line with the postulates of the Stockholm International Conference held in June 1988. Thus, in light of new knowledge, the Ministries of Health and Social Welfare complemented the Instruction in July 1988 so that it is now forbidden to use fresh sperm after only a single examination for HIV status. A repeated examination of HIV status is prescribed, therefore requiring that the sperm must be cryoconserved for at least 180 days.

Complete anonymity of the donor and the recipient woman and her spouse must be maintained. Thus the child has no 'right' to learn of his/her genetic origin. In this regard the Czechoslovak pattern differs intentionally from some other models — such as the Swedish or the West German.[30]

The second sentence of para. 2 corresponds to the general rules as to impediments to marriage, according to s. 12 of the Family Code. It should be noted that the Czechoslovak legal order does not recognize the *impedimentum affinitatis* to marriage. In respect of the last sentence of s. 2 it can be said that the consent of the donor's wife is not necessary although some foreign models (for example, the Australian) contain this condition and it is not without value. The requirement of an express consent by the donor to the use of his sperm for AI can be explained only if we admit that the Instruction also takes into consideration other possible uses of the sperm — for example, for research.

Since the promulgation of the Instruction in 1988 it is now clear that the cryoconservation of sperms is legally permitted by analogy with s. 26 of the Public Health Care Act 1966.[31]

S. 6

(1–2)   details as to procedure and competence

(3)   Whether AI is indicated shall be decided by the head of the department where the act is to be performed, at the request of the physician designated to perform the act. The department head will take into account the results of the gynaecological, androgen, and genetic examinations.

S. 7

(1)   All the circumstances connected with the AI are covered by obligatory medical secrecy.

(2)   AI is noted in the woman patient's health record. In this connection the name of the donor, by whose sperm the woman was fertilized, is not recorded.

The fact that, according to actual practice, the result of the blood analysis of the donor is not kept in the records causes difficulties for the position of the husband in affiliation denial cases.

S. 8

. . . A donor who applies for it will be granted a remuneration. . .

This remuneration is only small and is regulated by the governmental notices to implementation of the Labour Code 1965, from 1975, and represents only compensation for loss of time and payment of appropriate expenses.

S. 9

The present instruction shall enter into effect on 1 April 1983.

If this Instruction is compared with the AI-Draft Resolution of the Council of Europe,[32] it can be seen that there is general agreement between the principles of the Czechoslovak regulation and this Draft as to the first six sections of this document. The existing differences in s. 3, para. 2 and s. 6, para. 1 are not substantial. The content of s. 7 is realized by means of the Family Code Amendment Act 1982.

In Czechoslovakia no report on AI was published before the enactment of the Instruction. There was no public debate on the conformity of its principles with human rights documents (both Covenants on human rights were ratified by Czechoslovakia), and the Czechoslovak Constitution. However, objections were not raised to the same extent as, for example, in the Federal Republic of Germany and some other countries.

Administration of Fertilization in Vitro with Embryo Transfer or Replacement

As noted above, IVF has been practised in Czechoslovakia since 1982, but was carried out in the homologous variant only, without donors of ovocytes. Until now, no official guideline nor statute solving the legal problems of IVF + ET/ER and related matters has been published. Nevertheless, it cannot be said that a *vide juridique* exists. The Czechoslovak legal order knows the principle of analogy – expressed, for example, in s. 496 of the Civil Code – and recognizes not only *analogiam legis* but also *analogiam iuris*. So it is possible to solve the main problems of the legal consequences originating from the use of IVF + ET/ER in this situation. Judge-made law is not usual on the continent, but it can arise in an emergency. This was, for example, the approach of the French judiciary in the famous paternity denial case at the Toulouse Appellate Court on 21 September 1987: 'en l'absence d'intervention du législateur. . . .il incombe au tribunal d'assurer, en fonction du droit positif, le respect des droits. . . .' (It is here that my agreement with the Toulouse Appellate Court ends, and I do not wish to be associated with its other ideas.)

A number of problems concerning IVF + ET/ER have been discussed in Czechoslovakia and I have contributed a substantial amount to this debate. However, the last word on this issue was pronounced by a group of Czechoslovak authors[33] who suggested a 'Draft of Ethical Principles Regulating IVF + ET/ER and Related Problems' and published it in 1988. The acceptance of the Draft's ideas by the Czechoslovak Medical Associaton J. E. Purkyně (that is its gynaecological section) as an ethical guideline and its discussion as a basis for future legislation in the Scientific Councils of the Ministries of Health and Social Welfare should be the next steps. Since this Draft represents the core of current legal thinking in Czechoslovakia on problems of utmost interest, it is therefore worth commenting on it here.

Principle 1

> Realization of IVF + ET/ER in the *case of sterility* of the spouses and lack of other means to overcome it is ethically admissible.

On a worldwide scale this principle is not always accepted although it represents a majority approach.[34] Unlike AI in its heterologous (and most practical) variant, here the case of female sterility or other difficulties are preeminent and only in the second stage does the infertility of both spouses come to the fore. If we admit the use of AI by the sperm of the husband as well as by the sperm of a donor, then we cannot deny the use of IVF + ET/ER in all its forms in the converse situation. In the light of the Instruction to AI Administration 1982, it cannot be declared illegal. As with AI, this medical procedure should be used only in relation to married women and only as the last resort. As to the age of the woman patient and that of her husband, the above-mentioned Instruction should be used *per analogiam*.

Principle 2

> The spouses chosen for the IVF + ET/ER project as well as the prospective donors of gametes must be healthy. This state of health shall be proved by a medical testimony (e.g. in cases of suspicion of AIDS, hepatitis virus etc.). The *spouses and donors must undergo necessary medical examinations*, in particular genetical.

There is nothing surprising in the content of this principle itself and it can be fully deduced from the AI Instruction (as its counterpart).

Principle 3

> The spouses chosen for the IVF + ET/ER project must be instructed in the methods which will be applied to make them understand the particular steps of the therapeutic treatment. *The spouses shall give in writing their consent* to the medical procedure and before doing so they shall be informed about the risks connected with it.

This principle should be added to, so that it not only requires the informed consent of the woman patient and her husband to the medical treatment, based on sufficient knowledge of its character and risks, but also expresses that they knew the legal consequences as to affiliation of the desired child.

Both medical and legal information should correspond with the type of treatment intended by the physician.[35]

Principle 4

> If there is a grave disorder in the husband's spermiogenesis ability which makes fertilization impossible, fertilization of ovocytes *by a donor's sperm* shall be ethically acceptable.

Here the Czechoslovak doctrine is in harmony with the British Warnock Report[36] and the White Paper[37] and shares their reasons. There is nothing in the present law that would make this procedure illicit.

Principle 5

> *Ovocyte donation* to women who do not dispose of their own ovocytes in a natural way or are not able to have them replaced by the use of today's medical techniques, shall be regarded as ethically admissible.

Ovocyte donation is one of the more difficult problems for medical lawyers and has aroused much discussion. The pros and cons published elsewhere in the world were considered, but it was concluded that not only ethically, but also from the legal point of view, there are no constitutional or other obstacles to the acceptability of ovocyte donation.

Principle 6

> In connection with publicity given to IVF + ET/ER it is important that the physicians and all the persons involved preserve the *anonymity of the marital couple* participating in the project so long as the spouses desire.

This principle should be observed in relation to all the assisted fertilization procedures, and if it is emphasized in relation to IVF, the reason is that here the danger of tactless disclosure is the greatest. As to the ovocyte donor, the secrecy should be unlimited and unconditional, as in the case of a sperm donor.

Principle 7

> Donation of ovocytes by one woman to another for the sake of the so-called *maternal surrogacy* shall be considered in general ethically unacceptable.
>
> Only in extremely exceptional cases if arising from purely altruistic motives and with special guarantees for the future status and fate of the child, could such donation be ethically acceptable when carried out with the consent of a competent authority.

The first sentence, which should cover all the forms of ovocyte donation, is fully in conformity with the present Czechoslovak law. As I have repeatedly indicated,[38] all contracts between commissioning couples and prospective surrogate mothers must be regarded as void because of the provision of s. 39 of the Civil Code and cannot be enforced in any way. All payments or any other material advantages given or accepted in this connection could be argued to be undeserved profit on the basis of s. 457 of the Civil Code by the Prosecutor in civil proceedings. The practice itself does not constitute a criminal offence according to the present Penal Code. Perhaps the content of its s. 209 on injury to the rights of other persons or that of s. 212 on abandonment of the child could be taken into consideration in some situations, but the result is doubtful.

The second sentence on exceptional cases seems to refer to such cases as the French twin-sister surrogate mother case, or the South African grandmother surrogate case – both altruistically motivated.

However, there are two aspects: ethical or moral acceptability and legal admissibility. In my view the stipulations and preconditions contained in the final sentence are too complicated to be legally acceptable — what would represent a sufficient legal guarantee for the child's future and status? For this reason, I favour the complete legal illicitness of maternal surrogacy in family and civil law: lack of punishment if gainful motives are absent will be the manifestation of utmost tolerance; in other cases punishment should be introduced.

Those arguing for surrogate motherhood in Czechoslovakia[39] are quite exceptional, in contrast to Western Europe[40] or the United States,[41] although the opposition is not negligible.[42]

Principle 8

> Scientific *research on embryos* shall be ethically justified only under the condition that it is carried out during the period before the embryo reaches the stage normally suited for implantation. For this reason the 14-day period constitutes the extreme time-limit. Scientific research on embryos is permitted only in the framework of an approved official research project and with consent of the Scientific Council of the Ministries of Health and Social Welfare.

This problem is very complicated and controversial. Research cannot be unrestricted in those fields where it hurts or endangers the vital interests of society — and that is the case here. There are opinions radically against all research of this nature.[43] Even in national reports, opinion remained divided — as in the Warnock Report with *vota separata* against it[44] and in the Benda Report for it.[45] It is generally felt that the use of human embryos for research must be limited.[46]

It appears, however, that there are important arguments for the continuation of embryo research — notably to achieve improvements in fertility treatment and to detect genetic disorders. Thus, complete and unconditional prohibition of research could cause more harm than benefit, and it seems also inconsistent with legislation permitting abortion on non-health conditioned grounds.

Notable approaches to the solution of this problem can be found in *Principes provisoires*, AI, 1986,[47] the Warnock Report,[48] the English White Paper[49] and the Australian and the Canadian documents.[50] This is the principle that, except as a part of a specifically licensed project, it will be a criminal offence to carry out any procedures on a human embryo other than those aimed at preparing the embryo for transfer to the uterus of a woman, or those carried out to ascertain suitability of the embryo for the intended transfer. Licence should not be given to research on embryos beyond a certain stage of evolution. The licence should be given only if the licensing authority is satisfied that the aim of the project will lead to advances in diagnostic or therapeutic techniques, or in fertility control; that the project is scientifically valid and its aim cannot be achieved otherwise.[51]

As to the 14-day time-limit of the Warnock Report, despite several objections to it,[52] nothing better has been found.[53] The discussion as to at what moment human life begins does not seem to solve the problem: the core of the problem is in the question as to from what moment the embryo should be legally protected, and this moment could be identified with the beginning of cerebral life.

Principle 9

> *Cryoconservation of embryos* for future implantation to a woman from whom the ovocytes have been taken should not last for more than 5 years.

Up to now there is nothing to indicate the legal solution to this problem. I believe that we must seek a more general approach to the complex issues concerning cryobank operation.[54] We must take into account not only cryoconservation of embryos but also of gametes, and not only homologous replacement but also transfer of a partially (as to one of the gametes) or fully (as to both gametes) heterologous embryo.

The starting-point of our inquiry must be the complex of problems concerning collection, storage and distribution of human gametes. Until now, only cryoconservation of human sperm has been practised but now we must also consider cryoconservation of human eggs which the Australians announced had been successfully achieved at the end of 1985.

Cryoconservation of both types of gametes seems acceptable ethically as well as legally only for the following aims:

1. The autoconservation of the depositor, advisable in connection with an inevitable future medical treatment or danger to fertility caused by professional or similar activity (but not for convenience, for example in connection with voluntary sterilization not medically indicated);
2. The creation of a fund of 'donated' gametes for the sake of infertility healing.

It makes no difference if gamete cryoconservation is long-term or short-term. There are two general models establishing rights to stored gametes. The first one preserves the maximum of rights of disposal and use for the person from whom the gametes originate, the second one gives a superior position to the medical authority operating the storage. The second model seems preferable, signifying a general assignment of rights of disposal and use of the gametes to the cryobank or its successor, with some limitations. The rights of the cryobank should take force at the moment of taking over the gametes for storage.

In the case of intended autoconservation of the depositor, the cryobank's rights are restricted by the depositor's right to exclusive future use; they should be declared once and for all at the beginning of the storage, and should be time-limited and should finish *ex lege* with the depositior's death.

In the case of 'donation' (which cannot be regarded as transmission of property but only as assignment of the rights of disposal and use), no restriction of the rights of the cryobank by the rights of the donor should exist. However the rights of the bank should also be time-limited.

In both cases the storage should not exceed a 10-year period.

The production and storage of human embryos requires different rules: they should be admissible only in direct connection with the intended IVF + ET/ER. Artificial production of embryos for intended autoconservation and their subsequent storage in a cryobank should be prohibited. Only spare embryos remaining after an actual IVF + ET/ER should be stored, but no more embryos than seems advisable for the planned individual treatment should be produced. The possibility of 'donation' of embryos (that is, the transmission of the rights of disposal and use of the embryos) should be limited to superfluous embryos and should be admissible only if the embryos would otherwise be destroyed without using them for fertilization. Creation of a fund of human embryos by other means, and for other purposes, should be prohibited. At the beginning of the freezing process no embryo should be developed beyond the fourteenth day for the reasons mentioned in the foregoing Principles.

The period of storage of embryos should be limited to a maximum of five years.

In suggesting these rules I am aware that in current Czechoslovak law there is no regulation expressed in a statute or a decision: however, such rules would correspond largely to views already expressed nationally and internationally.

Principle 10

> For *donation of a cryoconserved embryo* to another recipient than the woman from which the ovocyte originates, the written consent of the man and woman whose gametes were used in the production of the embryo is needed.

This principle should be taken into consideration only in the case of a spare embryo produced in a manner and for a purpose stated in the comments to Principle 9.

Principle 11

Gametes and embryos not transferred or not used for research should be destroyed and this should be recorded in the minutes.

This should be done in a decent manner, and the maximum period of cryoconservation is always to be observed.

Principles 8–11 seem to be the most relevant; here the uncertainty of legal solutions is greatest and the necessity for legislation seems the most urgent.

Actual medical practice in IVF + ET/ER tries to avoid the procedures contained in the above-mentioned Principles, and this situation acts as a brake on the further development of assisted reproduction. This should be brought quickly to an end.

Legal Status of the Child Born after Assisted Fertilization

After long hesitation and much debate, the Family Code Amendment Act 1982 appeared. Its content as to the consequences of the use of assisted fertilization techniques was rather modest: the only new provision was contained in para. 2, interposed between the former two paragraphs of s. 58, which became paras 1 and 3. The new para. 2 has this wording:

Paternity may not be denied if the child was born between one hundred and eighty days and three hundred days after the administration of artificial fertilization with the consent of the husband. Paternity may, however, be denied if it can be proved that the mother of the child became pregnant in another way.

There were difficulties with translation of this paragraph into English. Sometimes the translators used the term 'insemination' but this is not adequate because the real meaning is 'fertilization'. Some other vaguenesses originated from an erratum in print, later corrected in the *Digest*. These obscurities were complicated by a mistaken interpretation by some Czechoslovak lawyers.

Nevertheless, the Amendment said nothing as to the problem of who should be considered legal mother of the child in cases of heterologous IVF + ET with the use of a donated ovocyte or embryo. We also find nothing as to the problem of whether or not legal affiliation of the child with the donor of the sperm or ovocyte can arise.

The only help in this situation is doctrinal interpretation, because judicial decisions — with exception of the formerly quoted decision D49/1990 — do not exist.

Maternal Affiliation

As demonstrated above, the Czechoslovak legal provisions do not include any definition of who is the mother of the child. As far as I know it was the same in all the European and the North American legal orders, and for a good reason: until the possibility of dissociation of the role of *mater genetrix* and *mater gestatrix* emerged, the Roman maxim *mater semper certa est* had occupied a quite firm and undoubted position. After 1978, this unshakeable sureness has seemed to tumble down.[55]

What followed immediately was a temporary confusion in the minds of some lawyers and among the public — caused partially by the mass media. There were several voices saying that a test-tube child can have two or even three mothers at the same time: the woman who had given the ovum, the woman who had offered the womb and possibly the third one who accepted the child after having it commissioned. More serious opinions centred upon the problem as to what is decisive — the biological fact of the provenance of the ovocyte or the fact of the birth.

I tried to explain the core of the problem in my articles published in 1985–86 and afterwards found with pleasure that more and more medical lawyers had accepted, or were ready to accept, the same method of reasoning. This reinforced my opinion, expressed in the maxim which I had formulated in Latin as follows: 'Partus-non ovum-facit maternitatem'. Here I will say only briefly that no legal order can dispense with the postulate of a clear and unambiguous legal relation between the mother and the child, otherwise there will be a danger that the foundations of family ties will be crushed. This fundamental relationship must therefore repose on a clear and patent fact. From time immemorial this fact has been the birth of the child by the pregnant woman. It must be admitted that the use of a donated ovocyte breaks the biological tie between the woman in child birth and the newborn. Cases of this nature are exceptional, and an overwhelming majority of child-delivering woman are simultaneously their biological ascendants. Let us hope that it will remain so, not only in the near future. The birth of a child by the use of a heterologous ovum is even more obscure than the paternity of a *vulgo conceptus* once was. The examination of biological ties between the woman in child birth and the newborn child cannot be taken as the basis for maternity in general. The only basis must remain the delivery, the birth. There are also subsidiary arguments for this opinion: such as the fact that the fertilized ovum becomes a part of the woman's body and the importance of its evolution in her womb for the future personality of the child cannot be underestimated.

The most that can be made by way of concession is that the fact of birth represents a rebuttable presumption of maternity, which can be denied or ascertained by a motion by the *mater genetrix* and *mater gestatrix*. However, I do not think that this concession is acceptable for Czechoslovak law. In the same way as in the other European 'socialist' legal orders its maxim continues in founding on the irrebuttable legal fiction — which only quite exceptionally fails to correspond with the objective truth — that the mother is always the woman who gives birth.

Some 'socialist' Family Codes have expressed this directly, among them the Bulgarian Family Code 1985, s. 31 of which states:

> Motherhood is determined through birth. The same applies also in relation to a child conceived with the genetic material of another woman.

This wording is so broad that it covers not only the use of a donated ovocyte but it would cover also, for example, transplantation of the whole ovary — once this is realizable.

Taking this approach, no motion to ascertain the provenance of the ovum, or the genetic link between the child and the woman who has borne it, has sense or legal importance, and in the Czechoslovak legal order should be regarded inadmissible. What remains is the possibility of motions of denial of the birth of a child by the woman who falsely appears as his/her mother in vital registers, or, on the other hand, determination of the fact of the birth of a child by a woman who did not yet figure in vital registers as his/her mother.

According to Czechoslovak laws the only way for a woman other than the *mater gestatrix* to acquire the legal position of the mother of the child is by adoption (s. 63 and following of the Family Code). Plurality of mothers is impossible in Czechoslovak law. Certainty of motherhood is also a fundamental prerequisite for paternal affiliation because the legal father of a child can be determined only in relation to an unquestionable motherhood.

Paternal Affiliation

The first presumption of paternity indicates paternity of the husband of the mother. The wording of s. 51 of the Family Code, which contains the old Roman principle *pater est quem nuptiae demonstrant*, has been referred to above. This maxim has retained its viability in modern times. On the one hand it works on the belief that the *consortium omnis vitae* is accompanied by fidelity of the woman, and on the other hand it conserves domestic peace and excludes suspicion from others as to legitimacy of the spouses' offspring. In the case where there is more than one husband, the second paragraph gives priority to the presumption of later husband's paternity. The application of new assisted reproduction techniques has changed nothing in the text of the quoted section, but the small verbal change in s. 58 of the Family Code has serious consequences.

According to present legal regulation the status of a child born to a married woman after the use of assisted fertilization techniques can be characterized as follows:

1. If the child is born during the marriage or up to the 300th day after its termination, the husband is always assumed to be the father of the child. In this regard the later husband replaces the former one. It makes no difference if the child originates biologically from another man *per viam naturalem* or by the use of assisted techniques, unless paternity has been successfully denied.
2. Denial of paternity is possible only under the regulations of s. 58 para. 2 of the Family Code in the amended version. The motion can be brought to the court either by the husband or the mother (or his/her curator if they are not legally capable) but the child is excluded from this possibility. No other person has this right with exception of the Prosecutor General.
3. This right remains time-limited to the relatively short period of six months after the birth of the child or the day of having learned about the child's birth, as stated in s. 57 of the Family Code.
4. The prerequisites of s. 58, para. 2 of the Family Code relate exclusively to the situation mentioned in s. 58, para. 1 of the Family Code which states:

> If the child is born in the period between the 180th day from the day the marriage was contracted and the 300th day following the termination or invalidation of the marriage, paternity may be denied only if there are circumstances precluding the possibility of the mother's husband being the father of the child.

The second paragraph excludes the general possibility of denial of paternity given in para. 1 for cases of children probably conceived during the marriage. Para. 2 itself is relatively strictly formulated, although its second sentence permits an exception. However, this second paragraph does not coincide with the situations in para. 3 and cannot be applied if the situation formulated therein arises, that is 'if the child is born before the 180th day from the day the marriage was contracted', because then the consequence is that

> . . .the mother's husband need not consider himself to be the child's father, provided he denies his paternity before a court; however, the foregoing provision shall not be applicable to cases in which the husband had sexual intercourse with the child's mother during the period of not less than 180 days and not more than 300 days prior to the birth of the child, or if he knew at the time the marriage was contracted that she was pregnant.

In such a situation the right to deny paternity remains unlimited by para. 2. But in practice such cases in relation to assisted fertilization can occur only after the remarriage of a woman who has been previously fertilized artificially during her former marriage.

5. If we return to the prerequisites of s. 58, para. 2 of the Family Code a more detailed comment must be added. The term indicated in the first sentence of s. 58, para. 2 of the Family Code must be calculated according to the rule of s. 104 of the Family Code in conjunction with s. 122, para. 1 of the Civil Code. This means that this term begins on the day which follows the day on which the event determining its beginning took place. A mere possibility of causal nexus between the conception of the child and the performance of the actual fertilizing act is sufficient to count as artificial fertilization. This is because those acts will usually be repeated until they are successful or until it becomes evident that the attempts will fail. Therefore the period referred to in para. 2 is calculated from the day following the medical treatment after which the beginning of conception is proved (testified normally by established lack of menstruation by the woman). The first sentence of para. 2 is based on the assumption of conception by assisted fertilization, and does not constitute evidence of a causal nexus between both the events. Lack of the nexus must be proved by the person who denies paternity.

The expression 'consent of the husband' causes several problems. This consent is a unilateral legal act of an exclusively personal character. It cannot be performed by a third person in the name of the husband and its absence cannot be replaced by a decision of a court. It must contain the qualities indicated in s. 37 of the Civil Code – that means it must be a serious, free, definite and understandable manifestation of will. It cannot be restricted by any condition but can be time-limited and lapses *ex lege* with the end of the marriage. This consent can also be withdrawn by the husband himself. The giving or withdrawal becomes effective at the moment it reaches the medical authority competent to decide on the performance of the fertilizing act. No form for the consent or its withdrawal is prescribed. A written joint declaration of the spouses to the medical authority according to the Binding Instruction only provides evidence of the request and of the consent of the husband and of the recipient herself. It is not permitted to infer the husband's consent from mere conduct (s. 35 of the Civil Code). A valid consent cannot be given by a person who is temporarily insane (s. 38 of the Civil Code), nor by a person permanently without full legal capacity (s. 10 of the Civil Code).

If the husband has not given a valid consent to the use of a fertilizing technique at all, or if it has lapsed, then para. 2 cannot be applied and paternity can be denied only in accordance with paras. 1 or 3 of s. 58 of the Family Code. Otherwise para. 2 applies to homologous as well as heterologous cases.

Prohibition of paternity denial in the case of a prior valid consent of the husband under para. 2 is subject to only one exception, viz. if it is proved that the child's mother has become pregnant 'in another way' – that is, *per viam naturalem*. The burden of proof is placed on the person alleging it and is very difficult to discharge. Evidence that the husband is not the biological father of the child is not sufficient in itself. Nor is the fact that the mother had sexual intercourse with another man in the critical period, because it does not exclude the possibility that the child had been conceived from the donor's sperm. Under these circumstances blood-group evidence or evidence of an expert witness can be of vital importance if the conclusion is to be reached that the donor's sperm was not the origin of the new life.

6. The practice of assisted fertilization of a widow with the deceased husband's sperm is not permitted by Czechoslovak law and would be illicit. Nevertheless, if it occurred it would have the following consequences:

    • if the child is born after the 300th day after the termination of the marriage by the death of the husband, it cannot be presumed to be the child of the deceased husband (s. 51 of the Family Code);

    • if the child was not in the uterus of his/her mother on the day of the mother's husband's death, he/she could not be regarded his legal heir and could not be declared heir by his will.

The second and the third presumptions of paternity   The second presumption of paternity by concurrent declaration by a man and by the child's mother comes into consideration only if the first one does not apply. The third presumption is the last in the sequence.

Both presumptions can also be applied in relation to a child born after the use of modern fertilization techniques. In this regard there is no legal barrier making this procedure impossible. But none of them has any relevance with respect to the donor of the sperm. The fact of sperm donation itself is juridically irrelevant as to the second and the third paternity presumptions.

In relation to the second presumption lack of sexual intercourse of the declaring man with the child's mother in the critical period does not form an obstacle itself to the validity of the concurrent declaration of paternity, and moreover there is usually no possibility of discovering the truth. If the child's mother (as an unmarried woman) was artificially fertilized by the sperm of the man later acknowledging paternity with the mother's consent, this would be sufficient for the application of the second presumption.   The third presumption will be used only if coitus between the child's mother and the defendant in the course of the so-called critical period is proved; the technological application of sperm or embryo is legally irrelevant for the third presumption.

We must remember, however, that the use of assisted fertilization in relation to an unmarried woman is not permitted and that only illicit performance of assisted fertilization by a third person or by autoinsemination could raise those problems.

The Donor's Position

The donor's position has been sufficiently elucidated in its main characteristics in the preceding text. It is identical in relation to a sperm donor, an ovocyte donor and to embryo donors. No legal rights or obligations from such a donation arise between the child and the donor. There is not only a lack of any legal affiliation between them, but also there is no opportunity for the creation of any other tie.

The donor cannot have parental rights, cannot claim the care of the child or visitation rights for this reason. On the other hand he/she cannot be found liable for maintenance of the child. This maxim could be expressed as follows: *Nullum est privilegium ac onus donatoris ex fertilisatione artificiali oriens.* As a rule such problems will remain only at the theoretical level, because the donor will remain anonymous.

There is no enforceable 'right' of the child to know his/her biological origin in Czechoslovak law. All the medical records are covered by obligatory medical secrecy for ever. Neither the legal parents, nor the child (even after reaching majority) are entitled to know the donor's identity; and no donor is entitled to know in respect of whom or with what result his/her gamete or embryo was applied.

PROSPECTIVE DEVELOPMENT

Prophesying is a very dangerous practice; it especially endangers the mental equilibrium of the prophets who may be forced to read their own predictions 10 years later! But, because this book seeks also to explore the question of what will happen in the future, I will undertake this risky task.

My response can be divided into two partial answers as detailed below.

Development of Medical Science in Czechoslovakia

A further increase in the use of AI, especially its AID form, is to be expected. Anxiety to avoid HIV/AIDS infection will place considerable pressure on the use of cryoconserved and sufficiently examined sperm, and this fact will lead to an increasing tendency to form more cryobanks. IVF is a well established technique in Czechoslovakia and its practice will expand to include the application of donated ovocytes and embryos. This will influence the growth of cryoconservation of ovocytes – if this is really possible – and the acceptance of cryoconservation of embryos. Their use for research projects will be limited although not outlawed. However, in general, the public has no inclination to support the wish of any woman to take on the role of a surrogate mother and 'martyrs' to this idea will not appear. Assisted fertilization methods will be also stimulated by the fact that adoption will become more difficult due to the lack of suitable children, and foster care, without the possibility of having a child of one's own with all the legal attributes of this status, is not attractive. The total number of assisted fertilization acts will be, however, lower than in Western Europe.

Further Development of the Legal Order

One basic fact seems certain: the increase indicated above in assisted fertilization medical procedures will have considerable impact on legal thinking.

The present legal regulation of AI seems likely to be only provisional for it does not take the form of an Act but only that of an instruction. Nevertheless it works, and gives a solid base for practice without fear. The application of IVF + ET/ER goes on without an express legal background – but many problems of a legal character can be solved by the use of analogy and doctrinal theories which influence the information of a common ethical approach in competent medical circles. A notable reinforcement for the formation of such opinions was not least the Eighth World Congress of Medical Law held in Prague in 1988.

It can be expected that one of the next steps will be the definite formation of ethical guidelines on IVF + ET/ER as a basis for a ministerial notice in respect of its practice, preparation of which will be one of the tasks of the Scientific Council of the Ministries of Health and Social Welfare of the Czech and the Slovak Republics. Within this framework, or separately, the legal problems of the operation of cryobanks will be solved.

The legal status of children born after the use of assisted fertilization techniques seems to be sufficiently secured by current judicial and doctrinal interpretation and it would be rather surprising if the remaining partial problems were stimuli for further amendment of the Family Code or the Civil Code. In relation to the latter we can expect that, in future, claims resulting from application of the new methods in respect of liability for damage will arise in a number of cases. However, such problems can arguably be dealt with on the basis of ss. 421 and 238 of the Civil Code.

In respect of liability it will become increasingly necessary to use the principle of objective responsibility and therefore to consider the gametes and embryos as 'things' in the legal sense – as this term is used in s. 238 of the Civil Code. The other kind of objective liability according to s. 432 of the Civil Code does not seem suitable for cases of this kind. Perhaps we could be led by further experience to the creation of new special provisions on medical liability.

At present a Penal Code Amendment Act is being prepared. It seems that its draft has not taken into consideration the new problems posed by the use of assisted fertilization techniques, although this occasion should not be missed.

It is also known that a new Vital Registers Act has been under preparation for several years but it does not seem to be intended to deal with the new methods of reproduction.

The new Abortion Acts have been a disappointment to a certain degree, for they have caused a substantial increase in the number of induced abortions. A return to the previous era is, however, unlikely. An effort to make contraception more readily available, and to dissuade from requests for abortion, will probably follow, but success is unlikely. Coincidence with a growing number of infertile women will be more patent. Nevertheless, a considerable proportion of people will go their own way, taking no interest in all the artificial methods; and, in Czechoslovakia, there is no danger of the 'Big Brother' world foreseen by Aldous Huxley. Traditional attitudes and moral convictions are more deep-rooted than seems possible at first sight. And this is good: the world of Sophocles' moral heroes seems more human than that of overtechnologized civilization.

POSTSCRIPT

The text of my foregoing contribution was finished in the beginning of 1989 and sets down the state of ethical and legal thinking, as well as the regulations of Czechoslovak legal order up to 1 January 1989.

The democratic revolution in my country in November 1989 has also brought changes in this regard and they make it necessary to add this supplement.

Czechoslovakia turns back to the group of the continental European civil law systems. Shortly after the fall of the totalitarian régime the reconstruction of the whole legal order in this sense has begun and this process is not yet completely finished.

For the purpose of our study we must note the following facts: The federal constitutional act containing the 'Charter of Fundamental Rights and Liberties' no. 1991-23 D.L. states that international treaties on human rights and fundamental liberties, ratified by Czechoslovakia and promulgated in D.L., are generally binding on its territory and have priority before the national (home) laws.

The Constitutional Court Act no. 1991-91 D.L. created this jurisdictional forum endowed with competence to deal — among other matters — with questions of conformity of national law in relation to the above mentioned international treaties.

Czechoslovakia signed on 25 February 1991 the European Convention on the Protection of Human Rights and Fundamental Liberties and has been admitted to full membership in the Council of Europe.

Czechoslovakia, signatory of the human rights covenants from 1966, acceded on 12 March 1991 to the Optional Protocol to the Covenant on Civil and Political Rights.

The Czechoslovak 'Charter', as mentioned above, accepts constitutional principles which are important for the inquiry contained in my contribution.

According to its art. 2, s. 3 everybody is entitled to do everything not expressly forbidden by the law. As stated in art. 6, s. 1, 'human life is worth protection already before the birth' — a formula found after lengthy parliamentary debates on the protection of unborn life. In art. 10, s. 2 the protection from unpermitted interference in private and family life is granted. Article 15, s. 2 protects liberty of scientific research. Article 12 deals with substantial aspects of the protection of the family, pregnant women and children.

All this gives new grounds to the prospective legislative deliberations on matters that I have considered in my contribution.

Czechoslovakia is creating new instruments for dealing with bioethics. In the Czech Republic the Central Commission for Medical Ethics was constituted in autumn 1990 (see an article by myself in *Bull. Med. Ethics*, London, 1991, 69, 18—19 June) and the web of local commissions will soon be completed. The autonomous Czech Medical Chamber will be formed in autumn 1991, according to the new regulation of the act 1991—220 D.L. A similar evolution in the Slovak Republic can be anticipated in the near future.

The parliamentary bodies, as well as the federal one and the national ones in the two republics, are overcrowded with drafts and bills, especially on urgent constitutional and economic matters. This situation has blocked till now the further evolution of legislation on medical law topics. In this field only abortions have won a priority. But the drafts of Abortion Acts Amendments are as yet not completely prepared. The pressures for changes are not so far-reaching as, for example, in Poland; more weight is given to sexual education, prevention and contraception, than to restrictions. The Family Code 1963 has remained till now unchanged. The partial amendments of the Civil Code 1964 do not affect matters referred to in my contribution but a general amendment act to this code is now in parliamentary committee. The amendments to the Penal Code and Vital Registers Notice accepted so far did not influence the questions of interest to us.

What is very important is the now completely free flow of information from abroad. The new legal norms, courts decisions and theoretical works, reports and so on originating from the period after 1989 are eagerly studied and I do not doubt that they will have an adequate impact on our future developments.

10 August 1991

NOTES

1   David R. (1978), *Les grands systèmes de droit contemporains*, Paris: Dalloz.
2   *Gillick v. West Norfolk and Wisbech AHA* [1985] 1 All.ER. 533. For discussion, see Lee, S. (1986), *Law and Morals: Warnock, Gillick and beyond*, Oxford: Oxford University Press.
3   For discussion, see Byk, C. (1986), *Ethique et droit en Amérique du Nord face*

aux développements des sciences biologiques et médicales, Paris: Ministère de la Justice.

4   Baudoin, J. L. and Labrusse Riou, C. (1987), 'Produire l'homme: de quel droit?', *Etude juridique et éthique des procréations artificielles*, Paris; Byk, C. and Galpin Jacquot, S. (1986), *Etat comparatif des règles éthiques et juridiques à la procréation artificielle*, vols 1 and 2, Paris; Byk, *Ethique et droit en Amérique du Nord*, op. cit., Byk, C. (1987), *Les aspects juridiques de la procréation artificielle au Royaume-Uni*, Paris; Bernat, E. et. al. (1985), *Lebensbeginn durch Menschenhand*, Graz: Leykamverlag; Corea, G. (1985), *Mother Machine*, New York: Harper and Row.

5   For discussion, see Haderka, J. (1987), 'Artificial reproduction in Czechoslovak law with special reference to other socialist countries', *International Journal of Law and the Family*, **1**, pp. 72–91.

6   For discussion, see Smith, G. P. Jr. (1983), 'The razor's edge of human bondage: artificial fathers and surrogate mothers', *Western New England Law Review*, **5**, pp. 639–66.

7   Cf. Pilka, L., Čupr, Z., Soška, J. and Štěpán, J. (1988), 'Vorschlag der ethischen Grundsätze der extrakorporalen Befruchtung und der damit zusammenhängenden Fragen in der Tschechoslowakei', *Prague Reports*, **2**, pp. 257–61.

8   For discussion, see Rubellin-Devichi, J. (1987), 'La procréation assistée', *Cahiers de médecine légale et droit médical*, no. 4, Singer, P. and Wells, D. (1988), Dzieci z próbowki i praktyka sztucznej prokreacji, (translation from English), *Wydawnictwo prawnicze*, Warsaw; Anon (1985), *Retortenbefruchtung und Verantwortung*, Urachhaus.

9   Haderka, J. (1985), 'Surrogate Motherhood Especially from the Legal Point of View', *Reports of the Seventh World Congress on Medical Law*, Ghent; see further: *Ghent Reports* (1985), **I**, pp. 152–70.

10 *Actes du colloque 'Génétique, procréation et droit'*, Actes de Paris, Paris: Nyssen, 1985.

11 Raymond, G. (1983), 'La procréation artificielle et le droit français', *La semaine juridique*, **57(23)**, p. 3114; Robert, J. (1984), 'La révolution biologique et génétique face aux exigences du droit', *Revue de droit international public*, **5**, pp. 1255–300.

12 Byk, C. and Galpin Jacquot, S. (1986), *Etat comparatif des règles éthiques et juridiques à la procréation artificielle*, vols 1 and 2, Paris; Bernat, E. *et al.* (1985), *Lebensbeginn durch Menschenhand*, Graz: Leykamverlag.

13 See, for discussion, Comité consultatif national d'éthique pour les sciences de la vie et de la santé, *Avis relatif aux recherches sur les embryons humains in vitro et à leur utilisation à des fins médicales et scientifiques*, Paris: CEDEX; Comité consultatif national d'éthique pour les sciences de la vie et de la santé, *Les recherches sur l'embryon humain in vitro: Rapport scientifique–Rapport éthique*, Paris: CEDEX; *Journées annuelles d'éthique pour les sciences de la vie et de la santé*, Paris: CEDEX, 1986; 'Directives médico-éthiques pour l'insémination artificielle de l'Académie suisse des sciences médicales', *Bulletin des médecins suisses*, **63** (11) 17 March 1982; 'Directives médico-éthiques pour le traitement de la stérilité par fécondation in vitro et transfert d'embryons de l'Académie suisse des sciences médicales', *Bulletin des médicins suisses*, **66** **(24)**, 12 June 1985; Ethics Committee of the American Fertility Society (1986), *American Law and the New Reproductive Technologies*: Ex: Byk, C. and Galpin-Jacquet, S. (1986), *Etat comparatif des règles éthiques et juridiques relatives à la procréation artificielle*, Paris: Ministère de la Justice.

14 *Bericht des Bundesministers für Wissenschaft und Forschung an den Nationalrat zu grundsätzlichen Aspekten der Gentechnologie und der humanen Reproduktions-*

biologie, Vienna, 1986, *Report on Human Artificial Reproduction and Related Matters*, vols 1 and 2, Ontario: Ministry of the Attorney General, 1985; Arbeitsgruppe des Bundesminister für Forschung und Technologie und des Bundesministers der Justiz (1985), *In-Vitro Fertilisation, Genomanalyse und Gentherapie*, The Benda Report, Munich: Schweizer-Verlag; *Informe de la Comisión del Estudio de la Fecundación 'in vitro' y la Inseminación Artificial Humanas*, Madrid, 1987; Barn Genom Insemination (1983), *Betakande av. Inseminationsuntredningen*, Stockholm; *Report of the Committee of Inquiry into Human Fertilization and Embryology* (Warnock Report), London: HMSO, 1984.

15   Anon. (1986), *Law and Australian Legal Thinking in the 1980's*, Melbourne.

16   *Human Fertilization and Embryology: A Framework for Legislation* (White Paper) London: HMSO, 1987.

17   Haderka, J. (1973), 'Moderní genetika a naše současné rodinné právo (Modern genetics and our contemporary family law)', *Československé zdravotnictvéi*, **21(3)**, pp. 119–25 and (1973), *Acta Univeristatis Carolinae Iuridica*, **2**, pp. 79–110.

18   *Procréation artificielle, Génétique et Droit* (Actes de Lausanne), Zurich: Schulthessverlag.

19   Haderka, J. (1987), 'Artificial reproduction in Czechoslovak law with special reference to other socialist countries', *International Journal of Law and the Family*, **1**, pp. 72–91.

20   Krzekotowska, K. (1985), 'Glosa do orzeczenia Sądu Najwyszego N S III CZP35/85 (Marginal note to the decision of Supreme Court III CZP 35/85)', *Państwo i prawo*, **11(11–12)**: pp. 187–90, Nesterowicz, M. (1985), 'Glosa do orzeczenia Sądu Najwyszego III CZP 35/85 (Marginal note to the decision of Supreme Court III CZP 35/85)', *Nowe prawo*, **41(2)**, pp. 113–16.

21   Cf. Krzekotowska, K. (1988), 'Inseminatio artificialis a situacja prawna dziecka (Artificial insemination and the legal status of the child)', *Państwo i prawo*, **43(6)**, pp. 101–9; Nesterowicz, M. (1985), 'Problemy prawne nowych technik sztucznego poczęcia dziecka (Legal problems of the use of new artificial conception techniques)', *Państwo i prawo*, **11(12)**, pp. 103–7; Radwanski, Z. (1986), *La filiation et la médecine moderne, Rapports polonais présentés au 12ième Congrès international de droit comparé*, Wroclaw: Ossolineum, pp. 75–89.

22   Council of Europe (1982), 'Artificial insemination of human beings: Not accepted resolution', *Medicine and Law*, Springerverlag, **1**, pp. 3–10; Comité des ministeres du Conseil Européen (1986), *Principes provisoires sur les techniques de procréation artificielle et sur certains procédés appliqués aux embryons en liaison avec ces techniques*; Ex: Byk, C. and Galpin-Jacquet, S. (1986), *Etat comparatif des règles éthiques et juridiques relatives à la procréation artificielle*, Paris: *Ministère de la Justice*.

23   *Bericht des Bundesministers für Wissenschaft und Forschung an den Nationalrat zu grundsätzlichen Aspekten der Gentechnologie und der humanen Reproduktionsbiologie*, Vienna, 1986; Bernat, E. *et al.* (1985), *Lebensbeginn durch Menschenhand*, Graz: Leykamverlag.

24   Haderka, J. (1986), 'K některým problémům určení a popření mateřství (On selected problems of maternity determination and denial)', *Bulletin Advokacie*, **1**, pp. 114–27.

25   For further information, see Drgonec, J. (1987), 'Nový zákon o interrupciách (The new Abortion Act)' *Právny obzor*, **70(1)** pp. 31–43; Haderka, J. (1987), 'Umělé přerušení těhotenství u žen, které nemají plnou způsobilost k právním úkonům (Artificial abortion on women lacking full legal capacity)', *Správní právo*, **20(8)**, pp. 500–7; Haderka, J. (1988), 'Czechoslovakia – two

partial statutory reforms and decisions to Family Code amendments', *Annual Survey of Family Law*, London–Louisville.

26 Haderka, J. (1973), 'Moderní genetika', op. cit., note 17 above and *Acta Universitatis Carolinae Iuridica*, 1973, **2**; pp. 79–110.

27 *Actes de Lausanne*, 1986, op. cit.

28 Drgonec, J. (1984), 'Právne aspekty umelého oplodňovania a ich úprava ČSSR (Legal problems of artificial fertilization and their regulation in the CSSR)', *Právny obzor*, **67(2)**, pp. 138–56; Haderka, J. (1985), 'Právní přípustnost a důsledky umělých inseminací a inovulací (Lawfulness and legal consequences of artificial insemination and egg donation)', *Československa gynekologie*, **50(6)**, pp. 431–5; Haderka, J. (1986), 'Czechoslovakia: the importance of recent changes in the law', *Annual Survey of Family Law*, **9**, London–Louisville, pp. 69–79; Haderka, J. (1986), 'Civilněprávní přístup k legalitě artificiální inseminace neprovdané ženy (Civil law approach to the legal character of artificial insemination of an unmarried woman)', *Československé zdravotnictví*, **34(1)**, pp. 20–32; Haderka, J. (1987), 'K některým otázkám umělého oplodňování (On several artificial fertilisation problems)', *Československá gynekologie*, **52(8)**, pp. 641–6; Haderka, J. (1987), 'Artificial reproduction in Czechoslovak law', op. cit., note 19 above; Hrušaková, M. (1985), 'Právní aspekty umělého oplodňování (Legal aspects of artificial fertilization)', *Medicína a právo*, Acta facultatis medicae Universitatis Brunensis, **89**, pp. 155–60; Sládek, M. (1985), 'Poznámky k problému umělého oplodnění (Note on the problem of artificial fertilization)', *Medicína a právo*, Acta facultatis medicae Universitatis Brunensis, **89**, pp. 149–54; Švarný, E. (1985), 'Povinná mýčenlivost při heterologní inseminaci (Obligatory confidence-keeping in relation to AID)', *Československá gynekologie*, **50(5)**, pp. 386–9.

29 Terré, F. (1984), 'Le droit inadapté', *Le Figaro*, 2 August; Vigy, M. (1984), 'Orphelin avant la conception', *Le Figaro*, 2 August. See also Haderka, J. (1986), 'Civilněprávní přístup', op. cit., note 28 above and Chapter 5 below.

30 The Benda Report, op. cit., note 14 above; Barn Genom Insemination, *Betankande av.Inseminationsuntredningen*, op. cit., note 14 above.

31 Haderka, J. (1988), 'Legal problems connected with the human genetic substratum cryobanks', (shortened version), *Prague Reports*, vol. II, pp. 273–80.

32 Council of Europe, 'Artificial Insemination of Human Beings', op. cit., note 22 above.

33 Pilka *et al.*, 'Vorschlag der ethischen Grundsätze', op. cit., note 7 above.

34 *Bericht des Bundesministers*, op. cit., note 14 above; *American Law and the New Reproductive Technologies*, Report of the Ethics Committee of the American Fertility Society, 1986.

35 Bernat *et al.*, *Lebensbeginn durch Menschendhand*, op. cit., note 12 above; Actes de Paris, 1985, op. cit., note 10 above; *Retortenbefruchtung und Verantwortung*, Urachhaus, 1985.

36 The Warnock Report, op. cit., note 14 above.

37 White Paper, op. cit., note 16 above; see also Human Fertilization and Embryology Act 1990.

38 Haderka, J. *Surrogate Motherhood*, op. cit., note 9 above; see further: *Ghent Reports*, op. cit., note 9 above; Haderka, J. (1986), 'Lze přijmout praxi používání tzv,náhradních rodiček k odstraňování bezdětmosti manželství? (Is the practice of the use of surrogate mothers for treatment of infertile marriages admissible?)', *Československé zdravotnictví*, **34(10)**, pp. 424–31; (1986), 'Surogační mateřství (Surrogate motherhood)', *Právny obzor*, 1986, **69(10)**, pp. 917–34.

39 Mitlöhner, M. and Bruthansová, D. (1988), 'Některé právní problémy, spojené s implantací plodu (Some legal problems associated with implantation of the foetus)', *Československé zdravotnictví*, **36(6–7)**, pp. 295, Prague: Avicenum.

40 Giraud, F. (1987), *Mère porteuse et droits de l'enfant*; Geller, S. (1988), 'La notion de projet d'enfant: un guide pour la solution des problèmes juridiques posés par la procréation artificielle', *Prague Reports*, vol. II, pp. 242–7; Parker, D. C. (1982), 'Legal aspects of AI and E', *Family Law*, **12**, pp. 103–7.

41 *Report on Human Artificial Reproduction*, op. cit., note 14 above; *American Law and the new Reproductive Technologies*, op. cit., note 34 above; Byk, *Ethique et droit*, op. cit., note 4 above; Dickens, B. M. (1985), 'Surrogate motherhood, legal and legislative issues, in Milunsky, A. and G. J. Annas, *Genetics and the Law*, vol. III, New York: Plenum Press; Dickens, B. M. (1987), 'Legal aspects of surrogate motherhood, practices and proposals', Cambridge: Papers of the UN National Committee for Comparative Law Colloquim; Krause, H. D. (1985), 'Artificial conception, legislative approaches', *Family Law Quarterly*, **19(3)**, pp. 185–206. See also Chapter 8 below.

42 Corea, *Mother Machine*, op. cit., note 4 above; Ince, S. (1984), 'Inside surrogate industry', in R. Arditi *et al.*, *Test-Tube Women: What Future for Motherhood?*, London: Pandora Press, pp. 99–115.

43 Haderka, J. 'Czechoslovakia – two partial statutory reforms', op. cit., note 25 above; Méméteau, G. (1988), 'La situation juridique de l'enfant/De la rigueur classique à l'exaltation baroque', *Prague Reports*, vol. II, p. 308, texte complet 27 pp; Sériaux, A. (1985), 'Droit naturel et la procréation artificielle, quelle jurisprudence?', *Chronique*, **10**, pp. 53–60; Sériaux, A. (1988), 'La procréation artificielle sans artifices/Illicité et responsabilités', *Chronique*, **26**, pp. 201–7.

44 Op. cit., note 14 above.

45 The Benda Report, op. cit., note 14 above.

46 *Recommendation no. 1046/1986 on the Use of Human Embryos and Foetuses for Diagnostic, Therapeutic, Scientific, Industrial and Commercial Purposes, of the Parliamentary Assembly of the Council of Europe*, Texts adopted by the Thirty-eighth Ordinary Session of the Assembly, Strasbourg, 1986; *Principes provisoires sur les techniques de procréation artificielle et sur certains procédés appliqués aux embryons en liaison avec ces techniques*, Comité des ministres du Conseil Européen, Strasbourg, 1986; *Bericht des Bundesministers für Wissenschaft und Forschung*, op. cit., note 23 above; *Journées annuelles d'éthique*, op. cit., note 13 above; *Informe de la Comisión del Estudio de la Fecundación*, op. cit., note 14 above; The Warnock Report, op. cit., note 14 above; Haderka, J. (1988), 'Ke snahám o mezinárodní deklarování principů reprodukční medicíny a génového inženýrství (On efforts aiming at declaration of reproductive medicine and genetic engineering principles)', *Praktický lékař*, **(68) 21**, pp. 777–80.

47 *Principes provisoires sur les techniques de procréation artificielle*, op. cit., note 46 above.

48 Op. cit., note 14 above.

49 Op. cit., note 16 above and the Bill.

50 Actes de Lausanne, op. cit., note 18 above; *Law and Australian Legal Thinking in the 1980's*, op. cit., note 15 above; *Report on Human Artificial Reproduction*, op. cit., note 14 above.

51 Haderka, 'Legal Problems', op. cit., note 31 above.

52 And the British Parliament is currently debating whether such research should not be permissible.

53 Baudoin and Labrusse Riou, 'Produire l'homme', op. cit., note 4 above; Knoppers, B. M. (1986), *Conception artificielle et responsabilité médicale*, Quebec: Cowansville; Lee, *Law and Morals*, op. cit., note 2 above; Rubellin-

Devichi, J. (1987), 'La procréation assistée', *Cahiers de médecine légale et droit médical*, (**4**).

54   I chose this as the theme of my contribution to the Eighth World Congress on Medical Law, held in Prague in 1988; Haderka, J., 'Legal Problems', op. cit., note 31 above.

55   See the presumption about maternity contained in Number 26 – now section 27 and partially 30 of the Human Fertilization and Embryology Act, 1990; for commentary see Morgan, D. and Lee, R. G. (1991), in Blackstone's Guide to the above-named Act, London: Blackstone Press Limited.

5 France: Law Reform and Human Reproduction

CHRISTIAN BYK

The important developments in biomedicine during the past 20 years have raised fundamental issues which question social principles and therefore the attitude of ethics and law. In particular, the new reproductive technologies have posed controversial questions. By dissociating sexuality and procreation, they demonstrate the power that man has acquired over his own kind, and emphasize the difficulty of defining what is a family in our industrial society.

The procedures applied to embryos *in vitro* have regenerated the debate concerning the status of the embryo and the right to life. They also require responses to certain important questions. Should we accept and realize all that is technically possible? Are current ethical guidelines or legislation adequate to ensure the 'good' practice of these new technologies? France was concerned very early with these complex questions. At the beginning of the 1970s, artificial insemination by donor (AID) became a common medical procedure to provide infertile couples with children. A number of factors, including the lack of children available for adoption, encouraged physicians and biologists to find new ways to solve infertility. While Edwards and Steptoe took the steps which led, in 1978, to the birth of Louise Brown, the first 'test-tube' baby in the UK, their French colleagues progressed in a similar way.[1]

During these first years, artificial insemination, even when undertaken using donor semen, was regarded as a private matter or a question of professional ethics. Public authorities shared this point of view when, in 1974, the Department of Health agreed to the creation of a national sperm bank network, CECOS (Centre d'Etude et de Conservation des Oeufs et du sperme). The Public Health Act 1978 provided that the cost of infertility treatments, including artificial insemination (AI), should be paid by the National Health Service thus giving an official, but discreet, legitimacy to the practice of the physicians working in connection with the CECOS.[2]

However, the intrusion of surrogacy[3] and posthumous insemina-tion[4] in the field of reproductive medicine catapulted these questions into the public arena, making it difficult for the public authorities to maintain a neutral position in this debate. Family law was ques-tioned; conflicts appeared between physicians and some of their patients who claimed the recognition of a new right — the right to procreate. Because the health system could have been questioned by this claim, as well as by the lack of professional ability of some of the medical teams involved in those procedures, the government, there-fore, decided to initiate a major debate on these questions and to give general and reasonable answers to the problems of reproductive medicine. It is now possible to draw from this debate some conclu-sions concerning the perspective of law reform in France.

This chapter will discuss the methodology adopted in France to prepare for law reform in this area, and will also describe the major principles which apply to reproductive techniques and related embryo research.

THE FRENCH METHODOLOGY

While agreeing that science is progressing faster than law, French lawyers were divided in their conclusions, some believing that repro-ductive medicine should be considered as an epiphenomenon which should not lead to any major change in law[5] and others urging such changes. According to the latter, it was too risky to leave fundamen-tal legal problems in the hands of scientists, who could impose their own rules which might be contrary to the provisions of the Civil Code.[6] The restatement of these two opposing attitudes shows how difficult it was to make choices related to bioethical issues.

The opinion of professionals was also very ambiguous.[7] While a majority would accept professional guidelines and required such guidelines to be approved by law,[8] a strong minority still believed that such questions should remain a matter for the individual rela-tionship between physicians and their patients.[9] Nevertheless, very few called for a real open debate on this matter. A large percentage of the public viewed with considerable respect the physicians and biologists who developed reproductive medicine.[10] Only a few groups opposed reproductive manipulations which deprive human embryos of their potential for life.[11] This confusion, coupled with the lack of a spontaneous and productive controversy on the major issues posed by reproductive medicine, left the government with the task of initiating the French debate.

To achieve this, the government proceeded in two stages. The first consisted in encouraging a wide discussion within the community to see how far it was possible to reach a consensus. The second, when opinion seemed to agree on some ethical principles, was to make an effort to take into consideration the necessary legislative reform.

From Discussion to Ethics

To clarify the complex debate on the question of whether or not to legislate, the government favoured two means : promotion of discussion on this issue; and the development of a specific forum where appropriate ethical guidelines could be established and supported by a large consensus.

The Promotion of the Debate

This was principally based on two governmental initiatives : the organization of a national colloquium and the formulation of a report providing a complete overview of the views expressed in the field of reproductive technologies by experts and members of the public.

Genetics, procreation and law   Although the government was firmly persuaded that some choices should be made in due course, it was also convinced that the different opinions should be clearly discussed before such choices could be made. The first concern, then, was to create the best opportunity for a debate. It was felt that the organization of a colloquium rather than the setting up of a National Commission was more appropriate as a method of reaching this goal. According to this point of view, only a colloquium could permit the terms of the debate to be publicly raised. The colloquium entitled 'Genetics, Procreation and the Law' and organized jointly by the Departments of Justice, Health and Scientific Research was duly held in Paris in January 1985.[12]   Mr R. Badinter, the Minister of Justice, explicitly declared :

> In a Democracy respectful of public liberties . . . it was necessary that the discussion could take place outside academic and professional institutions, outside Parliament, in every place where opinions developed. It was then necessary to follow a way which permitted a real discussion and a complete information of the public. . . . Organized by the Government, this colloquium is not a governmental colloquium. Ministers come here to be informed and not to express the Government's point of view.[13]

The need to be aware of the exact state of scientific knowledge in the field of genetics and reproductive medicine, and the urgent need to know their consequences for the law and society, constituted the principal focus of this colloquium. Nevertheless, the debate which took place during these two days largely concentrated on the question of law. Should we legislate? According to what principles should any future legislation be drafted? These were the principal questions in the debate which aimed to help French society to make collective and individual choices, as well as prepare sets of alternatives for legislation.

It was, therefore, decided to adopt a multidisciplinary and pluralistic approach, involving scientists, lawyers, but also philosophers and sociologists, as well as members of the public, who were invited to assist at the hearings and to put questions to the speakers. Over the two days multidisciplinary panels discussed four topics: the donation and use of gametes; the freezing of embryos; IVF and surrogacy; and predictive medicine. Each panel included a scientist – a physician, biologist or geneticist – to present the state of the art, and to introduce what were, in his/her view, the major issues posed by these new techniques. Following this introduction, a philosopher, sociologist and a lawyer gave their own views on the significance of such issues. In addition, politicians and representatives of churches or other influential groups participated, as did members of the public.

No direct conclusion resulted from the colloquium except an agreement that biomedical issues were not questions to be left solely to the decisions of scientists. From this perspective, the colloquium was perceived as favouring the expression of a liberal attitude in the field of reproductive medicine.

It should, in fact, be borne in mind that before 1985 *de facto* rules existed concerning reproductive technologies, which were effectively imposed by the physicians working in the field. The CECOS organization, founded in 1973 and responsible for almost 90 per cent of artificial inseminations, had voluntarily adopted guidelines such as the need to maintain the anonymity of donors, the gratuity of donation, the exclusion of single persons and a ban on surrogacy.[14] When the government announced, in July 1984, its intention to regulate reproductive medicine,[15] it probably had in mind the 'reasonable' principles adopted by the CECOS. However, this coincided with a case of posthumous insemination which was widely reported in the media and demonstrated that the young widow attracted wide public support, despite the attitude of the CECOS.[16] Thus, the government's initiative in promoting an open debate on these questions, which had already been apparently solved by physicians, was regarded by some people as a negative approach. Furthermore, the different public authorities underlined the moral necessity of considering reproductive techniques not only from the medical point of view but also from the perspective of human rights. Indeed, in his address to the conference, President F. Mitterrand stated:

> The history of Human Rights is the history of human personhood, human dignity, and human integrity. . . .All that concerns life concerns each of us and nobody should decide what is good or not for others than himself. . . [17]

A few weeks later, Mr R. Badinter further developed this theme at the first European Conference on Human Rights, held in VIenna on 19 and 20 March, when he declared:

> The right of every individual to use all means of procreation is beyond any legal control. To deny such a right to humanity will in fact deprive some human persons of a chance to realize their own well-being and will not create any advantage for other humans. [18]

The diversity of opinions expressed during the colloquium did not permit the reaching of immediate conclusions, except on two points. The first one concerned the social consequences of the new reproductive technologies. Sociologists and anthropologists reminded the conference of the existence of other family institutions in different human societies. [19] Human knowledge in this field shows that filiation is a purely social concept. Among these diverse situations some do lead to the same social consequences as would modern reproductive technologies, and so can be compared with AID, surrogacy or posthumous insemination. It may also have brought moral comfort to some to learn that what was thought to be new social behaviour was in fact an ancient practice, which could be accommodated quite happily when supported by social institutions.

The second point which arose from this conference was that the essential principles, on which the current French practice of reproductive medicine was based, were broadly questioned. For example, the access of single persons to reproductive technologies was approved by some lawyers[20] who observed that adoption law does not prohibit adoption by a single man or woman. The practice of maintaining the anonymity of donors was questioned for the reason that knowledge of biological origin was of a great importance for the identity of the child. [21] Even surrogate motherhood, although considered as a void contract from a civil law point of view, could, it was suggested, be accepted in some exceptional cases when no money was involved.

The requirement for legislation was not therefore felt to be so great, and in any event those who called for new laws did not seem to agree on the content of the reform they wished. For this reason Prof. J. Carbonnier came to the conclusion that it was wiser to wait, and proposed a moratorium on legislation.[22] However, in his view, this period of legislative abstention should be a positive procedure, during which the application of general principles of law to reproductive medicine should be tested. The government should also take advantage of this time to obtain a better knowledge of the numerous opinions of the different component parts of French society on questions which still appeared controversial. This should be done, not in an emotional, but in a research-based manner. Such a study should also try to find some explanation of the apparently overwhelming desire of infertile couples to have children. Why, for example, do people need so much recognition of the legal status of the family when just a century ago they seemed to be satisfied with some kind of *de facto* adoption?

It was also felt that comparative studies could be very useful in understanding why, in regulating the reproductive technologies, some countries have adopted principles which are very different from current French practice.[23]

It should also be noted that, at the same time, the Council of Europe had launched a programme of activities in order to study the legal implications of the development of the biomedical sciences.[24] In addition, in April 1985, President Mitterrand invited the seven most industrialized countries to a bioethics symposium in Rambouillet.[25]

Artificial procreation   The need to pursue the investigations suggested by Professor Carbonnier led the government to instigate a broad study of opinions. In July 1985 a group comprising two lawyers (Prof. C. Labrusse and Mr J. P. Rosenczveig) and three biologists (Mrs M. O. Alnot, Mrs S. Mandelbaum and Mrs Y. Pérol) was charged with coordinating this task. They reported to the Prime Minister in February 1986.[26]

Their mission was quite specific. They were to collect opinions from both the professionals involved and the different bodies of opinion in the religious and political fields. This way of proceeding was quite novel in French administrative practice. Usually, ad hoc committees are set up to assess a problem and to suggest proposals for reform. Here, the main task of the Committee was to give a 'snapshot' of opinions in the field of reproductive medicine.

Part I of the Committee's report, *Artificial Procreation*, presents a general analysis of facts and opinions. Following Chapter I, which describes the medical characteristics of reproductive medicine, Chapter II discusses the social and cultural context in which such techniques developed. It is observed that, from a general point of view, artificial reproduction is regarded as progress when it helps infertile couples to have children. Nevertheless, some opposition does exist in circumstances when it is necessary to use donors, except perhaps in the case of AID. The desire to have children appears itself to be complex and ambiguous. Chapter III deals with the important question of the social and economic cost of these techniques, noting the necessity to reduce their cost by an active policy of prevention for venereal diseases.

It appears that society is in search of the limits which should regulate the different powers involved in the new reproductive technologies : the power of science and research over man, the power of the individual over him or herself and the power of the State to interfere and to regulate these practices.

Part II presents some specific developments in respect of each of the reproductive technologies, focusing on those issues which could be considered as still raising some difficulties.

The conclusion of this analysis is that the positive aspects of reproductive technologies are minimized. If reproductive medicine brings real advantages, it also carries some risks and potential drawbacks. To find an adequate balance between the method and the results of such techniques will certainly require the imposition of some specific rules. These rules should not be inferred from the practice of biomedicine but rather should derive from a pluralistic view of society which broadly takes into account scientific facts as well as legal and moral opinions.

The difficulties involved, and the time needed to define these ethical principles, demonstrate the importance of the role which could be played by a specific forum such as a National Ethical Committee.

The National Ethical Committee

How could a pluralistic society agree on common principles concerning biomedical issues? A small group of scientists and philosophers tried to promote the search for consensus when they created, in 1974, the MURS (Universal Movement for Scientific Responsibility). Institutional Ethics Committees, such as the Medical Research Council (INSERM) Ethics Committee, were also created during the 1970s, but the activities of all these groups have been very confidential. Conversely, academic and professional institutions, such as the Academy of Medicine,[27] or the Corporation of Physicians, were heavily criticized for the conservative opinions which they expressed during the abortion controversy. Against this background, it was decided to set up a new and independent authority, which would act as a forum to discuss issues raised by medical research. The result of this decision was the creation, by presidential decree in 1983, of the National Ethical Committee for Life Sciences and Health.[28] President Mitterrand declared: '. . . the citizen is asking questions to the scientist about the risks of Science ... What is possible should not always be admissible'[29] and Prof. J. Bernard, who was appointed Chairman of the Committee, added: '...the new powers that biology gives to man imply new responsibilities for man.'[30] In calling for the emergence of a new morality, the President concluded: '...give yourselves time : time to think, time to discuss, and time to appraise the moral issues.'[30a] The mission and the membership of the Committee was to be guided by the principle: it is better to get it right later than wrong now.

In fact, the Committee has two main activities. First, it is to advise on ethical issues raised by research in the field of biology, medicine and health care. Questions can be brought to the Committee by members of the government, presidents of the two Houses of Parliament or by any public institution involved in research. But the Committee has also the opportunity to decide itself which particular important issues should be discussed.

Its area of competence is very wide, although limited to ethical questions posed by the development of research. The Committee is not designed or empowered to review individual experiments, which is the task of local ethical committees, but has only to consider major social issues. However, some advice may deal with specific experiments — for example, the new abortion pill mifepristone (RU 486) — when they can result in far-reaching effects.

The Committee acts as an advisory body and, as such, its advice is not enforceable. For example, the Medical Research Council has no compelling duty to subsidy or not to research on the basis of the agreement or disagreement of the Committee. A good definition of the role played by the Committee was given by the Prime Minister, L. Fabius, when he addressed the Committee in 1985:

> The statements of the Committee are only advice. That is the best safeguard for their credibility. Roles should effectively be clearly defined. The Committee has the mission to act as a scientific institution and to provide information in this field. The Government has the duty to administer the health system and to determine a public health policy. Parliament has to legislate and the judge to give application and significance to law.

He concluded:

> ... you are not a moral court, ... you are not judges of the scientific community... You are only men and women chosen by society to make understandable the consequences of biology for its future.[31]

Thus, the Committee is supposed to work as a moral authority, and its advice may be accepted by scientists, and may also be influential on the decisions of courts and the policy of public authorities. For this reason, its advice circulates widely in professional areas as well as in the public arena.

The Committee's second main activity is to function as a forum for discussion with both professionals and members of the public. Although when the Committee was set up, some clearly questioned its utility[32] (general practitioners were sceptical; some researchers saw it as a threat; others observed that ethics should be under the responsibility of the Corporation of Physicians), no one will now publicly contest the Committee's role. Indeed, in asking the Committee to advise them on major issues, researchers, and also physicians, have shown that they have accepted its role. And the Committee itself has developed specific relationships with researchers and scientific institutions. Many of them participate in the working groups set up by the Committee. Among these institutions, the Corporation of Physicians, which has no representative on the Committee, has been frequently associated with the Committee's work. Other useful relationships have been established, particularly with local ethical committees, and also with similar institutions in other countries.

However, a specific aim of the Committee is to try to establish a dialogue with the public. If each citizen is concerned with biomedical issues and has the right to make his or her own choices, he or she should be properly informed. Therefore, the Committee has the duty to explain the new medical procedures in language which can easily be understood. Misunderstandings which could create undue anxiety or fear should also be exposed to the public by the Committee. To provide this information the Committee organizes an annual two-day meeting where accomplished and prospective work is presented. These meetings are also used to allow public participation in the debate. Questions can be put directly to Committee members, and small workshops are organized to create appropriate fora for real discussion, encouraging the expression of critical views.

During the past few years, Committee days have been organized on the following topics : Children in Society (1985), International Ethics (1986), Educational Programmes in Bioethics (1987), Ethics and Knowledge (1988), Human Rights and Neurosciences (1989), Ethics and Pediatrics (1990) and Ethics and Eugenism (1991). Since 1986, some of these public conferences have been held outside Paris, in other major cities. All these meetings, which were well attended, proved that biomedical problems have generated increasing interest in society, and that it is possible to have dispassionate debate where everyone can freely express his or her own view.

The 37 members of the Committee belong to four categories and are appointed for two years. Half of the membership is renewed every two years. The Chairman is appointed by the President, the present chairman being Prof. J. Bernard, the well-known specialist in haematology. Five other members are also appointed by the French President, and represent religious and philosophical groups. The main four denominations established in France (Catholics, Protestants, Jews and Muslims) are members of this group, which includes also the director of the Institute of Marxist Studies. Sixteen members are chosen by different authorities in the light of their special competence in the field of bioethics. Two are Members of Parliament, one is designated by the Supreme Court (Cour de Cassation) and one by the Conseil d'Etat, which is the higher administrative court. The others are appointed by different ministers. The last 16 members belong to research institutes.

Such a composition makes the Committee 'a forum for debate on the consequences of the progress of biology and medicine which are assessed and criticized in a common work by theologians, philosophers, moralists, lawyers and scientists'.[33] This statement, however, does not entirely correspond to the reality of the membership of the Committee in which biology and medicine are widely represented (25 physicians and scientists, four lawyers, three theologians and philosophers, five persons of different professions). It should be observed that theologians and philosophers are a minority among the members representing the religious and philosophical groups. However, the philosophers and the lawyers who are members of the Committee have played an important and active role in the preparation and the explanation of the advice approved by the Committee.

To fulfil its task, the Committee benefits from an organization specific to each of its activities. Before being discussed by the Committee, each issue is studied by a permanent working group — the 'technical division' — which makes a complete assessment of the question raised, and with the contribution of consulting experts in the fields concerned. To conclude this work, two reports are written : one deals with the state of science, the other with the legal and ethical issues. They are presented with a draft advice for discussion at the plenary session of the Committee. In order to facilitate a potential consensus, the plenary sessions are not held in the presence of the public, and the attendance of half the members of the Committee is needed to take a decision. Although his vote has the same value as the vote of other members of the Committee, the President plays an important role in selecting the matters which will be discussed as a priority, and also in suggesting some possible ways to reach common proposals.

The bioethics information centre, which was founded by the Medical Research Council, has the responsibility of providing information about the work of the Committee and other ethical issues.

Many professionals (local ethical committees, hospitals, research institutes, universities) approach the centre, but it is also a place of reference for many students and their teachers, and also for members of the public who seek to obtain relevant information on bioethics.

The centre, which belongs to the European Association of Bioethics Centres created in 1985, receives researchers from other countries every year and contributes to the Committee's quarterly newsletter. Each year, the Committee reports to the government on its activities.[34]

During the past five years the Committee has issued twenty-four statements which consider the following topics:

1   Human experiment
    • general guidelines (1984);
    • patients under life-sustaining treatment (1986 and 1988);
    • research on embryos (1986, 1990);
2   The use of human tissues or cells
    • use of foetal tissues (1984, 1989, 1990);
    • use of human cells (1987);
3   The new reproductive technologies (1984, 1990, 1991);
4   Prenatal diagnosis (1985);
5   AIDS (1985, 1988);
6   The abortion pill (1987);
7   Local ethical committees (1988);
8   The testing of drug addicts in employment (1989);
9   Genetic fingerprints (1989, 1991);
10 Gene therapy (1990);
11 Commercialization of the human body (1990);
12 Euthanasia (1991);
13 and Epidemiologic databanks (1985).

In 1985 the Committee considered that the time had come to initiate a wider consideration of some major ethical issues. Three working groups have been created to respond to this task which has nothing to do with the preparation of advice. The Committee has also issued three major studies : Biomedical Research and Respect for Human Dignity; Ethics and Neurosciences; and Ethics in Pedagogy.[35]

The Committee is a rather unusual institution for a French administrative organization, being the first body which has the responsibility for considering major moral issues, rather than exclusively technical and specific matters. As such, its multidisciplinary membership is of real importance and contributes much to the success of its work. As one theologian said, he would have preferred the Committee's advice to follow more closely his own philosophy but, as a citizen, he recognized that its work is quite satisfactory.

As a consequence of this work, many groups in society became aware that a common position could be reached on those issues of artificial reproduction, due to the existence, in the national culture, of general principles on which many people could agree — that is, the identity between the human body and the legal existence of the person. Every person is entitled to have human rights because he or she is physically a human being. This implies that the body is the central point of the respect due to the dignity of the human person. As such, the integrity of the body should not be violated without the consent of the individual concerned.

The use of this philosophy as a basis made it obvious that some legal and coherent conclusions could be drawn in accordance with the existing French legal system. Moreover, the formulation of a framework for legislation could also be justified by the fact it should be helpful in proving the efficiency of this methodology to those who still doubted that these questions could be solved within a pluralistic society. To put it bluntly, it is better to have a law founded on a social agreement than to leave a status quo which could move suddenly to either a restrictive or a *laisser-faire* policy.

This is the reason why the government decided to proceed further down the same path. Consequently, as a second stage of the French methodology, a study was launched to see how it might be possible to translate into law the general principles of common morality which had been identified by the National Ethical Committee.

From Ethics to Law

In December 1986 while addressing the Conseil d'Etat, the permanent legal advisory council of the government, the Prime Minister requested a legal study which would take into account the work of the National Ethical Committee:

> A wider legal study seems necessary. This exhaustive work should particularly take into account the problems raised by:
> — the trade in human organs, tissues and fluids
> — genetic research and embryo research
> — prenatal diagnosis
> — the collection and preservation of human ova
> — the consequences of reproductive medicine on filiation law.[36]

In March 1988, the Conseil d'Etat reported to the Prime Minister. The proposals contained in the report[37] were considered by a governmental working group which prepared a draft Bill on 'bioethics and human rights' for submission to Parliament.

The Report of the Conseil d'Etat

As soon as the Prime Minister ordered this study, a working group was set up. It was exclusively composed of lawyers : members of the Conseil d'Etat; members of the Supreme Court (Cour de Cassation); law teachers; and the representatives of different government departments (Health, Justice,[38] Women's Affairs). The group maintained regular contact with the National Ethical Committee: the lawyers of the Committee were members of the group and the Chairman of the Committee contributed greatly to its work. The group did not hold public sessions but undertook many hearings and visits in order to become more familiar with the common practice of hospitals and research institutes.

At the beginning of 1988, the group finished its work and came to the firm conclusion that legal regulation was a necessity in this field. Its proposals concerning reproductive medicine cover nearly all the questions raised by the new reproductive technologies. The study reached the conclusion that the law, which is currently either absent or unclear on this matter, should face the bioethical issues. (At present, the law is still not involved with regard to the reproductive technologies themselves, and is unclear in the case of the status of the human embryo.)

The group concluded the discussion about the alleged legal no man's land with four arguments:[39]

1. Statute law, which can also be a good means to protect freedom of research, is definitely a better instrument in this field than case law.
2. Law is necessary to clarify family relationships and to secure public health.
3. The power over man that biology gives to scientists is not, in itself, legitimate and legal.
4. These issues are matters of international and European concern and, in order to have a clear approach in this debate, a national law should be adopted.

The study itself is entirely devoted to drawing conclusions from the principle of the integrity of the human body, which was firmly asserted by the National Ethical Committee. According to the report of the Conseil d'Etat, the legal relationship between an individual and his or her body, although not specifically covered by law, could be analysed from two points of view.[40]

First, a 'Civil Code' approach, which consists of discussing this problem as a question of contract, should be used. The question here is whether it is possible to make a contract in respect of the human body. Generally lawyers consider that no violation of the integrity of the human body could be based upon a contractual obligation. They interpret article 1128 of the Civil Code, which states that 'contracts should only deal with things which could be subject to trade', as banning the possibility of contracting about the human body, because it could not be categorised as a matter of property, goods or services. Nevertheless, one exception is admitted : some contracts can be legal when they pursue a philanthropic aim.

The second approach is based on a consideration of the limits of the right of the individual to dispose of his or her own body. In some cases, such as compulsory vaccination, the limit of individual freedom is very high. In other cases, such as organ or blood donations, the individual's right to dispose of his or her body as wished is very widely recognized. In fact, the real ground for these different limits to the individual's right to dispose of her or her own body is the promotion of the general interests of society. In interfering with individual privacy, state law is encouraging altruistic behaviour in the citizen. For this reason, the working group, which prepared the report, considered that these two legal approaches were complementary in that they both presupposed an individual will to act altruistically.

When seen as a contract, or as a way to dispose of his or her own body, donation should always imply a strong will to consent. The donation should be done *gratis* because the human body is *res extra commercium*, and because it is not possible to use one's freedom to reduce oneself to the status of slave. Therefore, donation should also be limited to some purposes and kinds. According to the report, these rules should constitute the basis of a legal public order which should prevent the occurrence of the potential risks implied by the new scientific technologies — in particular, those of scientific utilitarianism, a mercantile approach to the human body and the egocentric use of the right to dispose of one's body.

The report deals with three main topics : human experiment and organ donation (Chapter I), reproductive medicine (Chapter II) and the institutional context (Chapter III). Chapter II, which includes the problems of prenatal diagnosis and embryo research, particularly insists on some fundamental principles, as follows:

- Reproductive medicine should be considered as a way to remedy infertility.
- The child has an interest to be brought up in a biparental family.
- The right to individual autonomy should be recognized, but cannot be absolute.

- The legal status of the resulting child should be as similar as possible to the general status of children in general.
- *Prenatal diagnosis*[41] Eligibility for this technique should be strictly limited and the scientific qualifications of the centres practising prenatal diagnosis should be controlled. But the consequences of a diagnosis, which include information disclosure and decision-making should be left, as far as possible, to the physician and to the couple, respectively.
- *Research on the embryo in vitro* Law is necessary to protect a potential human being from the possible risks of scientific manipulation which could become a new form of eugenics. The creation of a human embryo for the sole purpose of scientific research should be banned and research on spare embryos should be strictly controlled.

A detailed discussion of the content of the proposed legal framework will be undertaken in the second part of our Chapter of this book.

Chapter III of the report deals with two other issues related to reproductive medicine : ethical committees, and the measures which are necessary to ensure that the proposed law will be enforceable.

The report calls for a clarification of the role and the structures of ethical committees in France. First, the National Ethical Committee should acquire new functions, such as the control of research on human embryos and the agreement of institutional ethics committees. Members of the National Committee should be appointed for a longer term.

Second, the local committees should be reorganized. Multidisciplinary institutional committees should be set up in each University hospital to review research projects. Other, task-specific, ethical committees should only be permitted to pursue their activities if they are organised in conformity with relevant guidelines.[42]

With regard to the best way to implement these proposals, the working group developed a specific methodology for the setting up of guarantees and sanctions.[43] Four categories of guarantees exist:

1. Many of the proposals are founded on general principles of law (*principes généraux du droit*) — for example, the integrity of the person. These principles, although not explicitly mentioned in the French Constitution, could nevertheless be regarded as constitutional principles. As such, courts have the responsibility of ensuring that they are respected.
2. The hierarchy of rules which exists in the French legal system offers another guarantee, because a large number of the suggested measures could only be implemented by statute laws.
3. The role of the judge is the natural safeguard of individual

liberty. In recent years, courts have already dealt with some of the issues raised by biomedicine and they will certainly find in the proposed regulations assistance in reaching relevant answers in other cases.

4. The advice of the National Ethical Committee could also be considered as specific guarantees.

The working group also agreed that it will be necessary to establish sanctions, especially in respect of those constitutional principles aimed to protect the human person. They recommended that administrative sanctions should apply to medical institutions involved in the practice of reproductive techniques. The Health Department should have the power to withdraw licences from physicians who seriously infringe the law.

In addition, codes of professional ethics should include new powers to punish physicians and biologists who fail to respect the limits imposed on the use of reproductive techniques and embryo research. In their view, general principles of civil law and tort law should be used every time damage occurs as a consequence of the use of these new techniques.

Finally, criminal penalties should only be used in two main cases. The first case concerns procedures which will be strictly forbidden by law. The second case occurs when some major requirements, such as the obtaining of informed consent or the gratuity of the donation of gametes, are not respected.

Thus, the approach of the Conseil d'Etat is much more than a simple elaboration of general principles. It is already a relatively precise framework which can be translated into law. This task was realized during the year 1988–89 by a joint working group under the auspices of the Department of Health and the Ministry of Justice. The draft Bill,[44] which was published at the beginning of 1989, contains 89 sections and six chapters proposing to introduce law reform in virtually all the biomedical fields discussed in the report *From Ethics to Law*.[45]

However, the main interest of this text is the constant reference both to the general principles which govern the human body in the Civil Code system and to the concept of human rights. Chapter I proposes to introduce into the Civil Code five new articles, clearly establishing what kind of respect is due to the human body. These principles will then constitute a kind of public order.

- Article 1   outlines the principle of respect for the human body.
- Article 2   states that no violation of this right should be

          permitted without the prior consent of the person
          concerned.

- Article 3   limits the violations of the integrity of the human body to situations where there is a legitimate interest.
- Article 4   specifies that any part of the human body is *res extra commercium*.
- Article 5   gives to the court the opportunity to take any measure in order to prevent or to stop illegal violations of the human body.

Two chapters particularly concern reproductive technologies. Chapter II, which deals with prenatal diagnosis, proposes to limit the use of this technique to serious diseases, and recommends that only licensed hospitals should provide prenatal diagnosis. Chapter V is concerned with all the reproductive techniques, including IVF, artificial insemination, gamete donation, surrogacy and embryo research. It provides specific provisions which will be referred to below. Thus, the French methodology seems to have encouraged the emergence of specific regulations applying to reproductive medicine by proceeding in different steps : the encouragement of a social debate on biomedical issues, the development of ethical considerations, the setting of principles which could commonly be accepted as a basis for any future legislation and the writing of appropriate statutes in this field. In following this method, two elements were important. First, there was no major social opposition to the development of the reproductive technologies; and, second, the government permitted a new independent authority — the National Ethical Committee — to define what was possible social agreement in the field of bioethical issues. It is, therefore, now possible to affirm that France has a coherent opinion as to what should be the strategy of the law in these matters.

In order to achieve the latter step in this methodology, the government should have presented the draft bill to Parliament, but it appears that there was a lack of political will to take this step. Given that the present government has no majority, it may be that it was unwilling to risk Parliamentary debate, but in fact a better explanation may be found within French society itself.

As there was no strong debate in respect of reproductive medicine and embryo research, it is difficult to say how the general public would act if a Bill did come to Parliament on this matter. On the one hand, the different institutions in charge of the question of law reform in respect of reproductive issues have not even tried to involve some members of the public in the elaboration of their views, so that it is impossible to know whether there is even a minimal consensus on these views.[46] On the other hand, it is quite clear that some lobby groups of professionals and academics would influence Members of Parliament to oppose the bill.

A large part of the scientific community would oppose such a Bill because they believe that researchers are themselves humanists and, as such, they are responsible to the community for proposing ethical solutions to solve the problems raised by the progress of science.[47] In contrast, others would oppose legislation because the Bill would leave too much power to scientists, particularly in respect of embryo research. Human rights would not, according to them, be sufficiently preserved.[48] All the opponents also wanted to widen the debate to include other issues, such as a possible ban on patenting biotechnologies which would have created major difficulties for industry. Moreover opponents to law reform benefited from the support of the Minister of Research[49] and only the Minister of Justice pronounced himself for law reform.[50] The Minister of Health and the Deputy Minister for Foreign Affairs more prudently declared that the President would decide in due course.[51] The consequences of this situation are likely to be that, for some time to come, lawyers will have to wait for more precise answers to the questions raised by reproductive technologies. However, in a 1991 report titled 'For a French approach in the field of biomedical sciences',[52] Mrs N. Lenoir, a member of the Conseil d'Etat, suggested that legislative reform should only be realized when a general consensus exists. Consequently limited proposals have been made in the report to prohibit the selling of human body parts, to regulate the practice of DNA fingerprints and to authorize the use of personal medical data for epidemiological studies. Reproductive medicine and embryo research are still considered by the report as a too sensitive field to allow regulations at the present time.

ETHICAL AND LEGAL RULES APPLYING TO REPRODUCTIVE MEDICINE AND RELATED EMBRYO RESEARCH

For a clear understanding of this study, it will be useful to distinguish the legal framework applying to reproductive techniques themselves, and the system of control which will regulate related embryo research. The reader should also take into consideration that, at the present time, statutes have not been passed in many areas, so that this legal study deals both with the actual position of law as it exists, and the proposed legislation.

Rules Applying to Reproductive Techniques

First, we should discuss a question of principle : who is eligible for participation in an artificial conception programme? Second, additional issues related to the practice of reproductive techniques will be considered.

Eligibility for Participation in an Artificial Conception Programme

At the beginning of the debate on reproductive medicine, the approach to this question seemed to be more liberal than it currently is.

The legitimacy of the use of reproductive techniques   This questions was widely discussed. Some lawyers observed that, from a purely medical point of view, it is not possible to distinguish between artificial insemination aimed at therapeutic finality and artificial insemination intended to respond to the desire of a couple, because insemination does not treat infertility.[53] Those who express their personal opinion in favour of the use of reproductive techniques for reasons of infertility generally agree that this question should remain a matter of privacy and medical deontology.

However, the most explicit support for the recognition of a right to procreate was expressed by Mr R. Badinter, Minister of Justice, when he declared to the first European conference on Human Rights, in March 1985 in Vienna, that choice should be derived from our conception of human rights:

> ... shouldn't the right of privacy have a wide application and give guarantee to the liberty of each human being to take fundamental decisions by himself? Is the right to privacy a limit imposed on the intrusion into the private life of the individual or the recognition of an individual right to decide for oneself? If this second opinion is prevailing, every human being could dispose of the freedom of choice in those areas which fundamentally affect the human person and particularly in the matter of procreation.[54]

Such a position, founded in articles 8 and 12 of the European Convention on Human Rights could also be based in the precedent of French adoption law which permits adoption by single persons.[55] In 1984, a district court recognized the right of a widow to be inseminated with the sperm of her dead companion who had consented to posthumous insemination but in 1991 another district court denied such a right to a widow whose husband was affected with AIDS.[56] The 1985 interim report showed that public opinion was largely divided. If a large majority (76 per cent) approved the use of reproductive medicine for the benefit of infertile couples, a strong minority was also in favour of its use for single women (42 per cent for, and 46 per cent against).[57]

The decision to restrict the use of reproductive technology to the treatment of medical conditions (either the infertility of the couple or the risk of transmitting incurable diseases) was, however, adopted in the report of the Conseil d'Etat and in the draft Bill for three reasons:

1. only a minority of opinion approves the recognition of a right to procreate;
2. no legal rule exists; and
3. this question is not a matter of absolute individual rights but should be resolved by a balanced compromise between the legitimate desire of a couple to have children and the best interest of the unborn child.[58]

The importance of the individual desire to have children   This is recognized but should not be absolute. The report clearly states that 'the desire to have children. . . should be recognized as a legitimate aspiration of the couple. Reproductive medicine is a medical way by which Society helps the infertile couple.'[59] Reproductive techniques and adoption have the same social purpose — that is, to give a positive response to the desires of the future parents. Such an approach proves how important it is for French society to encourage people to have children.

The first step in the development of artificial insemination took place when a new article was introduced in the Public Health Code providing that the cost of infertility treatment, including artificial insemination, could be entirely paid by the National Health Service.[60] The counterpart to this public policy in favour of artificial reproduction was the organization and development of these techniques under medical control. The limits fixed by law are merely a mean to give more credibility to this system.

Without saying that every child has a right to have both a mother and a father, it appeared necessary to propose a model of family for assisted reproduction. This proposal has two main consequences. First, a family should only be composed of two parents and no more. So the legislation should not encourage the rights of a donor vis-à-vis the future child. Second, a family should be composed of two parents and no less. Single women and widows should therefore be excluded from artificial reproduction programmes as should married couples who are no longer living together. This last case shows how far the working group has gone along the road towards exluding from reproductive medicine monoparental, and even potentially monoparental, families. For the same reasons, homosexual couples will not be regarded as eligible for artificial reproduction.

Nevertheless, recourse to reproductive medicine is permitted both for unmarried and married couples, although the report mentioned three conditions which are required in the case of a cohabiting couple:

1.   the couple should live in a stable relationship;
2.   the consent of the male partner should be required in the same way as if he was married;
3.   the couple should apply to a court for authorization.[61]

This last condition, which is designed to permit an assessment of the genuine existence of a stable relationship, would certainly have intruded on the couple's privacy and would have constituted discrimination against cohabiting couples. This is probably why the draft Bill does not take it into account.

Proposed Rules for Governing the Practice of Human Artificial Reproduction

The proposed rules which will govern the practice of human artificial reproduction largely derive from consideration of the finality of the techniques. Some general considerations address the couples; others address medical practitioners.

General considerations applying to couples[62]   Although not absolute, the will of each member of the couple should be respected. A free, informed, consent and proper medical, social, and legal information for the couple appear to be essential obligations. To fulfil this obligation, the French system largely relies on the responsibility of the physicians who practise reproductive medicine, and no specific rules will advise them of the way in which they should give the information and obtain consent.

Concerning consent given by the members of the couple to the 'treatment', the proposed rules contain a difference between AID and homologous insemination (the same distinction is made in the case of IVF).

In the case of AID, only the woman needs request the use of reproductive techniques, while in the case of homologous insemination, all applications should be presented by both the woman and her husband or companion. This distinction does not seem justified because, if it implies that a woman should not be inseminated without her consent, this should be true in all cases. However, the draft Bill does not distinguish between the two cases.

In the report, no special form was required when obtaining consent, except from the husband or the companion in the light of his consent having consequences for the status of the future child. The draft Bill specifies that consent should be written and is required for each cycle during which a woman is inseminated.

As mentioned previously, the 1991 report 'For a French approach in the field of biomedical sciences' does not support any specific law reform concerning reproductive medicine. The report only proposes that a general debate should be organized in Parliament and that three points should be considered. These points are the medical finality of reproductive technologies, the interest of the future child and the respect due to human dignity in regard to embryo research.

General conditions applying to practitioners   Very few people contested the necessity to practise artificial reproduction under medical control, and the draft Bill clearly specifies that medically assisted reproduction could only be carried out under the responsibility of a qualified physician.

The main problem is concerned with the licensing system. The National Ethical Committee, as well as the different reports issued in this field, proposed that these techniques should only be used by licensed physicians. As a result of this consensus, the government issued, in April 1988, two decrees which oblige IVF and AID centres to be licensed by the Minister of Health.[63] In addition a National Board for Reproductive Medicine and Biology has been set up to advise the Minister of Health.

The Board has now completed its work and 86 centres have been granted a licence by the Minister of Health.[64] This task has been made difficult by the incredible number of applications: nearly 300 were received. This situation can be explained by the rapid and widespread development of IVF techniques, with more and more medical teams deciding to commence the provision of IVF. Among this group, a large number had never before practised in the field of reproductive medicine, but they may have been enthusiastic about the status to be achieved by so doing.

The problem is quite different with AID because AID centres, including the French sperm banks, were organized very early in the 1970s in the private, non-profit institution, CECOS. This institution has in fact a very close relationship with public hospitals and has adopted, as mentioned earlier, strict guidelines which prevent the proliferation of AID centres outside the control of health authorities.

Today, more than 95 per cent of the children born through AID are 'CECOS children' and only a few general practitioners routinely provide AID privately. The fact that frozen sperm has always been used by the CECOS organization was also a great advantage when it was decided, in 1985, to screen donors for HIV antibodies.

There is a further reason which might explain the large number of hospitals wishing to develop IVF programmes – money. Some years ago, a study undertaken for the Department of Health showed that the cost of a child born through IVF was about 150,000 F (approximately US$30,000 or £15,000).[65] The fact that a large part of this sum is paid by the National Health Service facilitates the wish of a couple to have an IVF child and consequently increases the potential market for 'test tube babies'.

However, two decrees approved in 1988 probably came too late. In 1984, when the government first announced its desire to submit IVF centres to a licensing procedure, only 20 centres were functioning, but there were more than 150 when the Minister approved the Commission's proposal to license only 86 of them. It is, however, far from certain that the unauthorized centres have now stopped their activities. The 1991 report therefore proposed to reinforce the powers of the Commission which could become an independent authority, very similar to the UK Human Embriology and Fertilisation Authority. New provisions have been finally adopted by Parliament at the end of 1991 to ban the use of fresh sperm and to reaffirm that the donation of sperm is made gratis.

Suggested Answers to Other Problems Raised by Reproductive Techniques

The Preservation of Gametes and Embryos

The cryopreservation of sperm raises both medical problems and the potential risk of consanguinity (although this is in fact very low) when the sperm of the same donor is used to inseminate different women. The existing regulations, which impose screening tests for donors, in fact imply the freezing of the donated semen. In addition, the law will fix a limit to the use of the sperm of the same donor (the present limit adopted by the CECOS is six donations).[66]

The legal and ethical problems are much more acute with the freezing of embryos. Although this technique makes the procedure of IVF for women and couples easier, it also creates risks for both children and society as a whole. In addition to the medical risks of harm to the embryos, a psychological risk exists when it is noted that this technique could lead to a gap of generation between children born from embryos created at the same time. Legal problems could appear when parents divorce or disagree on the use of these embryos. In Australia two embryos were stored for four years after the parents died in an air crash, before the public authorities found a solution to this problem. The development of uncontrolled and numerous banks where frozen embryos could be stored indefinitely is also an important issue for society. (A French study has confirmed Australian findings according to which babies conceived through IVF appear to have a higher risk of congenital malformations than babies conceived through normal intercourse.)[67]

The debate in this field seems largely to have concluded that recourse to cryopreservation of gametes and embryos is legitimate, but that it should be carried out under strict conditions which permit neither couples nor physicians to do exactly as they like.

The suggested answer of the French report to this difficult question is as follows:[68] the will of the couple should be respected when the gametes or the embryos are stored for their own use. They can ask for the preservation of the gametes and the embryos and they can freely decide when they want to use these gametes or embryos. Two conditions are nevertheless required : the first condition is necessary to ensure respect for the rules that only couples can have access to reproductive techniques and implies that no use can be made of frozen gametes and embryos when the members of the couple are divorced or do not cohabit, or when one of them is dead. The second condition restricts the freedom of the couple's choice to a five-year period. This limit, which is longer than the two years proposed by the National Ethical Committee, is a balanced compromise between respect for the couple's privacy and the necessity for the public authorities to prevent the development of banks for embryos.

At the end of these five years, the gametes or the embryos should no longer be stored. The wishes of the couple concerning their disposal can nevertheless be taken into account if they have given their consent to the donation of their embryos for the use of another couple, or for legal research purposes.

The Use of Donated Gametes and Embryos

Recourse to donors is generally well accepted by public opinion. An important reason, which may explain this fact, is certainly the role played by the CECOS institutions in the development of AID in France. From early on, strict guidelines were applied to the recruitment of donors. They should be married men, having one or two children, and their wife must consent to the donation. They are also very carefully tested in order to prevent the transmission of diseases and genetic abnormalities. Except for a very small minority of lawyers[69] and moralists[70] who were influenced by religious points of view, no major debate occurred on the question of the legitimacy of using sperm donors.

The French report is particularly clear on this point when it proclaims that : 'Reproductive medicine does not exist without the practice of sperm and even oocytes donation.'[71] Such a statement is of real importance because the question of oocyte donation has long been under debate. Some opposed this type of donation because the method of collecting oocytes creates higher risks for the woman and because it seems that it would be more difficult to preserve the anonymity of the donors.

The National Ethical Committee considered it unethical to collect oocytes for the sole purpose of research.[72] The use of donated gametes is now regarded as a *sine qua non* for the practice of reproductive technologies.

In the view of the working group, this legitimacy is not a consequence of the necessity for donated gametes, but is founded rather on the altruistic aim which should inspire donation.[73] Like blood or organ donation, gametes donation is viewed as philanthropic activity and, as such, it should be respected. This approach to the problem of donation has two main consequences:

1.   The donation should be made *gratis*.[74] This principle is implied by article 1128 of the Civil Code which states that : 'Man can only contract about things which could be subject to trade.' It also applies to blood and organ donations.
2.   No parental responsibilities should be established vis-à-vis the donor[75] because the donation is supposed to be carried out in order to permit an infertile couple to become parents. This consideration justifies the principle of anonymity adopted in France by the CECOS institutions.

      Although, there was a major debate on the benefits and disadvantages of this rule, the French report[76] favoured this choice which is both a condition for safeguarding the family in which the AID child will live, and a counterpart to the altruistic contribution of the donor. In addition, the working group thought that the interests of the child were better served by the enforcement of the principle of anonymity than by recognition of an alleged right to know about his or her biological origin.

      Appropriate provisions will modify the Civil Code to specify that the donor of gametes will not be considered as the father or the mother of the child.

Embryo Donation

In 1986, the National Ethical Committee was unable to reach a consensus opinion on embryo donation but urged the legislator to take a decision.[77] The French report also observed that no social consensus was reached on this question. Those who are opposed to embryo donation point out the risk of developing some kind of eugenics. Embryo donation involves choosing the 'best' spare embryos for implantation, but the question remains, according to which criteria should this choice be made, and who should decide?

On the other hand, proponents consider that it is better to give spare embryos to other couples than to destroy them. According to this view, embryo donation should be compared with the giving up of a child before birth.

The proposed legislation suggests that embryo donation could be admitted under the following conditions[78] – it should be a 'last-resort' solution when the embryos are no longer needed by the couple for whom they were created; it should also comply with the principles applying to gamete donation.

Surrogate Motherhood

As in many countries, this question has drawn passionate reactions from many areas of public opinion. During the first stage of the debate some sociologists and lawyers pointed out that surrogate arrangements were common to the history of humanity.[79] African societies are still practising some forms of surrogacy and the recourse by infertile couples to surrogate arrangements, including sexual relationships between the husband and the commissioned woman, was also frequent in nineteenth-century Europe.

According to this view, surrogate arrangements, which can now benefit from the progress of reproductive medicine to rule out the connotation of adultery, do not question our conception of family.[80]

Moreover, it could seriously be questioned whether surrogacy is not a matter of privacy and individual freedom. When presenting the French report concerning human rights and biomedicine at the first European Conference on Human Rights, the Minister of Justice, Mr R. Badinter said:

> Should we reasonably sanction such a contract and consider that the recipient and the surrogate mothers as well as the father of the child are potential criminal offenders? According to our point of view, it is sufficient to repeat that the surrogate arrangement is void and could not be enforced by the judge.[81]

However, professionals and moral authorities very rapidly opposed these views. While, in 1985, a majority of opinion opposed the payment of the surrogate mother[82] and only 30 per cent of women supported altruistic cases of surrogacy exposed in the media,[83] medical and ethical institutions wished to prevent the risk of development of commercial surrogacy.[84]

In October 1984, the National Ethical Committee proclaimed that

... the recourse to this practice is at present illegal. Surrogacy implies the sale of a child. Such an agreement is void and contrary to adoption law which supposes the decision of a court based on the interest of the child and the opportunity of adoption ... Moreover, the intermediary, either a physician or not, is guilty of criminal offences for having incited a woman to give up her child.[85]

In 1987, the government decided to put an end to the activities of private agencies working in the field of surrogacy. Actions were brought to the courts by the government, and all of the judgements responded positively to the requests of the public authorities. Although those involved in the work of the private agencies claimed that they were working on a non-profit basis in order to help infertile couples and to prevent the existence of a black market in this field, the courts decided that surrogacy was illegal for two major reasons.[86] First, the agreement concerns the human body and, as such, is prohibited by article 1128 of the Civil Code. Second, any kind of contract by which prospective parents give up their future child constitutes a criminal offence.

The French report supported this legal analysis but expressed the view that surrogacy should clearly be banned. The three following proposals were made in this report:[87]

1. Any kind of contract under which a woman, who is carrying a child, agrees to give up her child is void even in the case where the child has been produced using the gametes of the commissioning couple.
2. Any person who acts as an intermediary between the surrogate mother and the infertile couple may be sued in court for civil damages.
3. No legal action, either to secure the giving up of the child or the reimbursement of any money paid, can be taken against a woman who refuses to give up her child

    However, two decisions of the Paris Court of Appeal in June 1990 considered that a surrogate arrangement did not prevent the commissioning parents from adopting the child born as a result of such a procedure. Finally, the Supreme Court of Appeals (Cour de cassation) ruled that surrogacy was unlawful because it violates the principle of inalienability of the human body and because it was contrary to the legislation on adoption.[88]

Other proposals which suggest considering the surrogate mother as the legal mother of the child will now be considered with the problem of parental rights.

Parental Rights

The view that reproductive techniques should be a medical reponse to the infertility of couples implied, in the opinion of the French working group, that the future child should have, as far as possible, the same legal status as that of children conceived by 'natural' methods.[89] Therefore, no parental responsibilities should be established in respect of any donors. Surrogate motherhood, which is regarded as an illegitimate practice, is excluded from this legal approach.

The maternity of the child   The present state of the law provides that the woman who gives birth to a child is the legal mother of the child.[90] The French report saw no reason to change this law, which means that the recipient woman, even in the case of a surrogate mother, should always be the legal mother of the child. Although the law governing maternity will remain as it is, the legal mother could nonetheless choose not to assume her parental responsibilities by refusing to be registered as the mother, or by giving up the child after birth. Therefore, some forms of surrogacy, when no money and intermediary are involved, can still be legally realized. In practice, the commissioning husband, who gave his sperm to inseminate the surrogate mother, will be registered as the legal father of the child. Then his wife will adopt the child. This procedure, which presupposes no payment is made to the surrogate mother, is legal, but adoption should be decided by a court. Usually no information is given to the court on the fact that the child has been born as the result of a surrogate arrangement.[91]

The paternity of the child   The report came to the conclusion that it was necessary to enforce some specific rules to take into account the problem of the use of sperm donors. According to the present state of law, when the couple is married, the man is presumed to be the father of the child but this presumption is rebuttable.[92] If he can prove that he is not the genetic father of the child, he will always succeed in denying his paternity. The majority of court decisions have not agreed to give weight to his consent to the artificial insemination of his wife because it is contrary to public order to abandon the right to deny a child.[93] A change of this occurred when a first instance court, in 1990, held that the husband could not disavow the child.[94]

When the couple is not married, the man can legally recognize the child,[95] but can afterwards also deny his paternity. Nevertheless, one case is interesting because the judge declared that a man who consented to artificial insemination was therefore civilly liable for the child.[96]

According to the 1989 proposed draft Bill, no one will be permitted to contest the filiation of a child born through reproductive technologies, except the husband or the partner of the mother when he did not give consent to the insemination or when he can prove that the child was not in fact born through artificial insemination. Already the Paris Court of Appeals decided in a unique case that a man who has accepted the insemination of his wife could not deny the child on the ground that he was born through AID.[97]

An important difference should be noted between married and unmarried couples in the draft Bill. In the first case, the husband will be presumed the father of the child, while in the second case the partner will have to declare himself to the registrar as the father of the child. The working group did not want to change the present state of law in the sole case of children born through reproductive techniques.

However, the Bill made clear that a partner who consented to the insemination of his wife, and does not register the child as his child, could have to pay damages both to the mother and the child.

Research on Human Embryos

This problem, which everybody recognized as fundamental, did not arouse in France the same passions which polarized the debate in Australia, the United Kingdom or in the United States. French people seem so compliant and admiring vis-à-vis scientists that they did not seem concerned about embryo research which is aimed at developing reproductive techniques.They also seemed not to believe that French biologists would create hybrids or manipulate the human genome.

The 'Pro-Life' groups, although opposed to embryo research, were not very active in their opposition, except in the campaign which they launched in 1983 to stop medical research, including treatment of children affected with immunodeficiency diseases, which involved the use of foetal tissues obtained from aborted foetuses.[98]

In 1985, Prof. R. Frydman and his medical team called the attention of the public to the question of the status of fertilized embryos which were no longer wanted by the infertile couples for whom they were stored. The tremendous development of IVF centres led to a situation in which superfluous embryos can be stored indefinitely. On receiving no answer as to the future of spare embryos from the local ethics committee, Frydman asked the National Ethical Committee to consider this problem.[99]

Prof. J. Testard, the French biologist who first developed in France the technique of IVF and embryo transfer, declared in 1986 he would now stop his own research as a result of its implications.[100] He thought that the increasing use of screening techniques to detect abnormal embryos would lead to unacceptable new forms of eugenics which he considers dangerous for humanity. He is also strongly opposed to sex selection and the potential application of predictive medicine on embryos *in vitro*.

No real solution can be expected from the present state of law either on the status which should govern the human embryo or the limits which should be imposed on research. Aware of the necessity to reach some conclusions on this difficult debate, the National Ethical Committee issued comments, and the work accomplished by the Committee helped the working group to present, in the French report, some proposals for legislation.

The Status of the Embryo

If the embryo is traditionally entitled to some rights,[101] such as the right to inherit, these rights are subject to the condition that the embryo should be born viable. Moreover, specific offences apply to the killing of an embryo, which is always punished by a lesser penalty than the homicide of an adult.

In addition, the abortion law of 1975 abolished penal offences when an embryo is aborted during the first 10 weeks of pregnancy.[102] Consequently, the question of the status of the embryo needed to be clarified.

The first comment of the National Ethical Committee, which was devoted to the question of the use of foetal tissue obtained from dead foetuses, stated that 'the human embryo should be considered as a potential human being and as such should be respected'.[103] Such respect implies that no living embryo should be submitted to research *in utero*, except when the aim of the research is the promotion of the well-being of the embryo in question.

In 1986, the National Ethical Committee reaffirmed the statement that the embryo should be considered as a potential human being.[104] In the view of the Committee, this opinion does not imply that no research should be carried out *in vitro* on the human embryo, but that, in consideration of its human origin, experimentation should be strictly limited.

Rules and controls are necessary to ensure that the power of science over the origin of life will be used in the best interests of mankind. They are also needed for scientists themselves to remind them of their responsibilities. The content of such regulations should take into account both the fundamental requirements of ethics and the benefits and the disadvantages of embryo research. There is, of course, a potential conflict between research which is carried out benefiting future children and that which is not. Predictive medicine can bring real advantages to children, but its development can also lead to the practice of eugenics. Because numerous examples of such ambiguities exist, the Committee suggested strict guidelines to control the real aims of research, particularly in the field of genetics, and to prevent the carrying out of research which has no medical interest but which has biological and ethical risks.

Guidelines Concerning Experiments on the Human Embryo *in vitro*

Embryos Intended to be Implanted

Experiments with potential individual benefit, which means benefit for the infertile couple, could, it was agreed, be practised in accordance with the following conditions:

1. These experiments can only be carried out if biologists have sufficient information to believe that there is a reasonable chance of success.
2. The experiment requires the consent of each member of the couple, who should be duly informed of the procedures involved in it.
3. The experiment should be conducted by licensed professionals working under the direction of a biologist and a physician. The experiment should be reviewed by a local ethics committee.

These guidelines mean that research concerning the stimulation of the ovary, and those aimed at facilitating fertilization and the development *in vitro* of embryos at the early stages, should be permitted. Research aimed at predicting embryo abnormalities or determining the sex of the embryo should, however, not be practised.

Research without direct benefit for the couple can only be carried out if relevant tests on animals can prove it would result in real progress for the techniques of reproductive medicine. This is the case with research applied to the freezing of embryos, but not with research which involves micromanipulations of the embryonic cells.

Spare Embryos

The Committee is opposed to the creation of embryos for the sole purpose of research, but considers that the donation of spare embryos could be permitted if a couple, who have no more parental plans, consent to their use in this way. Further conditions will then apply:

1. Embryo research should be the only means to acquire this specific knowledge.
2. Physicians and biologists participating in this research should not have treated the couples who agreed to donate the embryos.
3. The National Ethical Committee should authorize such research.
4. The storage of embryos should be limited to the number strictly necessary for the purpose of the research in question.
5. The results of the research should be published and no therapeutic practice should be undertaken without the consent of the National Ethical Committee.
6. Research should only be carried out on embryos *in vitro* at the early stages of development.

The Committee considered that the suggested limit of 14 days for research had no strong scientific basis, and that it could lead some people to believe that, under 14 days, the embryo is not a potential human being. They therefore proposed that no embryo should be used after the time of implantation, which effectively means after seven days.

Research under Moratorium

The Committee suggested a three-year moratorium on research which aimed to select the sex of the embryo or to predict abnormalities, believing that such procedures could lead to recourse to IVF for reasons other than infertility. In their view, the temptation to choose the characteristics of a future child could be seen as contrary to the dignity of man.

Consequently, the Committee suggested that, during the time of the moratorium, further studies should be carried out to assess the risks and the consequences of this type of research. However, in 1990, it suggested that the moratorium should be extended.[105]

Research Which Should Be Banned

Taking into account the views offered by scientists the Committee proposed that any kind of research which could modify the germinal cells should be prohibited.

Research Without Scientific Interest

The Committee proposed to ban the transfer of a human embryo into the womb of another species and considered that ectogenesis, parthenogenesis, and male gestation have no scientific interest.

What will happen now that the Committee has extended the

moratorium: a prohibition or specific regulations? The problem is that virtually no discussion has taken place since the Committee asked for a scientific, social and legal study of this problem, probably because scientists recently created their own professional associations.[106] Ethical and scientific studies are in progress within the committees specially set up by the professional institutions, but it will be some time before conclusions will be reached.

Consequently, no social agreement exists on the question of having law applying to embryo research. Some think that any general regulation in this field is contrary to the freedom of research and to the right of patients to benefit from the progress of science and medicine.[107] Conversely, others consider that embryo research questions the right to life of existing human beings.

The legal study made by the working group of the Conseil d'Etat is, however, proposing to regulate research on embryos *in vitro*.[108] The group considered that the fact that IVF is becoming a procedure routinely practised by an increasing number of medical teams makes it difficult not to reach solutions to the problems which are inherent in this everyday practice.

The need for legislation has become urgent not only because we should instruct biologists on the disposal of spare embryos, but also because the planning of research programmes and the future of humanity relies on the attitude which is adopted.

The report suggested four recommendations:[109]

1. The working group considered that the best way to define the status of the human embryo *in vitro* is to pass statute law. This statute should not define when life begins, but should address the process of life and offer an appropriate protection to the embryo, in consideration of the fact it is not just material but a potential human being.
2. The creation of embryos for the sole purpose of research should be banned. Furthermore, the process of life should not be reduced to the acquisition of material for the purpose of research. Patenting the human embryo should be prohibited, as well as experiments implying the alteration of the human genome.
3. Other research should be submitted to an agreement procedure.
    The working group approved the approach of the National Ethical Committee, which distinguished permitted research about which sufficient scientific information is known from research which should be covered by a moratorium until a better knowledge about its risks and feasibility has been acquired. However, the working group considered that it would be difficult to translate the idea of a moratorium into law. It suggested

therefore that all research programmes should require the agreement of the National Ethical Committee.

Taking into account the example of the legislation adopted in Victoria (Australia),[110] the working group thought this would be the best compromise between a total prohibition, which would deprive societies of medical progress, and a *laissez-faire* policy which would endanger individual integrity and the future of mankind.

4.   A limit should be imposed beyond which no research on embryos should be permitted. A 14-day period, which is generally accepted in many countries, was proposed as a suitable limit.

The report also proposed some draft regulations for the use of dead embryos.[111]

1.   Statute law should state that the use of dead embryos should only be permissible for diagnostic purposes and, in limited cases, for therapeutic reasons.
2.   The embryos or foetuses used should have been born non-viable, and the experiment should be submitted for approval, to a local ethics committee.
3.   The use of foetal tissues should involve no payment, and no member of a medical team should be obliged to participate in these experiments.

The draft Bill contains only general provisions on embryo research, and states that only spare embryos may be used for research purposes, with the consent of the couple. No embryo *in vitro* should be developed after seven days, or less if the couple explicitly asks. In exceptional cases, the seven-day period may be doubled if the National Ethics Committee specifically agrees. Each protocol should be authorized by the National Ethics Committee. No research will be permitted if it could endanger the integrity of the human species or if it aims at eugenic purposes.

Anyone breaking these proposals would be liable, on conviction, to a sentence of up to three years' imprisonment.

CONCLUSION

Much work has been accomplished since biomedical issues became matters of public concern. The problems raised by the new reproductive techniques have been widely discussed: the National Ethical Committee has helped the emergence of a social consensus on some ethical guidelines; and lawyers have progressed towards translating these ethical principles into a framework for legislation which is in accordance with the French legal system. How could we have done better than to have a dispassionate controversy, a rational process of legislation and reasonable principles to protect the human being and to preserve the freedom of science?

However, a potential danger threatens this neat ethical landscape in that Parliament has never had the opportunity to debate on these questions, and the attitudes of these elected representatives are not clear.

In fact the 1988 discussion on a Private Member's Bill concerning human experiments shows that, with the exception of some Members of Parliament,[112] a large number of French representatives have no precise idea of what they would like to regulate in the field of bioethics and how they would like to do it.

The suggested debate which should take place in 1992 will probably show if French MPs are satisfied with the existence of relevant national ethical and legal institutions and if they are ready to endorse the draft legislation that the Government will propose to them in the very limited areas stated above.

We could then know if France is still facing a centralizing attitude which makes it difficult to create powers which could counterbalance governmental initiative. Bioethics could then be regarded as in good hands but it is in the hands of a new class of professionals. Should these professionals become a new class of powerful men? The future will tell us if France will be the first country to create an ethicocracy.

NOTES

1   David, G. (1982), 'L'insémination artificielle', *Ed. Economica*; Alnot, M. O. *et. al.* (1984), *L'insémination artificielle humaine, un nouveau mode de filiation*', Paris: ESF; Testart, J. (1984), *De l'éprouvette au bébé spectacle*; Brussels: Ed. Complexe; Clarke, R. (1984), *Les enfants de la science*, Paris: Stock.
2   Law 78–730 of 12 July 1978 (article L 286–1 of the Public Health Code).
3   Andréani, G. (1983), 'Jumelles : un bébé par procuration', *Elle*, 3 May (the story of the first baby born in France through a surrogate arrangement, 27 April 1983).
4   Mrs C. Parpalaix, a 23-year-old widow was refused insemination by a CECOS centre in December 1983.
5   Raymond, G. (1986), 'La procréation artificielle et le droit francais', *Semaine Juridique*, **(23)** 8 June; Carbonnier, J. (1985), 'Rapport de synthèse (première journée des travaux)' in *Actes du colloque génétique, procréation et droit*, Paris: Ed. Actes Sud, p. 79; Rubellin-Divichi, J. 'Congélation d'un embryon, FIV et mère de substitution', in *Actes du colloque*, p. 307.
6   Gobert, M. (1985), 'Les incidences juridiques des progrès des sciences biologiques et médicales sur le droit des personnes', in *Actes du colloque*

génétique, procréation et droit, Paris: Ed. Actes Sud, p. 161; Avocat, G. (1986), 'Analyse des opinions des juristes sur une législation relative aux nouvelles techniques de reproduction humaine', in *Les Procréations Artificielles*, Paris: La Documentation Francaise, p. 161.

7   Blanc, M. (1985), 'L'opinion des scientifiques et des praticiens de la procréation assistée', in *Les Procréations Artificielles*, Paris, p. 144.

8   David, G. (1985), 'Don et utilisation du sperme', in *Actes du colloque*, op. cit., p. 203.

9   Bourson, P. A. (1983), 'Comité National d'Ethique ou Comité d'Ethique Nationale?', *Le quotidien du médecin*, 12 December.

10 Opinion poll, SOFRES, *Le Monde*, France Inter, 22–26 June 1985 in *Les Procréations Artificielles*, op. cit., p. 121.

11 Association Internationale contre l'Exploitation des Foetus Humains, 17 rue F. Bonvin, 75015 PARIS.

12 *Actes du colloque génétique, procréation et droit*, Paris: Ed. Actes Sud, 1985.

13 Badinter, R. (1985), 'Intervention du garde des sceaux, Ministre de la Justice', in *Actes du colloque*, op. cit., p. 17.

14 David, G. (1985), 'Don et utilisation du sperme', *in Actes du colloque*, op. cit., p. 211.

15 Communiqué officiel du Conseil des Ministres, 12 July 1984.

16 'L'enfant impossible de Corinne', *Le Point*, **(617)**, 16 July 1984, p. 47.

17 Mitterrand, F. (1985), 'Message du Président de la République', in *Actes du colloque*, op. cit., p. 13.

18 Badinter, R. (1985), *Les droits de l'homme face au progrès de la médecine, de la biologie et de la biochimie*, First European Ministerial Conference on Human Rights, Vienna, 19–20 March, p. 13.

19 Héritier-Augé, F. (1985), 'Don et utilisation de sperme et dovocytes. Mères de substitution. Un point de vue fondé sur l'anthropologie sociale', in *Actes du colloque*, op. cit., p. 237.

20 Gobert, M. (1985), 'Les incidences juridiques des progrès des sciences biologiques et médicales sur le droit des personnes', in *Actes du colloque*, op. cit., p. 161.

21 Tomkiewicz, S. (1985), 'L'insémination artificielle par donneur', in *Actes du colloque*, op. cit., p. 546.

22 Carbonnier, J. (1985), 'Rapport de synthèse (première journée des travaux)', in *Actes du colloque*, op. cit., p. 79.

23 Byk, C. (1986/88), 'Etat comparatif des règles éthiques et juridiques relatives à la procréation artificielle', Paris: Ministère de la Justice.

24 Hondius, F. (1988), 'Législation et éthique européennes', *Forum*, September, p. 29.

25 Réunion Internationale de Bioéthique, Rambouillet, 18–22 April 1985.

26 Alnot, M. O., *et. al.* (1986), *Les Procréations Artificielles*, op. cit.

27 'L'éthique médicale selon l'Académie', *Le quotidien du médecin*, 14 December 1983.

28 Décret 83–132 du 23 février 1983 portant création d'un Comité consultatif national d'éthique pour les sciences de la vie et de la santé.

29 Mitterrand, F. (1983), 'Address to the inaugural session of the National Ethical Committee, Paris, 2 December 1983', in *Le généraliste*, 9 December.

30 Bernard, J. (1983), 'Address to the inaugural session of the National Ethical Committee, Paris, 2 December 1983', in *Le généraliste*, 9 December 1983.

30a See note 29.

31 Fabius, L. (1986), 'Address to the inaugural session of the Committee national conference, Paris, 6 December 1985', in *La lettre d'information du Comité*, January, p. 111.

32   Valadier, P. (1983), '"Comité d'Ethique" et Technocratie', in *Le Monde*, 14 October.

33   Bernard, J. (1984), interview in *Le Monde*, 8 December.

34   Comité consultatif national d'éthique pour les sciences de la vie et de la santé, *Rapports annuels 1984, 1985, 1986, 1987, 1988, 1989, 1990*, Paris: La Documentation Française.

35   Comité consultatif national d'éthique (1987), *Recherche biomédicale et respect de la personne humaine*, Paris: la Documentation Française (December 1987); *Ethique et Neurosciences* (1989); *Ethique et Pédagogie* (1989).

36   Chirac, J., letter to the Vice-President of the Conseil d'Etat, 19 December 1986.

37   Conseil d'Etat, *De l'éthique au droit*, Paris: La Documentation Française, 1988.

38   The author represented the Department of Justice and wrote the comparative law study which is included in the report.

39   La nécessité de la loi', in *De l'éthique au droit*, op. cit., p. 50.

40   'Quel droit?', in *De l'éthique au droit*, op. cit., p. 15.

41   'Le diagnostic prénatal', in *De l'éthique au droit*, op. cit., p. 69.

42   'Les comités d'éthique', in *De l'éthique au droit*, op. cit., p. 113.

43   'Garanties et sanctions', in *De l'éthique au droit*, op. cit., p. 121.

44   As a working document, the draft Bill has not officially been published but informal copies have circulated, in particular among lawyers and journalists.

45   The different chapters are: The integrity of the human body; Prenatal diagnosis; Ethics committees; Organ transplants; Human artificial procreation; Epidemiological data banks.

46   With the exception of the annual two days' public session of the National Ethics Committee, no public hearings have been held while the Conseil d'Etat and the working group prepared their work. No pre-report has been released. Such practices are extremely rare in the French administrative system.

47   Interview of Professor F. Gros, colloque, Patrimoine Génétique et Droits de l'Homme, *Le Monde*, 26–27 October 1989.

48   Proposition de loi 1156 déposée par Mme C. Boutin, député et tendant à assurer le respect de l'intégrité de la personne, 19 December 1989.

49   Address by M. Curien, Minister for Science, colloque, Patrimoine Génétique et Droits de l'Homme, Paris, 26–27 October 1989.

50   Inaugural address of M. P. Arpaillange, Minister of Justice, Public Session of the National Bioethics Consultative Commitee, Paris, 15 December 1989.

51   Address of Mme E. Avice, Minister of Foreign Affairs, Conseil de l'Europe, First symposium on Bioethics, Strasbourg, 5–7 December 1989; interview of M. C. Evin, Health Minister, *Le Monde*, 11 November 1989.

52   Mme N. Lenoir, *Aux Frontières de la Vie. Pour une Démarche Française en Matière d'Ethique Biomédicale*, La Documentation Française, Paris, 1991.

53   Gobert, M. 'Les incidences juridiques des progrès des sciences biologiques et médicales sur le droit des personnes', in *Actes du colloque*, op. cit., p. 161.

54   Badinter, R. *Les droits de l'homme*, op. cit., note 18 above, p. 11.

55   Loi no. 76–1179 of 22 December 1976 (art 343–1 of the Civil Code).

56   *Parpalaix* v. *CECOS*, Tribunal de Grande Instance de Créteil, 1 August 1984, *Gazette du Palais*, 16–18 September 1984, p. 11. *Gallon* v. *CECOS*, Tribunal de Grande Instance de Toulouse, 26 March 1991.

57   Opinion Poll, Sofres – *Le Monde* – France Inter, 22–26 June 1985, in *Les Procréations Artificielles*, op. cit., p. 129.

58 'Affirmation de la valeur des structures naturelles de la parenté', in *De l'éthique au droit*, op. cit., p. 57.

59 'La procréation médicalement assistée remède à la stérilité du couple', in *De l'éthique au droit*, op. cit., p. 53.

60 See note 2 above.

61 'La procréation assistée au sein du couple non marié', in *De l'éthique au droit*, op. cit., p. 67.

62 'La procréation artificielle pur soi-meme et sur soi-meme', in *De l'éthique au droit*, op. cit., p. 66.

63 Décret 88–327 du 8 avril 1988 relatif aux activités de procréation médicalement assistée; décret 88–328 du 8 avril 1988 portant création de la commission nationale de médecine et de biologie de la reproduction, *Journal Officiel, Lois et Décrets*, 9 April 1988.

64 Vigy, M. (1988), 'Fécondation "in vitro" : stricte réglementation', *Le Figaro*, 25 November, p. 10.

65 Athea, N. (1985), 'La fécondation "in vitro" ', *Direction Générale de la Santé*, February, p. 54.

66 'Le don de sperme, d'ovule ou d'embryon', in *De l'éthique au droit*, op. cit., p. 63.

67 *The Age*, 28 April 1988.

68 'Droit de disposition des auteurs de gamètes ou d'embryons "surnuméraires" ', in *De l'éthique au droit*, op. cit., p. 64.

69 Sériaux, A. (1985), 'Droit naturel et procréation artificielle : quelle jurisprudence', *Recueil Dally*, chron, p. 53.

70 Moretti, J. M. and de Dinechin, O. (1982), *Le Défi Génétique*, Paris: Ed. du Centurion.

71 'Reconnaissance de la valeur de la contribution au projet parental d'autrui', in *De l'éthique au droit*, op. cit., p. 55.

72 *Avis du Comité National d'Ethique relatif aux recherches sur les embryons humains 'in vitro'*, 15 December 1986, p. 20.

73 See note 70 above.

74 'Gratuité et objet du don', in *De l'éthique au droit*, op. cit., p. 64.

75 'Absence de liens de filiation entre l'enfant issu de la procréation artificielle et les donneurs de sperme, d'ovule ou d'embryon', in *De l'éthique au droit*, op. cit., p. 64.

76 'Anonymat du don et confidentialité de son objet', in *De l'éthique au droit*, op. cit., p. 64.

77 *Avis du Comité National d'Ethique relatif aux recherches sur les embryons humains 'in vitro'*, p. 11.

78 'Droit de disposition des auteurs de gamètes ou d'embryons "surnuméraires" ', in *De l'éthique au droit*, op. cit., p. 64.

79 See note 19.

80 Papiernik-Berkhauer, E. (1984), 'Porter l'enfant d'une autre, le débat sur les "ventres d'emprunt" ', *Le Monde*, 29–30 July.

81 Badinter, R., *Les droits de l'homme*, op. cit., note 18 above.

82 Opinion poll, SOFRES – *Le Monde* – France Inter 22–26 June 1985, *Les Procréations Artificielles*, op. cit., p. 126.

83 Public opinion poll, IPSOS, *Femme pratique*, September 1985.

84 An IPSOS poll dated 12 and 13 October 1987 shows that 56 per cent of the French do consider that a surrogate mother who has agreed to give up her child for money to a commissioning couple should fulfil the arrangement concluded with the couple (*Le Journal du Dimanche*, 18 October 1987).

85 *Avis du Comité National d'Ethique sur les problèmes éthiques nés des techniques de reproduction artificielle*, 23 October 1984, p. 3.

86   Association Nationale pour l'Insémination Artificielle, Tribunal de Grande Instance de Paris, 20 January 1988; Association Les Cigognes, Conseil d'Etat, 22 January 1988; Association Sainte Sarah, Tribunal de Grande Instance de Créteil, 23 March 1988; Association Alma Mater, Cour d'Appel d'Aix-en-Provence, 29 April 1988.

87   'Les conventions de procréation ou de gestation pour le compte d'autrui', in De l'éthique au droit, op. cit., p. 65.

88   Paris Court of Appeal, 15 June 1990, SCP 1990, Actualités, 25 July 1990, pp. 29–30; Procureur Général v. Mme Guichard, cour de cassation, Plenary Assembly, 31 May 1991.

89   'Souci de s'écarter le moins possible du droit commun de la filiation', in De l'éthique au droit, op. cit., p. 61.

90   This rule is inferred from article 341 of the Civil Code.

91   Hauser, J. (1987), 'L'adoption à tout faire', Recueil Dalloz, chron, p. 205.

92   Article 314 of the Civil Code.

93   Article 316 of the Civil Code : Tribunal de Grande Instance de Nice, 30 June 1976, D 1977, p. 45.

94   Tribunal de Grande Instance de Bobigny, 18 January 1990, D 1990.

95   Mme Catherine, G. c. Madame et Monsieur V., Tribunal de Grande Instance de Nanterre, 8 June 1988.

96   M. Jean Claude, B c. Mme G. Fontaine, Cour d'Appel de Toulouse, 21 September 1987, Recueil Dalloz 1988 jurispr., p. 184 and Sériaux, A. (1988), 'La procréation artificielle sans artifices', Recueil Dalloz, chron, p. 202.

97   J.L.B. v. N. F., Paris Court of Appeals, 29 March 1991.

98   Jacquinot, C. and Delage, J. (1984), Les trafiquants de bébés à naître, Paris: Ed. O.M. Favre.

99   Frydman, R. (1985), 'Quel destin pour les embryons congelés?', La Croix, 8 July.

100   Testard, J. (1986), 'Les risques de la procréation artificielle en le monde de la médecine', Le Monde, 10 September.

101   Théry, R. (1982), 'La condition juridique de l'embryon et du foetus', Recueil Dalloz, chron, p. 231; Raynaud, P. (1988), 'L'enfant peut-il être objet de droit?', Recueil Dalloz, chron, p. 109; Baudoin, J. L. and Labrusse, C. (1988), 'La situation juridique de l'enfant conçu', Revue Trimestrielle de Droit Civil, 1988.

102   Loi 75–17 du janvier 1975 relative à l'interruption volontaire de grossesse (articles L 152–1 et s du Code de la santé publique).

103   Avis du Comité National d'Ethique sur les prélèvements de tissus d'embryons ou de foetus humains morts, 22 May 1984, p. 1.

104   Avis du Comité National d'Ethique relatif aux recherches sur les embryons humains 'in vitro', 15 December 1986.

105   Avis du Comité National d'Ethique sur les recherches sur l'embryon soumises à moratoire, 18 July 1990.

106   BLEFO for 'Biologistes des Laboratoires d'Etude de la Fécondation de l'Oeuf' and GEFF for 'Groupe d'Etude de la Fécondation en France'.

107   Rubellin-Devichi, J. (1985), 'Congélation d'embryons, fécondation "in vitro", mère de substitution', in Actes du colloque, op. cit., p. 321.

108   'L'intervention du droit', in De l'éthique au droit, op. cit., p. 82.

109   'Embryons "in vitro" ', in De l'éthique au droit, op. cit., p. 89.

110   A Parliamentary study commission on bioethics was set up in 1990.

111   'Embryons morts', in De l'éthique au droit, op. cit., p. 88.

112   Proposition de loi adoptée par le Sénat relative à la protection des personnes dans la recherche biomédicale, Assemblée Nationale, Journal Officiel, Débats, 25 November and 2 December 1988.

6 New Zealand: Regulating Human Reproduction

MARK HENAGHAN

New developments in human reproduction provide the opportunity for a society to enter into open and vigorous debate about one of the fundamental issues of life. After an 'Issues' paper[1] was aired in 1985 by the law reform division of the New Zealand Justice Department for public debate, the reaction was neither vigorous nor intense. One hundred and sixty submissions were received and they were primarily from two groups – those with avowedly religious beliefs and the medical profession. Parliament's reaction was to show more 'faith' in the medical profession than in itself. The law reform message has been spelt out that we shall wait and see rather than declare our legislative hands. Doctors can look after things in the meanwhile and the legislature will chip in when required (by whom is not made clear) and when overseas trends indicate that it is necessary to do so. This chapter analyses the consequences of such a law reform stance for human reproduction issues in New Zealand. This law reform position is held at a time when there have been unprecedented changes and reforms in New Zealand's economic structure. What has been termed 'market'[2] philosophy has been the order of the day, and it may well be a reflection of such ideology that human reproduction is left largely unregulated.

The term 'human reproduction' has an element of mechanism about it which does not capture the miracle and uniqueness of a conception and birth and the personal effects such an event has on pregnant women. Yet when writing about how law reform bears on 'reproduction' there is an unavoidable element of depersonalization and generalization.

At a New Zealand Law Society Conference[3] learned professionals from all over New Zealand and overseas gathered to discuss the issue of surrogate motherhood. The arguments for and against were put with clarity, the data was analysed, the overseas approaches were explored and the minds of all those in the room were buzzing with the possibilities. Then, a surrogate mother was asked to address the assembled group. Her insight, wisdom and personal dignity made the rest of what had been said seem like clever rhetoric — words in space, divorced from any reality. Those in the room felt like voyeurs looking into a deeply personal aspect of this woman's life. The gap between experience and theory was painfully obvious.

Yet when legislative policy is formed about 'human reproduction' it is not the likes of that surrogate mother who will be consulted and who will have a major input. Rather it is the likes of all the other people in the room, including myself, who are likely to influence policy. Human reproduction has been taken over by professionals who control it, define it and debate it. If that is taken as a given, then it becomes of intense interest whether or not law reform puts in place rules which control the say and power of professionals. Terms such as 'intervention' and 'non-intervention' are often used in intellectual debate to test a particular legislative strategy.[4] Professionals often win both ways. Intervention means that they are given legislative endorsement to control someone's else's life; non-intervention means they are left free of legislative restraint to pursue their own interests and goals. The actual participants in the process are conditioned to accept intervention in their lives by professionals. The surrogate mother at the law conference looked apologetic and, at times, frightened of the professional group she spoke to. She spoke of a deeply personal experience to a group of people who were used to hearing other people's personal problems and calling them 'case histories'. All of us in the audience had been given the power to make moral, legal and social judgements on this woman's experience.

When it becomes accepted by professionals that we control other people's lives in many recognized and unrecognized ways, then law reform may be more directed at controlling professionals or protecting others from their influence. That is not to say that professionals and experts are not vitally important to the well-being of our society but, rather, reveals that we sometimes overlook the log in our own eyes while carefully dissecting the splinters in the eyes of others.

Because human reproduction has not been the subject of major law reform in New Zealand, the emphasis has been on non-intervention, which means that certain professionals have almost total, unregulated control. The New Zealand Court of Appeal in *Wall* v. *Livingstone*,[5] where a paediatrician challenged an abortion decision made by another doctor, sums up both the judicial and legislative attitudes towards issues of human reproduction:

The Courts are ordinarily entitled to ... determine whether the statutory criteria under any legislation have been or will be met in particular cases. But if that principle is to be applied to this statutory scheme what will always be difficult will be to isolate underlying and strict legal questions from what will be the heavy overlay of straight-out medical judgement.[6]

The primary focus of this chapter will be on the legislative response to what has been called in New Zealand 'new birth techno-logies'.[7] A theme that will be pursued is that the concern of the legislature with status has left the medical profession with free rein to make its own rules. This is consistent with legislative non-intervention on the issue of sterilization of the mentally handicapped when such opportunity was readily presented with the passing of the Protection of Personal and Property Rights Act 1988.

NEW BIRTH TECHNOLOGIES

Who has a Stake?

New Zealand probably identifies itself as having a history of what may be termed 'social' legislation. Right from the heady days of the creation of the welfare state in the 1930s New Zealand has portrayed itself as an egalitarian society where there is an equality of oppor-tunity for all. Social legislation, such as the Family Protection Act 1955 to provide protection for members of a family who were not treated fairly in a will, the Status of Children Act 1969, which eliminated the distinction between legitimate and illegitimate chil-dren, the Matrimonial Property Act 1976, which recognizes the equal contribution to the marriage partnership by men and women, the Accident Compensation Act 1982 (first passed in 1972) which spreads the burden of personal injury accidents across all members of the society, has represented the ideal of equality. Therefore it comes as no surprise that New Zealand's legislative reaction to new birth technologies has the declared purpose of putting children born as a result of such technologies on the same legal footing as children born as a result of 'normal' processes. The legislation is aimed at status and has been described as a 'technical measure'[8] to take children born as a result of new technology out of a 'legal limbo'.[9] The term 'new birth technologies' is the one used by the New Zealand government in putting out an 'Issues' paper for public discussion although there are of course many other ways of describing the process – such as 'alternative human reproduction' or 'modern reproductive tech-niques'. It may be that the term used best reflects the way New Zealand sees the issue: one of technology rather than reproduction; one of birth rather than conception.

When the legislation is measured against its own politically dec-lared goals it becomes clear that it is not 'legal limbo' generally that the Act is concerned with, but rather the 'legal limbo' of certain children born in certain situations as a result of certain birth techno-logies. These children and their parents are given legal equality while other children and their parents are not. The legislator is more concerned with protecting certain technologies and reinforcing certain kinds of relationships. The unarticulated premise behind the New Zealand legislative response is that it is built on the idea of an infertile married couple going to a medical infertility clinic to receive aid to start a family. The legislation is a direct response to the medical profession's desire to ensure that couples who can afford to, and who are approved of to use their birth technologies, will not be treated any differently by the law than couples who have children in the traditional way. Although the New Zealand legislative response to new birth technologies is superficially concerned with the status of parenthood, it is really about reinforcing the status of the medical profession as guardians of the new technology – and, because this is done covertly, there is less likelihood of any threat to the status of the medical profession. The legislation is open to another power broker or entrepreneurial group staking ground for itself in what could be seen as a potential industry.

Law reform in New Zealand on the issue of new birth technolo-gies is based on the idea of reacting when necessary, but otherwise leaving matters to develop. In other words, let the scientists and doctors and others who may stake their claim make their progress and Parliament will provide legal back-up when needed. Public debate on the issues has been neither heated nor noticeable; the moral, social, cultural and personal issues have barely been con-sidered.

A surrogate mother went public in New Zealand because she was paid less than she had been promised. The baby was born three months prematurely. Media reaction highlighted how under-debated the issues are in New Zealand – 'New Zealand has yet to experience the public furore provoked by court battles over the fate of children conceived under surrogacy agreements which later go sour' (*Otago Daily Times*, Friday 5 April 1991). Only one surrogacy case has been before the courts in New Zealand. The case of Re P (Adoption: Surrogacy) [1990] NZFLR 385 was a test case on the issues of whether or not adoption by surrogate parents was a breach of section 23 of the Adoption Act 1955 which makes it unlawful to give or receive any payment or reward in consideration of an adoption or proposed adoption, and section 26 of the Adoption Act which prohibits advertisements showing desire to adopt a child. The presiding judge held that ss.25 and 26 'only go to the determination as to whether applicants are fit and proper persons' to have custody and to be adoptive parents. There was no evidence (which is hardly surprising) that, at the time of the surrogacy arrangement, the parties intended to adopt the child. The Judge also commented that s.26 was an inappropriate and outdated provision to deal with the issue, as surrogacy was not contemplated at the time of its enactment. All parties and the Department of Social Welfare favoured adoption. There was no tension in the case and therefore no need to analyse the difficult issues as to whether surrogacy arrangements are in the best interests of children. There was some opportunity to do this because the adopting parents had been involved in earlier difficulties when trying to adopt because of their health and their age. The issue was not analysed because Social Welfare found them at the time of the hearing to be suitable.

Because of the lack of public debate the scientists, doctors and others who strike a claim (who well may be legal academics like me) will shape and sharpen the issues. Those most affected — women and children — are not likely to be heard: their world will be created for them by others. New Zealand's response of a single piece of legislation — the Status of Children Amendment Act 1987 — and its description as a 'technical measure', demonstrates that New Zealand's reaction to new birth technologies is to be found more in the gaps and what is left undone than what is done. But first, what has been done?

Doctor in Charge

The Minister of Justice, when introducing the Status of Children Amendment Bill, indicated that the need for such legislation 'arises because children concerned through the use of donated gametes are in a legal limbo'.[10] The examples of this 'legal limbo' given by him predominantly revolve around fatherhood. Without the Status of Children Amendment Bill the sperm donor would be the 'legal' father. The 'social' father (the man who is married to, or lives in a marital-type relationship with, the woman having the child) would have none of the legal rights and responsibilities of a father. Examples are given of 'no legal standing' to exercise rights over the child, such as consenting to a change of name, consenting to adoption or consenting to the child's marriage.

Before the Status of Children Amendment Bill there was, according to the Minister of Justice, 'no clear legal rule' defining the mother when a donated ovum was used; it may be 'either the woman who contributes the ovum or the woman who bears the child'.[11] The Bill was described as a 'technical measure' of the greatest importance because it protected children born as a result of new birth technologies by giving them 'the same security with respect to their parents as children have who are conceived in the usual way'.[12] The other purpose of the legislation was to 'protect' the donors. The Bill is premised on the assumption that 'it is the donors' intention and that of the couples concerned that the donors should be excluded from legal paternity or maternity'.[13]

The response to the objection that the new birth technologies should be opposed anyway was that it is too late to do so, because the practice exists and there are already some people who are in what is described as an 'anomalous' position and who had no say in the manner in which they were conceived.[14] The developed technology in Australia, particularly in Victoria, is cited[15] as a further reason for the need for legislation, because even if new birth technologies were banned in New Zealand there is the strong possibility that a child could be conceived by the new technology in Australia and then born in New Zealand.

The social purposes of the new technologies do not feature centrally in the declared aims of the new legislation. Both the Minister of Justice and the opposition spokesperson on Justice do indicate how they see the social purpose. The Minister of Justice spoke of the 'gift of parenthood'[16] that the donor was giving to a childless couple. The opposition spokesperson welcomed the Bill 'because it further encourages the family unit in our society' by giving 'hope and encouragement'[17] to childless couples. Those social purposes exist in the context of infertility programmes run by the medical profession. The Minister of Justice cites the 'legislation needs of infertility programmes' as the 'policy commitment'[18] behind the Bill. That is the real reason behind the legislation.

The New Zealand legislative response to new birth technologies is based on the assumption that infertile couples (married or living in a marital-type relationship) have a right to use new birth technologies and that the medical profession requires the legal issue of parenthood status to be clarified, so that there are no legal complications following from the use of such technology. The Minister of Justice, when introducing the 'Issues' paper that was to provide a forum for public debate on new birth technologies, put the issue more in terms of the needs of doctors than of infertile patients. The human urge to procreate was looked at in terms of how that urge is made manifest to doctors and what doctors can do to cope with it: 'What matters to doctors now though is the number of distressed persons who are suffering because of their infertility.'[19]

The Status of Children Amendment Act 1987 (the result of the Status of Children Amendment Bill) further reflects the emphasis on perceiving the issue as a medical one. The long title to that Act states that it is 'An Act to amend the Status of Children Act 1969 in relation to the status of persons, conceived as a result of certain medical procedures'. By comparison the Status of Children (Amendment) Act 1984, which was enacted in the Australian state of Victoria, Australia, uses the phrase 'conceived by certain means'. The Justice and Law Reform Committee, which considered the Status of Children Amendment Bill, called a professor from the Wellington infertility clinic to give evidence. The committee chairman commented that the committee was 'very impressed' by the professor, stating that 'he is the kind of qualified medical practitioner who would be ideal for dealing with infertile couples'.[20]

Before the Status of Children Amendment Act 1987 the only matter outside the control of doctors using new birth technologies was the ability to change the legal status of parenthood. All other matters, such as who had access to such procedures, who would be appropriate donors, and what records would be kept of the donor for information in the future, were left entirely in the hands of the medical profession. In that context, by clarifying the status issues and leaving the other issues untouched, the legislative response has further reinforced the power which doctors will have in the use of this new technology in New Zealand. In the introduction to the 'Issues' paper, the Minister of Justice had no hesitation in making it clear that

> ...there is no reason to doubt that AID and AIH and IVF are performed in New Zealand according to the highest ethical standards. It is most unlikely that any further developments would fall below these standards. The kind and degree of legal intervention that is required must be determined having regard to the controls that doctors already place on themselves.[21]

No research or evidence was cited for this statement, which can only be categorized as an assumption based on what it is hoped doctors will do, rather than any clear idea of what they in fact do.

The real reason for the New Zealand legal response to new birth technologies (to meet the 'needs' of medical infertility programmes) means that the broadly stated goals of protecting children from 'legal-limbo' and providing security for children born in circumstances over which they have no control are only met to the extent necessary for such programmes. Needless to say, the interests of women in the process are completely overlooked.

The Enfranchised

Where the legislative response is placed sets the tone of how the issues are likely to be seen in New Zealand. The Status of Children

Amendment Act 1987 is an amending Act to the Status of Children Act 1969 which was passed so that there would be no difference in law between children born inside marriage and children born outside marriage. Its prime purpose was to do away with the concept of illegitimacy — 'to remove the legal disabilities of children born out of wedlock'.[22] This was a field in which New Zealand has been described as producing 'a considerable amount of legislation, generally in advance of England and many other Commonwealth jurisdictions'.[23] The common law had been harsh on the illegitimate child, giving him or her inferior status — *filius nullius* (no-one's child). In the New Zealand context, the Maori Affairs Act 1953 had provided[24] that, in the will of any Maori, the term 'child' or its equivalent was to include a legitimate or illegitimate child unless there was a contrary intention. The legitimacy of the child did not affect the child's status. This was to recognize the Maori perspective on family relationships. Cameron and Webb in a comprehensive article on 'Illegitimacy', which preceded the passing of the Status of Children Act 1969, came to the conclusion that 'the only explanation for the many inroads that have been made by parliament into the rules discriminating between legitimate and illegitimate children must be a policy that no child ought to be penalised on account of the misfortune of its birth'.[25]

The Status of Children Amendment Act 1987 comes on the heels of this pattern of reform and, in many ways, bears the marks and patterns of its predecessors in the issue of illegitimacy. In other ways it can be seen as the beginning of these processes on a different, and perhaps more complex, issue. The issue is different because new birth technologies affect the status of both the child and those involved in the process. Illegitimacy principally affected largely the status of the child; although it did have effects on the father's rights but not on his status as father. A more accurate title for the 1987 amendment would be 'the Status of Children and Persons involved in conceiving a child by new birth technologies'. The biological contributor is deemed not to be the legal parent and the social parent is deemed to be the legal parent.

History[26] before the Status of Children Act 1969 shows that it was a gradual process from the Adoption Act 1881 (which legitimized children by adoption) and the Legitimates Act 1894 (which legitimized children on marriage of the parents) through to the final recognition of equal status set out in s. 3 of the 1969 Act. The Status of Children Amendment Act 1987 is really at the other end of that process as it only overcomes legal impediments in some situations and leaves others still in legal limbo. The Status of Children Amendment Act 1987 does not meet the test that 'there is no reason to apply different rules to children solely because of circumstances over which the children have no control'.[27] By its very deeming provisions, the 1987 Act does apply 'different rules'. The biological donor of sperm, who traditionally has been seen by the law to be the father, is no longer the father. While illegitimacy was done away with, amongst other reasons to ensure that children could make claims against their father's estates, the 1987 amendment works in the opposite direction. The medical student donor is protected from a claim against his estate by the legislation. This is justified on the basis that he was providing the 'gift of parenthood'[28] to others and therefore, as a *quid pro quo* for this social service, he is relieved of any obligation of legal paternity. The same applies to a woman who donates her ovum to another woman. Legal approval is given to such acts by this legislation.

Couching the legislation in terms of children's 'legal limbo' obfuscates the fact that this legislation disenfranchises other groups in New Zealand society from exercising their particular choice of human reproduction. There is no evidence of malice or intent in this outcome, nor any obvious conspiracy of forces or vested interests who have manipulated the result. It is more likely a reflection, as most things are, of the ways of the world, of the haves and the have nots, the powerful and the powerless, the rich and the poor. Certain values predominate, and are controlled by those who have the most say.

The Disenfranchised

The Surrogate Mother, Contracting Father and Surrogate Child

Although the majority of the submissions to the 'Issues' paper were on the issue of surrogate motherhood, that issue is not addressed overtly in the legislation. However, the legislation does have a bearing on such arrangements. Section 5 of the Act states that where

> . . .a married woman becomes pregnant as a result of artificial insemination and she has undergone the procedure with the consent of her husband — the husband shall for all purposes be the father of any child of the pregnancy and any man not being the husband who produced the semen used for the procedure for all purposes not be the father.

The consequence of this wording for a surrogate arrangement is that any husband who consents to his wife being artificially inseminated for the purposes of surrogacy becomes the father of the child. The contracting party, who presumably wants the child and donates the sperm for that purpose, will not be the father. Before the 1987 amendment there was a presumption that the child was a child of the woman and her husband but that presumption could be rebutted by a person who had entered into a surrogate arrangement and donated sperm for that purpose. Such a presumption still applies if the surrogate arrangement is performed by 'natural', rather than 'artificial' means. Where artificial means are used there is a blanket rule that the donor is not the father.

Applying this provision to *Baby M*,[29] the highly publicized US case on surrogate motherhood, would mean that Mr Stern, who donated the sperm which impregnated Mrs Whitehouse, could not be recognized in law as the father (unless he married Mrs Whitehouse, or adopted Baby M). The result of the *Baby M* case was that it was in the child's best interest to remain with Mr and Mrs Stern because they were seen as the best parents. However, if Mr Stern had applied for custody of Baby M in New Zealand, he would be applying as a stranger in law to the child. Of course, that would not necessarily prevent him from obtaining custody as the outcome depends on what arrangements best meet the welfare of the child. However, if custody were granted then, although he is the biological father, he can only be recognized in law as the legal father by adopting the child. Mr Whitehouse is the child's legal father.

Baby M ends up in the kind of 'legal limbo' that this legislation declares it was designed to eliminate. The parents caring for the child have no legal relationship to the child even though one of them is biologically related to the child. Security and protection is given to children born as a result of certain medical procedures but not to children born as a result of a surrogate arrangement. Is there a difference between such methods of conception? In an AID procedure a male donor gives sperm and thereby, in the words of the Minister of Justice, gives the 'gift of parenthood'. In a surrogate arrangement a woman provides her ovum and her body to give the 'gift of parenthood' to others. While legislation is passed to ensure that, in the first situation, all legal impediments to the desired outcome are removed, that same legislation creates legal impediments to the desired outcome in the second situation. There is no evidence to suggest that this was a designed outcome of the legislation. However, whether it was or not does not really matter.

What the legislation signifies is a priority to put in place rules which protect desired legal outcomes when certain medical procedures, including donor ovum transplant, are used. Such procedures are normally only available to those who can afford them and are normally only available through a medical clinic. Surrogate motherhood may be entered into for monetary return, or it may be entered into purely for the gift of parenthood to others. Whatever the reasons, it is usually an arrangement made outside the confines of a medical infertility clinic, and it is probably that fact which leaves such an arrangement out in the legal cold. Those considering surrogacy are best advised to achieve the conception by natural rather than artificial means, so that the spirit of the arrangement is not lost by the wording of the Status of Children Amendment Act.

Immediately after the recent public exposure of a surrogacy arrangement which had caused friction over price, the medical profession went public with a donor egg plan which would 'reduce the need for surrogates' (*Dominion Sunday Times*, 7 April 1991). There is then a shift in focus from the rhetoric of fights over surrogate babies, to the rhetoric of clinical judgement and tricky ethical questions. Control is taken back by the medical profession with the help of the media.

The Single Woman, and the Non-consenting Husband

Where the woman is married or living in a marital-type relationship and her husband or partner consents, then the man who produced the sperm shall not be the father 'and the man who consented to the arrangement' shall be the father.[30] There is a presumption of consent[31] in the Act. As there is no requirement to record the consent in writing it may be very difficult to rebut consent some years after the event. In such cases the consenting man will be deemed to be the father. By doing nothing at the time the procedure is carried out, he is presumed to consent. A man who does not wish to consent and thereby take on the rights and liabilities of fatherhood would be well advised to record that in a statutory declaration or some other formal record as some evidence upon which the presumption can be rebutted. Where that presumption is rebutted, or when the woman is not married or living in a similar arrangement, then the man who produced the sperm no longer is declared not to be the father. Rather, in that case, the sperm donor no longer has the 'rights and liabilities' of a father — which is different from deeming him not to be a father at all.[32]

Where there is consent and the woman is married or in a relationship in the nature of marriage, then the legislation replaces one father for another. When there is no replaceable father, the law has chosen to leave the donor as father but relieve him of the 'rights and liabilities' of that status. One of the goals of the legislation was to exclude donors from 'legal paternity'. What that means is not clear. Depending on by whom and how the donation is used, a donor may be a father without 'rights and liabilities' or not a father at all.

What does it mean when a person is a father without rights and liabilities? Being a father *per se* does not give a person any meaningful rights. The rights flow largely from the fact that, by virtue of s.6 of the Guardianship Act 1968, a father is a natural guardian of a child if he is married to the mother or living in a marital-type relationship at the time of birth.[33] A guardian has a 'right of control over the upbringing and education of a child' and 'a right to possession and care of a child subject to any custody order made by a Court'.[34] Paradoxically a father is called a 'natural'[35] guardian in the Guardianship Act and, by the use of the Status of Children Amendment Act, a person who is not the natural father at all is deemed to be the father and becomes a 'natural' guardian.

A non-cohabiting father has no automatic rights of guardianship as it is left to the discretion of the court, on application, to decide whether or not such a person should be appointed a guardian. A sperm donor will not normally be married to the woman who becomes pregnant, so to declare that such a donor does not have the 'rights' of a father is more narrow than it seems. All that is being taken away is, arguably, the 'right' to apply as father to be appointed as guardian of a child. There is one other provision that may be argued to be a 'right' of a father and that is s. 7(3)(b) of the Adoption Act 1955 which provides for the court to require the consent of an unmarried father to adoption if, in the opinion of the court, it is expedient to do so.

The liabilities that are taken away are largely those for maintenance set out in the Social Security Act 1969[36] and the Family Proceedings Act 1980.[37] Whether liabilities extend as far as provision in a will is not clear from the legislation. The Family Protection Act 1955 allows for claims by a child against a parent's will if that will has not provided as a wise and just testator should for that child.

The term 'rights and liabilities' does not omit the duties of a parent. The Crimes Act 1961 specifies that a parent is under a legal duty to provide 'necessaries' for any child under 16.[38] The duty only applies when the child is in the actual custody of the parent and therefore is not likely to have major impact on a sperm donor parent unless the child is in that person's custody. A parent is also given the power of discipline over children in their care provided that the use of force is reasonable in the circumstances.[39] The Accident Compensation Act 1982, which as a general rules prohibits court action for personal injury, limits the possibility of tortious actions by a child against a parent.

The emphasis in the legislation is on the need for a child to have a legal father. If there is no other person to be deemed a father, then the donor retains that status without its rights and liabilities. It may well be asked whether or not it is necessary to have a legal father when new birth technology is used. In a situation where a woman wants to have a child of her own accord, then, if the law is to reflect that fact, it should deem the donor not to be the father. This may be threatening to men in that they are legally eliminated from the process. But is it not the intent of the legislation to eliminate the donor as father in certain situations? Different rules for single women and women who do not have the consent of their husbands further enhance the view that there is a preferred and set way of having children. Values emerge in the guise of 'technical' legislation to take children out of 'legal limbo'.

The Non-consenting Mother

It is well known that in the biological process there is a difference between how men and women bring children into the world, but should there be such a difference where artificial methods are used? Under the legislation a non-sperm donor becomes the father by consenting to the woman to whom he is married, or with whom he is living in a marital-type relationship, using one of the birth technologies. That consent is presumed unless proved otherwise. However, there is no indication that, if the woman does not consent to the new birth technologies, she will not be the mother. This may seem an obvious point — how could a woman go through this process without consenting? Therefore the consequences of not consenting are not spelt out. In fact the assumption that the woman who gives birth to the child is the mother, no matter what the process, is very strong. Where donor ovum, donor embryo implantation, donor ovum intrafallopian transfer and embryo intrafallopian transfer procedures are used, the woman who becomes pregnant shall be the mother, not the donor.[40]

The likelihood of a woman becoming impregnated by the use of new birth technology without her consent is reasonably remote. However, it is possible that a situation could arise where a donor embryo implantation operation is performed on the wrong patient by mistake. As the Status of Children Amendment Act stands, that woman will be the mother even though she has not consented to the implantation. Motherhood arises from the time of becoming pregnant according to the Status of Children Amendment Act.[41] New birth technologies are called technologies because of the use of the procedure involved: the possibility of mistake is a reality with any technology.

The fact that there is no provision for what happens where the technology is used on a woman by mistake, or perhaps even in a situation where there is no truly informed consent, suggests that the legislators have overlooked that this legislation will more often than not involve a number of persons in the process of impregnation. If motherhood is deemed to arise at impregnation then it is crucial that safeguards are put in place to ensure that the person who is impregnated desires this. The value that emerges is that there is no choice about motherhood even when it is created by the mistaken use of medical procedures — biology is destiny. This fact should alert legislatures to the need for careful control of the use of such technology.

Children Born who have no Access to their Past

There is no provision in the Status of Children Amendment Act for children to have a right of access to the identity or even to the medical history of a donor. There was concern expressed in the submissions to the 'Issues' paper[42] that a deeming provision, such as has been enacted, would eliminate a child's biological origins. The majority of submissions[43] felt that this was less important than the protection of anonymity for the donor since, without anonymity, it was thought that there would be a decline in the number of donors. This is a surprising view to hold and legislate for, given that one year before the Status of Children Amendment Act 1987, the New Zealand Parliament had passed the Adult Adoption Information Act 1986 to allow more access to information by those who had been involved in the adoption process.

The real fear is that if no records are kept and there is no law requiring them to be kept (as there was with adoption) then if a demand for information does surface, that demand may not be able to be met. Before the passing of the legislation, the only way to protect a donor from possible future liability was to destroy the record or to use a system which protects anonymity. Now that the donor is protected by the legislation, the need for those practices has gone. Anonymity is not necessarily threatened by making provision that medical records of donors be kept. Failure to do this may be an oversight, but nevertheless reinforces the view that the legislation is to further empower the medical profession in the use of the new technology. Rather than suffering legislative imposition of any possible fetter upon the exercise of their power, infertility clinics are left to make their own arrangements, safe in the knowledge that any problems of legal status have been resolved.[44]

Children Born Outside the Legislative Scheme

The Status of Children Amendment Act 1987 deals with what have been described as the 'six main medical practices used to deal with infertility.[45] These are:

- artificial insemination by the donor placing donor semen in the uterus with fertilization within the body of the female;

- the donor semen implementation procedure with the ovum from the woman and donor semen, with fertilization taking place outside the body;
- the donor ovum or donor embryo implantation procedure, with the ovum from a donor and semen from either a donor or the husband, fertilization taking place outside the body, and the embryo then being implanted in the uterus of the woman;
- the donor semen intrafallopian transfer procedure with an ovum from the woman transferred from the ovary to the fallopian tube and donor semen being used;
- the donor ovum intrafallopian transfer procedure whereby a donor ovum is placed in the fallopian tube and fertilized inside the body by the semen of the husband;
- the embryo intrafallopian transfer procedure whereby both ovum and semen are donated and fertilization takes place outside the body, and the embryo is then placed in the uterus of the woman.

By listing a finite variety of medical techniques in the Status of Children Amendment Act, the technologies control the legal outcome rather than the needs of the children and their parents.[46] There were other options open to Parliament. For example, it would have been possible to put in place general principles which could cover any future developments. The exhaustive listing of specific technology says a great deal about the lobby behind this legislation. Although it is politically declared to be about taking children out of legal limbo, the way in which the legislation is written shows that it is a catalogue of birth technologies available. The technologies provide the headings to the provisions, and, behind those technologies, is the medical lobby who will no doubt add new technologies as they become available for public display. In effect, the technologies control which children will be taken out of legal limbo. If a new technology is used, outside those specified, the child will remain in legal limbo until the technology is given legislative endorsement.

Maori and Polynesian Families

The Maori Affairs Act 1953,[47] which removed the distinction between illegitimate and legitimate children for Maori people well before the Status of Children Act 1969, recognized that Maori people had a different view of family relationships than *pakeha* (the Maori term for European settlers). The Nuie Act 1966 (every person shall for 'the purposes of the law of Nuie be deemed to be the legitimate child of each of his parents') is an example of recognizing a similar difference for Polynesian people. It is not a simple matter to capture the differences today due to the pressures which the 'dominant' culture have put on the Maori and Polynesian people. This 'dominant' culture has gathered its values largely from its British background. Although that in itself is a gross oversimplification, it provides the necessary contrast here since, apart from the odd concession to cultural difference, as exemplified, law reform in New Zealand has normally proceeded on the assumption that values within the country are homogeneous.

In recent years that assumption has been challenged, and two events sharply focus the current climate of values in New Zealand. The New Zealand Court of Appeal in *New Zealand Maori Council and Latimer* v. *Attorney General*[48] were faced with defining the 'Principles of the Treaty of Waitangi' in the context of an Act of Parliament. Before this case, the Treaty of Waitangi, signed between chiefs of Maori tribes and the British Crown, had not been recognized as part of New Zealand municipal law.[49] Parliament's placing of an express legislative reference to 'Principles of the Treaty of Waitangi' in the context of the State Owned Enterprises Act 1986 faced the Court of Appeal with the task of giving those words some meaning. The President of the New Zealand Court of Appeal, Sir Robin Cooke, made the observation that 'this case is perhaps as important for the future of our country as any that has come before a New Zealand Court'.[50]

Although the issue in that case was about land, the ideas expressed by the New Zealand Court of Appeal set the benchmark of how Maori/*pakeha* relations should proceed. It was made clear in the case that 'neither the provisions of the Treaty of Waitangi nor its principles are, as a matter of law, a restraint on the legislative supremacy of Parliament'.[51] Sir Robin Cooke made the statement that '[n]ow the emphasis is much more on the need to preserve Maoritangi, Maori land and communal life, a distinctive Maori identity'.[52]

The effect of this change in values is most clearly reflected in the law reform process concerning the Children and Young Persons Act 1974. This is legislation which is quite familiar in other parts of the world and which deals with child abuse, child neglect, children in need of care and juvenile offending. Reform had been a slow process but had largely centred around recommendations to involve more professional expertise (child protection teams) and control. By the end of 1987 there had been a fundamental change in the criticism of the reforms. A working party attacked the proposed approach as 'monocultural' — particularly the emphasis on the welfare of the child being treated as 'the first and paramount consideration'. The following submission by a Maori summarizes the thrust of the objection:

The paramountcy accorded to the child . . . subsumed the importance attached to the responsibility of the group through tribal traditions and lore which took precedence over the view of birth parents. Thus children's interests could only be determined after having regard for and giving due consideration to the views and concerns of the child's whanau and hapu . . . .[53]

Atkin in an article in the *Journal of Family Law* captures the essence of what family relationships mean for the Maori people:

In traditional Maori terms the important concepts for personal relationships are the whanau, the hapu and the iwi. A rough translation which fails to do justice to these words is respectively 'extended family', 'sub-tribe' and 'tribe'. The phrase 'extended family' is in fact quite misleading since it suggests an extension of the nuclear family. For the Maori it is the other way round: the whanau is the basic family unit from which the parent–child relationship develops. The whanau involves at least three generations and is likely to have twenty-five to fifty members. The responsibility for bringing up children does not rest solely about the birth parents but is shared by adult relatives. Indeed, the parenting will often be done primarily by uncles, aunts or grandparents. The hapu will have between one hundred and one thousand members, all having common ancestors going back six generations . . . the iwi is a much larger kinship linkage where members share a common ancestor. The iwi will be associated with a certain territory which traditionally will have been protected and defended.[54]

In this context, legislation which is concerned with giving particular children a legal father and mother and with excluding other people from that legal status seems a very *pakeha* way of addressing the issue of new methods of human reproduction. The nuclear family image is very strong in the mind's eye of the legislature, as is the idea of parental legal tenure of children. Since the values of individual liability and individual rights and duties with regard to children are reflected in our legislative scheme concerning child and parent issues, it comes as no major surprise that the Status of Children Amendment Act 1987 follows this trend. However, it may well be an incident of time which dictates such an outcome; the tide has begun to turn and it is no longer possible for legislation to proceed on the basis of one set of values. The Children and Young Persons and their Families Act 1989 is testimony to the fact that Parliament is prepared to pass legislation which emphasizes a broader view of family relationships than previously considered. The mix and outcome is not necessarily well thought through nor widely accepted.[55] The debate has been more at the level of political compromise than well reasoned social policy.

Further law reform in the area of human reproduction is likely to have to face the different values which that event represents for different groups within the community. It may be that, in confronting that issue in rational exchange, a more rich understanding of what human reproduction means for New Zealanders will emerge.

The Present-day Guardians of New Birth Technologies

Doctors are the guardians of new birth technologies, and it is not easy to get a comprehensive picture of what is being done. In 1985, in order to discover the extent of AID practice in New Zealand, a postal survey of obstetricians and gynaecologists was carried out[56] which produced a disturbing variation in practice. All 20 of the practitioners who replied as being AID practitioners were males. The recruitment of donors was seen as a major problem, medical students and the husbands of obstetrics patients appearing to be the most commonly used source.

There were considerable variations in the number of conceptions allowed per donor. Six practitioners set no limit; five limited to five conceptions; three to four conceptions; one to three conceptions; two to two conceptions; and one to one conception. The practice of the remaining two gynaecologists varies. Two-thirds of the practitioners keep records to indicate which donor's sperm has been used for a particular couple, while the remainder keep no real record. Only 45 per cent of the practitioners felt that it was desirable for a child conceived as a result of AID to be told of its origins. Concern was expressed at what had happened in the adoption field and the need for a family's honest relationship with each other. Approximately one-third of the practitioners did not feel it was desirable for children to know of their origins; a quarter were unsure of what was best for the child.

AID was described as a biopsychosocial intervention and, because of this, 80 per cent of the practitioners assess the psychological suitability of a couple before deciding to proceed. Sixty-five per cent also assess the social circumstances of the couple. Some of the literature highlights the importance of psychosocial assessment of suitability for AID. At present the majority of assessments are carried out by the practitioners themselves.

The concept of maintaining centralized control via the Health Department was strongly rejected by the practitioners. Although termination of pregnancy, sterilization, and adoption are all subject to some notification requirements, practitioners were concerned with the question of secrecy and the possibility of more and unnecessary work.

The survey shows that, at present, new birth technologies are controlled by the medical profession and are used as treatment for infertile couples who are in a stable relationship. Whilst there are general ethical guidelines, individual practitioners are using the process as a form of treatment in the way that is believed best for individual patients. Apart from the efforts of individual practitioners, New Zealand currently has operating an AID clinic in Wellington, an IVF programme in Auckland, and a private infertility clinic also in Auckland.

The survey established that there is more demand that there are services available.

The Royal New Zealand College of Obstetricians and Gynaecologists have also issued ethical Guidelines for Artificial Insemination Using Donor Semen.[57] These guidelines show the broad social issues which doctors are prepared to assume that they should exclusively determine. It is stated that 'the primary requirement for couples requesting AID is a stable relationship'. Are doctors well qualified to measure the indicators of a stable relationship? It is also stated that 'donors should be of acceptable appearance and intelligence'. This probably explains why medical students are a popular form of donor – the medical profession can trust their own pedigree. The discussion paper on In Vitro Fertilisation,[58] put out by the same Council, opens with the quite revealing statement that 'there appears to be general medical agreement that in vitro fertilisation and embryo replacement within a stable heterosexual relationship is ethically acceptable'. So it is 'medical agreement' which determines what is ethical and what is not. No broader considerations seem to be relevant.

It would appear that the controls exercised really depend on those running the infertility programmes. There is no evidence of community consultation as to appropriate safeguards, nor is there evidence of collective assessment by the medical profession of the need for standard safeguards. The discussion paper mentions the need for 'management' of the 'highest standard' but there are no specifics.

Should doctors be able to decide who has access to fertility programmes? The power to decide who can use new birth technologies is really a power to decide who has the right to have children. The particular personal values of a doctor or team of doctors are inherent in the process.[59] While this may have pragmatic appeal, in that it prevents a whole screening bureaucracy from being set up to deal with the issue of eligibility, it also has the potential to diffuse any possible analysis of the issues involved. The door is not closed to further debate as there is an interdepartmental committee whose brief is 'to act as a repository of information on the techniques to monitor the issues and to advise the Government as required'.[60]

However, the lobbying strength of persons wanting to use new birth technologies, but who have been refused medical access to them, is not likely to be strong.

Just what a doctor is doing in providing new birth technology for a patient has not been the subject of careful scrutiny. Is the doctor providing essential treatment for a particular condition or is the doctor not really involved in treatment but more involved in providing an extra service for those who the doctor considers can best benefit from such a service? It has been argued that there is a 'right to reproduce'.[61] If there is such a right, and a doctor has the means for the right to be carried out, does a doctor have the 'right' to refuse because of a belief that the person wanting to exercise the right is not living in the appropriate type of relationship or is not likely to be able to parent the resultant child adequately?

By leaving these issues untouched by legislation, the New Zealand government is clearly signalling that these are matters of private concern not to be regulated by the state. If new birth technologies are a health service, then they are a service whose operation lies with the individual doctor, patient and donor who decide how they are going to operate. Given the fact that New Zealand has quite clear regulation in other – arguably similar – areas of medicine, such as the Contraception Sterilisation and Abortion Act 1977, and the Human Tissue Act 1964, it does seem anomalous that there is such a big gap in the area of new birth technologies. Part of the explanation is that it has not been perceived as a major issue in current New Zealand society.

Nevertheless, at the same time, the ethical standards of the medical profession have become a public issue: some New Zealand doctors have been publicly challenged and, after a major public enquiry, their ethical standards have been found wanting. The issue of this challenge was cervical cancer and it arose due to the fact that some doctors were using experimental regimes without telling the patients about this fact. Judge Cartwright, after hearing evidence from many medical personnel and patients during the inquiry, identified the following themes about ethics and patients' rights:

- a failure to offer generally accepted treatment to certain classes of patients;
- a failure on the part of colleagues to ensure that generally accepted treatment was offered;
- failure on the part of other health professionals to provide protection for the patients;
- failure to ensure that patients were informed of the nature of

their condition and that the treatment offered was not generally accepted treatment;

- patients, neonates and foetuses were included in research trials
  with almost no attempt to seek appropriate consent;
- some teaching and clinical practices were outmoded, disre-
  spectful to women patients or unmindful of their feelings or
  desire for privacy;
- preventable health measures were discouraged by failing to
  give women or their general practitioners accurate information about their condition and by the active downgrading
  of the value of screening for cervical cancer;
- the doctrine of clinical freedom was observed to a dangerous
  degree.[62]

In the context of human reproduction these are disturbing findings. There has been no legislative response, although a bioethics
centre[63] has been set up at Otago University Medical School and the
first ethics lecturer[64] in medicine been appointed. Yet these are small
changes. They have the potential to promote public debate but also
the potential to keep the firm control of that debate in the hands of
the medical profession. As I write this the medical profession has
reacted to what has been described as 'fall-out' from the Cartwright
report: a private fertility clinic has alleged that its desire to move into
a donor egg scheme for women with early menopause has been
inhibited by the reluctance of any ethical committee to approve it.[65]

Questions as to the acceptability of creating surplus embryos,[66]
the freezing of surplus embryos,[67] research on surplus embryos,[68] the
allocation of health care resources,[69] and the prevention of infertility[70] have not been the subject of legislative action or major public
debate. New Zealand has taken the approach set out by the law
reform decision of the Department of Justice that 'New Zealand can
afford to wait and watch developments'.[71] It was felt that there are
currently in place two non-governmental forms of control to which
government policymakers must have regard, namely 'the ethical
guidelines which bind medical practitioners and researchers' and
'public opinion'. The problem is that, when entering new fields, these
guidelines may be neither adequate nor sufficiently subject to
scrutiny and therefore accountability. Public opinion is really dependent on knowing what is going on, and, if what is going on is in the
hands of medical professionals and researchers, public opinion is
likely neither to be informed nor very active. Much of what is
written about new birth technologies in the media in New Zealand is
based on the sensational cases that happen overseas.[72] We look afar
without questioning within. An encapsulated summary of the New
Zealand law reform response on new birth technologies is found in

the following analysis of access to information for those born as a result of certain methods.

> The area of access to information may prove to be one where a legislative response is necessary. At present, however, this issue requires monitoring only. This is because we do not yet know whether the people concerned will want information or if they do, what kind of information they will require . . . there is room for the development of guidelines by the medical profession on the matter.[73]

By the time something is done, the information required may not be available.

STERILIZATION OF THE MENTALLY HANDICAPPED

The issue of sterilization of the mentally handicapped has been the subject of judicial analysis.[74] The first case to come before the New Zealand courts on this matter (*Re X*)[75] decided in favour of leaving the issue in the hands of the parents and the doctors. The Guardianship Act 1968, which applies to children under 20, was read as providing the necessary authority for parents of handicapped children to give consent on their behalf to sterilization. The wording of the crucial section, s.25(3) is ambiguous: it allows a guardian of the child to give consent to the medical procedures where that consent is 'necessary'. This seems to beg the question. There is no definition of when consent is 'necessary'. Hilleyer J, in *Re X* had no problem with holding that the provision gave parents of intellectually handicapped children the power to consent to a sterilization operation. Full power was not left in the hands of the parents, because 'doctors will appreciate that they have an obligation to ensure that the operation they are carrying out is a proper one, and that the consent given is a proper consent.'[76] What this means is that the doctor must be satisfied that parents give informal consent, and also in the view of Hilleyer J the doctor must be sure the consent is for the 'benefit of the child'.[77] Failure to do this, according to Hilleyer J, could make the donor liable 'under civil law' (presumably assault) or to medical disciplinary proceedings, or possibly even to criminal charges (assault again).[78] Two assumptions lay behind the decision to leave the matter to doctors and parents. First, that 'the medical profession as a whole is a responsible caring and professional body, and that their interest is in what is best for the patients'.[79] Second, the cost of court proceedings, delays, and the trauma of court proceedings, were seen to place too heavy a burden on parents having to come to court in each case. While this may be so, there are still no publicly debated criteria for the situations where sterilization may or may not be appropriate. Without legislative guidance the most Hilleyer J could do was provide a list of factors from decided overseas cases which may be helpful as a guideline.[80] The difficulties with this open ended, unregulated approach is that it will depend very much on the views of those involved in the particular decision to sterilize.

The planned vasectomy of a 16-year-old intellectually handicapped youth received wide press coverage in New Zealand[81] and the different views reported show how confused the issues become. The National Director of the Society for the Intellectually Handicapped said that his main concern was whether there was informed consent by the youth. 'I have been told and am relaxed in the fact that he was aware of what the operation was about and knew what he was in for – he said he knew it meant he would not be able to "make babies".' The youth's mother reported as seeing little of her son, but had requested the vasectomy because the youth had been sexually active and she feared unwanted pregnancies. The legal advice to the Mental Health Foundation said, 'We would probably see what you are describing as an abuse.' A man who knew the youth called it a 'forced sterilization'. A Christchurch paediatrician said that from what he knew of the case 'it was probably in the best interest that the youth did not become a father'. But in the best interests of whom? A case is cited in the press report of an intellectually handicapped man being told he was going to hospital for a toe operation when a vasectomy was planned. When parliament abdicates its responsibility to give clear direction in such areas the matter is left to chance. The National Director of the Society for the Intellectually Handicapped said that if there had been more time the Society would probably have taken the case to the Director General of Social Welfare and on to the High Court.

The Protection of Personal and Property Rights Act 1988, which was passed to provide for the protection and promotion of the personal and property rights of persons over 20 who are not fully able to manage their own affairs, was an opportunity for the New Zealand Legislature to address the issue of sterilization, at least for those over 20.

The Family Court is given power under the Act to make personal orders on behalf of such persons relating to medical advice and treatment. Any medical action taken as a result of a court order will have legal authorization. The phrase 'medical advice or treatment' is distinctly unclear since, arguably on a broad interpretation, anything done by a medical practitioner in the course of his or her practice is medical. A narrower view would limit the meaning to diagnosis and care of specific ailments. Atkin, who is the New Zealand authority on this legislation, has come to the conclusion that, because of the seriousness of the consequences of sterilization, a judge may be unwilling to grant an order unless it was very clearly related to some other diagnosable condition (for example, a hysterectomy might be ordered where the patient is suffering from cancer).[82] Section 8 of the Act mandatorily requires the Court to make the last restrictive intervention possible, having regard to the degree of the person's incapacity, and to encourage the person to exercise and develop such capacity as the person has to the greatest possible extent. Such principles show a clear emphasis on a cautious approach to interventions. The development of capacity leaves open the value question which is sometimes argued to be at stake in sterilization decisions – the capacity to freely enter into relationships vs the risk of unable to be coped with pregnancy.

The Family Court has power to appoint a welfare guardian.[83] Such a person will have power to control a certain aspect of the handicapped person's life and will have all such powers as may be reasonably required to enable the welfare guardian to make and implement decisions for the person . . . . The court has overriding power to impose conditions on the guardian.[84] The Act specifies certain issues over which the welfare guardian has no authority. For example, a guardian cannot give consent to the adoption of the mentally handicapped person's child. On the issue of sterilization the legislation is again ambiguous. The Act states that a guardian cannot withhold consent to standard medical treatment intended to save the person's life or to prevent serious damage to health.[85] That suggests that if sterilization was necessary to prevent serious damage to the mentally handicapped person's health then the guardian has no power to stop it. The converse is not necessarily true. If there is no threat of serious damage to the person's health, there is no clear power to consent in that circumstance. Sterilization of the mentally handicapped is a complex and difficult issue which Parliament had the chance to address directly in this legislation.

CONCLUSIONS

For the legal academic, human reproduction is a complex issue which raises a number of interests. The interests of the women, the expected child, the family and the society in which all this occur need to be considered closely. Sometimes – for example, on the issue of abortion – those interests are balanced against one another and a law is passed which allows abortion if certain criteria are established. But even that law will depend largely on the judgement of those who have the most say in the application of the criteria and whether the law is prepared to hold them accountable or hand over the responsibility. New Zealand, like many other countries, has limited abortion on the statute books and liberal abortion in practice[86] provided that the appropriate doctor can be found. Because issues of human reproduction invoke personal choices, and because we live in a society which values personal autonomy, there is a great reluctance to be too intrusive into how individuals go about human reproduction. Unfortunately such an analysis overlooks the fact that, in human reproduction, there is not always personal choice but rather much of the control is exercised by professionals. When proposing law reform about human reproduction the role of professionals must be built into the analysis of interests involved rather than be seen as a separate non-partisan controlling device, a non-elected legislature.

The reasons why issues of human reproduction have not been the focus of public debate are difficult to find. We have had no Warnock enquiry[87] into the issues. We have had a public 'Issues' paper which received very little public reaction. We have had a major public enquiry into the ethics of certain doctors. This latter did receive a great deal of public attention and provided an insight into how the interests of professionals, disguised as 'research', can easily override the interests of the patient and the wider community. It would be a terrible waste of the courage of the victims of that episode if, when New Zealand does decide to address the issues of human reproduction fully, the practice and procedures of those who practise the 'technologies' are not brought under close scrutiny. In the meanwhile New Zealand seems prepared to adopt what may be termed a 'Nero' approach — sit and watch the rest of the world develop their legislative schemes and practices.

Germaine Greer in her work *Sex and Destiny*[88] cites the following passage by Clellan Stearns Ford:

> Human reproduction is effected by biological processes assisted by learned behaviour. The customs which are thus in adjustment to the imperfections of human biological processes of reproduction arise from a desire to bear children. This wish for offspring is not an innate component of human nature; it is not a basic drive. On the contrary, it is an acquired motive which is constantly being reinforced by social rewards and punishments. Promises of security, approval and prestige support the desire for children; threats of insecurity, punishment and ridicule block incipient wishes to escape the fears and pains of childbirth and parenthood.[89]

Greer's own work in *Sex and Destiny* is testimony to the idea that whole ideological systems have been built on 'the achievement of parenthood and how child-bearing has been motivated in traditional familial societies'.[90] The difficult paradox in the matter of human reproduction is that, because of its very personal nature, there is a general reluctance to take it into the public domain – to legislate about it.

Yet by leaving many matters in the private sphere, an ideology is formed by those who control reproduction and those who have access to that control – the doctors and those who can afford their services. Weber[91] captures the irony of what to do about such a situation. The goal of 'equality before the law' requires a formal and rational objectivity of administration and rules. Yet if this is done, as is shown in this chapter, the substantive justice of particular claims collides with this formalism and rule-boundness. The formal rules of status set out in the Status of Children Amendment Act 1987 collide with the substantive claims of those who do not fit into that mould of status. Informalism does not necessarily provide the answer because, as the analysis of the medical profession's current practices with the new birth technologies shows, that informalism can 'be very easily subverted by the powerful to their advantage'.[92]

The argument of this chapter has been to shift the roles. The formal rules should be directed at those who use the technology – the medical profession – to 'inhibit power and afford some protection to the powerless'.[93] It may also be a relief to the medical profession to have the burden of self-regulation lifted. Informalism should be left for individuals or groups to choose their own particular form of reproduction.

Oliver in the process of writing an historical overview of social policy in New Zealand makes the following poignant comment:

> Since the beginning of the century an increasing concern with national efficiency had made health policy a more urgent matter. Horror at the 'fertility of the unfit' and at the prospect of deepening 'degeneracy' together with a fear that 'white' (and especially British) supremacy was under threat from hardy Asians focused attention on the nurture of children and so upon the social focus of women.[94]

A comprehensive analysis of social policy was carried out by the New Zealand government in 1988.[95] Issues of reproduction are not specifically addressed anywhere in the four-volume report. The best explanation of the lack of open and public debate on the issue is that New Zealand does not yet see reproduction as a 'social' issue.

NOTES

1   Law Reform Division Department of Justice (1985), *New Birth Technologies – An Issue Paper on AID, IVF and Surrogate Motherhood*, March ('Issues' Paper).
2   'Rogernomics' is the term which has been used after a Minister of Finance, Roger Douglas.
3   Christchurch, New Zealand, 1987.

4   See, for example, McLean S. A. M. (1989), 'Women, Rights and Reproduction', in S. A. M. McLean (ed.), *Legal Issues in Human Reproduction*, Aldershot: Dartmouth.
5   *Wall* v. *Livingston and Roborough* [1982] NZFLR 418.
6   Ibid., p. 425.
7   See 'Issues' paper, op. cit., note 1 above.
8   *Hansard*, vol. 473, 13 August 1986, p. 3870, per Geoffrey Palmer, Minister of Justice.
9   Ibid. p. 3869.
10 Ibid.
11 Ibid.
12 Ibid.
13 Ibid.
14 Ibid.
15 Ibid.
16 Ibid.
17 *Hansard*, vol. 473, 13 August 1986, p. 3871, per Jim McLay MP.
18 Op. cit., note 8 above, p. 3869.
19 Op. cit., note 1 above, p. 8.
20 *Hansard*, vol. 479, 2 April 1987, p. 8370, per Bill Dillon MP.
21 See 'Issues' paper, op. cit., note 1 above.
22 From the long title of the Act.
23 Cameron, B. J. and Webb. P. M. (1967), 'Illegitimacy', in B. D. Inglis and A. G. Mercer (eds), *Family Law Centenary Essays*, Wellington: Sweet and Maxwell, p. 133.
24 Section 115(1) Maori Affairs Act 1953.
25 Cameron and Webb, op. cit., note 23 above.
26 This is well traced in detail in Cameron and Webb, loc. cit.
27 This was the essence of the Minister of Justice's speech on the second reading of the Status of Children Amendment Bill, *Hansard*, vol. 482, pp. 10104–5.
28 Op. cit., note 8 above.
29 *Baby M* (1987) Fam. L. Rep., **13**, (US) 22 2001 at first instance. Supreme Court of New Jersey reversed the ruling in the lower court on the issue of visitation and also disregarded the analysis of surrogate contracts (*New York Times*, 4 February 1988.)
30 Sections 5(1), 7(1), 9(1), 11(1), 13(1), 14(1), 15(1) Status of Children Amendment Act 1987.
31 Section 17 Status of Children Amendment Act 1987.
32 Sections 5(2), 7(2), 9(2), 11(2), 13(2), 14(2), 15(2), Status of Children Amendment Act 1987.
33 Re. in *the Guardianship of B* (1986) 4 NZLR 673 Judge Mahoney took the view that 'married' in s.6 Guardianship Act 1968 includes living in a relationship in the nature of marriage.
34 Section 3 Guardianship Act 1968.
35 Heading used in s. 6 Guardianship Act 1968.
36 Known as the 'liable parent scheme', ss. 27 I - 27 ZH Social Security Act 1964.
37 Part VI Family Proceedings Act 1980.
38 Section 152 Crimes Act 1961.
39 Section 59 Crimes Act 1961.
40 Sections 9(3), 13(3), 15(3) Status of Children Amendment Act 1987.
41 Sections 9(3)(a), 13(3)(a), 14(4)(a) 'The woman shall for all purposes be the mother of the pregnancy whether born or unborn.'

42 'Issues' paper, op. cit., note 1 above. Law Reform Division Department of Justice (1986), *New Birth Technologies. A summary of submissions received on the Issues paper*, December, p. 10 ('Submissions' paper).

43 See the Submissions' paper, op. cit., note 42 above.

44 Even the Adoption Act 1955 allowed access to records in special circumstances: s.23 Adoption Act 1955.

45 *Hansard*, vol. 479, 2 April 1987, p. 8271, per Paul East, MP.

46 It has been said that New Zealand's slow approach has helped us because 'while other legislatures have been passing legislation, new birth technologies have developed'. See 'Submissions' paper, op. cit., note 42 above. On this reasoning we would not pass any legislation just in case a new technology emerged.

47 Section 115(1).

48 (1987), 6 NZAR 353.

49 *Hoani Te Heuheu Tukino* v. *Aotea District Maori Land Board* [1941] A.C. 308 – the Privy Council held that treaty rights cannot be enforced in the courts except insofar as a statutory recognition of the rights can be found.

50 Ibid., 355 per Cooke P.

51 Ibid., 399 per Somers J.

52 Ibid., 370 per Cooke P.

53 Department of Social Welfare, *Report of the Working Party on the Children and Young Persons Bill. Review of the Children and Young Persons Bill 1987.*

54 Atkin, B. (1988–89), 'New Zealand: Children versus families – Is there any conflict?', *Journal of Family Law*, **27**, p. 231.

55 See ibid., pp. 236–7.

56 Carried out by K. R. Daniels (a senior social worker) and reported in full in the 'Issues' paper, op. cit., note 1 above.

57 These are set out in the Appendix to the 'Issues' paper, op. cit., note 1 above.

58 Set out in the Appendix to the 'Issues' paper, op. cit., note 1 above.

59 A submission by the *Ministry of Women's Affairs to the Report of the Royal Commission on Social Policy April 1988, te Komihana, A Te Kaurauna, Mo Nga Ahautanga A Iwi* sums up the consequence of such an outcome: 'The decision makers, that is those who have the power, are the same people who design the systems and they also decide the criteria for eligibility to enter them and to operate and succeed. They base their decision on their value systems and beliefs about what is important and what is not', vol. 1, p. 627.

60 See the 'Submissions' paper, op. cit., note 42 above.

61 McLean, S. A. M. (1986), 'The Right to Reproduce', in *Human Rights – From Rhetoric to Reality*, Oxford: Basil Blackwell, p. 99.

62 Cartwright (1988), *The Report of the Committee of Inquiry into Allegations Concerning the Treatment of Cervical Cancer at National Women's Hospital and into Other Relevant Matters.*

63 Under the guidance of Professor Gareth Jones and a steering committee.

64 A neurosurgeon who has a degree in Philosophy from Oxford University.

65 *Eye Witness News*, Monday 21 August 1989.

66 See 'Submissions' paper, op. cit., note 42 above, pp. 26–7.

67 Ibid., pp. 27–8.

68 Ibid., p. 28.

69 Ibid., pp. 36–7.

70 Ibid., p. 36.

71 Ibid., p. 40.

72 For example, the case of the 'jointly owned' embryo which is being fought over in the USA. *Otago Daily Times*, Dunedin, 16 March 1989.

73   Ibid., p. 39.
74   In *Re B* (a minor) Sterilization [1987] 2 All ER 206 (C.A.), *Re B* (a minor) [1976] 1 All ER 326. *Re Eve* (1986) 2 SCR 407. In *Re F* (Mental Patient: Sterilization) (1989) 2 WLR 1025.
75   [1991] NZFLR 49.
76   Ibid., 57.
77   Idem.
78   Idem.
79   Ibid., 60.
80   Ibid., 61–3.
81   *Otago Daily Times*, Dunedin, 2 October 1987.
82   Butterworths, *Family Law Service*, New Zealand, Butterworths, para. 7.818. See also Butterworths, *Family Law Guide*, 4th edition (1991), (eds Webb, Adams, Atkin, Henaghan, Caudwell), New Zealand: Butterworths.
83   Protection of Personal and Property Rights Act 1988, s. 12.
84   Idem.
85   Protection of Personal and Property Rights Act 1988, s. 18C.
86   Kennedy, L. A. (1987), 'Abortion – Society's Midwife', unpublished LLB(Hons) dissertation, Otago University.
87   Committee of Inquiry into Human Fertilization and Embryology, Cmnd 9314/1984 323.
88   Greer, G. (1985), *Sexual Destiny – The Politics of Human Fertility*, London: Picador, p. 380.
89   Cellan, Sterns Ford (1985), *A Comparative Study of Human Reproduction*, New Haven: Yale University Press, p. 86.
90   Greer, op. cit., note 88 above.
91   Weber, M. (1946), *Essays in Sociology*, ed. and trans. H. H. Gerth and C. Wright-Mills, copyright 1946 Oxford University Press Inc., reviewed 1973 by Hans. H. Gerth, cited by M. D. A. Freeman in 'Questioning the Delegalization Movement in Family Law', in J. M. Eekelaar and S. N. Katz (eds) (1984), *The Resolution of Family Conflict*, Toronto: Butterworths, p. 9.
92   Freeman, op. cit., note 91 above.
93   Thompson, E. P. (1975), *Whigs and Hunters*, London: Allan Lane, pp. 262–3.
94   In The Report on Social Policy, op. cit., note 59 above, vol. 1, p. 23.
95   Ibid.

7 United Kingdom: Legal Regulation of Human Reproduction

KENNETH McK. NORRIE

INTRODUCTION

Human reproduction has traditionally been a process that requires two individuals only – one man and one woman. It is a process which, in its 'natural' form, commences with the most intimate physical experience between the two. The law in England and Scotland has long recognized the intimacy and the privacy of that physical experience and has, on the whole, seen little role for itself to play in regulating it.[1]

However, human reproduction has never been wholly unregulated by the law, and the legal consequences arising from the process can easily be manipulated in such a way as to promote a particular policy. So, for example, the common law in both England and Scotland stigmatized a child born outside marriage as illegitimate, this in pursuance of a centuries-old, and church-led, policy of discouraging licentiousness outside the marriage bed.[2] The legal consequences of the unacceptable mating were severe (for the child). Similarly, and more directly, the law continues to prohibit marriage between persons within certain degrees of relationship,[3] and punishes, as the crime of incest, sexual intercourse between specified categories of person.[4] These provisions are designed to prevent the reproductive process commencing for certain individuals; if the process does commence then at common law it could not be interrupted legally. So abortion was a common law crime in both England and Scotland, and indeed remains a criminal act in both jurisdictions today (subject to the defences that are available for certain people performing the abortion).[5]

As restrictions to freedom of choice in reproduction these provisions are fairly minor, for the law in Great Britain has tended to regard the process as one that is so private as not to be appropriate for detailed regulation. Within the marital bed the law leaves it up to the individuals themselves to decide whether their relations are to be fecund,[6] and there have never been the legislative attempts that were seen in other jurisdictions to prohibit, for example, the use of contraceptives,[7] or to limit their use to married couples.[8] The dissemination of knowledge concerning contraceptives was prosecuted in England as obscenity in 1877, but the conviction obtained was quashed on appeal[9] and there has since then been no challenge to the legality of such dissemination. It has never been suggested that the use of contraception, or sterilization, are common law crimes,[10] in the way that, for example, abortion was. Statute would therefore be required to prohibit these activities, and there has never been any such statute. While it cannot be denied (although it is seldom asserted) that some people are quite unsuited to parenthood, the law will allow them to become parents nevertheless, and only in the most exceptional circumstances will children be removed from their parents.

Human reproduction, as well as being an essentially private process, is one that raises many important moral issues concerning the nature of marriage, the nature of parenthood and the nature — indeed origin — of life-creation itself. But the British legislature has always attempted to avoid these sorts of issues if it can, preferring to deal with absolutes that can be stated in the form of legal rules that are black and white both in their terms and in their justification. While life remained simple this approach was acceptable and, in most situations, provided sensible solutions. Couples were left to procreate how and if they chose, and their so doing posed no threat to the basis of society itself.

But human reproduction today is no longer necessarily the exclusive concern of the two parties involved. Certainly it remains so for most couples; but there are a significant number of people who, without medical intervention, are and would remain infertile. Infertility is a problem that, when it prevents those who wish to procreate from so doing, causes real and lasting distress to affected individuals. Until relatively recently that distress had to be borne, but medical science has now made it possible to alleviate that suffering in a number of different ways, both by curing the infertility itself and by providing means of circumventing it. Parenthood can now, through the intervention of a third party, be open to those for whom it was previously closed. There are a number of new techniques that can be employed, such as AID, egg donation, embryo transfer, surrogacy, and many combinations of these.[11]

These new techniques have disrupted the traditional view of human reproduction in two ways. First, and most obviously, the principles governing the law in relation to parent and child were developed in the context of the traditional private method of reproduction (that is, heterosexual — presumptively marital — sexual intercourse). The application of these principles to reproduction following one of the new techniques, where the basis upon which the normal principles are founded often does not exist (for example, a genetic link between 'parent' and child), would inevitably produce anomalies and sometimes absurdities. Second, because the techniques are dealing with the creation of life itself, and may potentially involve the intentional destruction of some form of life, the feeling arose that those who were providing these techniques ought not to be allowed to act totally without any control. The individual submitting her or himself to medical science may be in a highly vulnerable condition, desperately wishing to reproduce, confused at the inability to do so, and potentially little more than raw material for the scientist's research project. Society, too, requires protection from the scientist motivated only by her or his quest for knowledge, to the exclusion of considerations of ethics, morals and the law. There is no doubt that medical technology has been able to bring great happiness to large numbers of people who would have been unable to become parents otherwise, but, in the process of developing that technology, knowledge has been acquired that can be used for less benign purposes. In other words, human reproduction can have directly public consequences as well as the purely private ones.

The reality of this disruption to the traditional view of parenting burst onto the public consciousness in July 1978, with the birth in England of Louise Brown, the first child whose fertilization had taken place outside her mother's body, and who had been implanted into her womb for successful gestation. Until then, society seemed able to cope with (or at least be content to ignore) the reproductive techniques previously available, such as artificial insemination. But the birth of Louise Brown brought people to the realization that many very different things were suddenly possible, such as the freezing of gametes and even fertilized eggs, the removal from one woman of a conceptus for reimplantation in another, and the donation of gametes for the creation of embryos to be used in the creation of children for 'parents' who have no genetic link with the children whatsoever. Similarly, *in vitro* fertilization has allowed scientists to examine and to experiment with the *in vitro* conceptus, with various diverse aims, such as improving medicine's understanding of — and ability to cure or eliminate — some of the genetic defects that cause so much suffering to those born with them. Greater understanding of the very early embryo, observed under scientific conditions, is hoped to lead to better, easier, cheaper and more reliable contraception, which, in terms of the sheer numbers of people involved, might validly be regarded as the single most important development to come out of the sort of embryological study made possible by the development of *in vitro* fertilization.

It quickly became clear that the law could not simply ignore these developments, nor attempt to solve the problems they created for the existing rules. It became clear also that there was strong public anxiety at the thought of scientists being completely uncontrolled in particular fields of endeavour. Stories of hybrids, mutants, clones, monsters, are the staple of horror science fiction; only strict control could prevent them becoming science fact. The fears may not all have been realistic, but they were undoubtedly real, and they were directed more to scientists than to science — we fear Frankenstein more than we fear his monster.

Legal writers were discussing the potential legal problems of new reproductive developments long before they became reality,[12] but it was the public concern at the lack of control which existed that persuaded the British Parliament that the law had to step in, even though many of the issues raised were moral ones, and therefore anathema to most British politicians. Thus, in July 1982 the government set up the Committee of Inquiry into Human Fertilization and Embryology (the Warnock Committee), and that Committee reported back to the government in June 1984[13]. A government Consultative Paper was published in December 1986,[14] followed by a White Paper[15] in November 1987. The Queen's Speech two years later announced that legislation would shortly be introduced, and on 29 November 1989 the Human Fertilization and Embryology Bill was introduced in the House of Lords. It received the Royal Assent on 1 November 1990.

The Human Fertilization and Embryology Act 1990 is one of the most comprehensive (and may well be one of the most permissive) statutes concerning reproductive technology anywhere in the world. It does not, however, cover anything like all the issues raised by artificial human reproduction. As will be seen, some changes in the law would have occurred in any event, and some legal problems are still not covered by any statute. The motivations behind all the different provisions in the Act are not precisely the same, and they will therefore be dealt with separately. It is impossible to deal with all the issues here, and the following pages represent a personal choice of the most important aspects of the legal provisions concerning human reproduction that exist in Scots and English law today.[16]

THE STATUS OF THE CHILD

In a very important sense, it is right to consider the position of the child first. The end result of infertility treatment — if successful — is the birth of a living child. Yet it is terribly easy to overlook this fact since the initial problem lies with the parents, and the science and technology is all directed towards them. Couples who long for a child do not usually worry about the status of any child they acquire and, given the chance of becoming parents, they may well be tempted to do whatever is required without regard to such 'secondary' matters as the child's status in law. But the law itself has to be concerned with the child's status, whether or not its parents give any consideration to the issue.

The status of children has recently undergone radical changes, which were taking place independently of the development of reproductive technology. Until recently, the status of children was determined not exclusively by the relationship between the child and its parents, but rather by the relationship between the parents themselves, and in particular by the question of whether the parents were married to each other. There were many differences in law between the legitimate child and the illegitimate child (that is, the child born within wedlock and the child born outside wedlock),[17] relating to such things as parental rights and duties, liabilities for maintenance, and succession. In all these areas the illegitimate child was severely disadvantaged in comparison with the legitimate child. The imposition of these disadvantages was part of the law's attempts to discourage extramarital intercourse and, in particular, extramarital procreation.

Throughout the twentieth century, however, British society's disapproval of non-marital relationships has been progressively weakening, and the law has been steadily acquiring a new policy of enhancing freedom of choice in personal relationships.[18] The legal consequences of illegitimacy disadvantaged the child and not the parents who had committed the disapproved act; moreover, these consequences were increasingly becoming anomalous and becoming seen as draconian and unjustifiable. Various pieces of law reform legislation therefore attempted to reflect this by removing many of the more serious differences. Today the express status of 'illegitimacy' is all but abolished, although a child's legal relationship with its parents will still be affected by the question of whether these parents are married to each other.

The development of reproductive technology to alleviate or bypass infertility was not the major impetus towards these changes in the law, which had been mooted for many years in any case,[19] but that development did threaten to heighten and highlight the anomalies which the status of illegitimacy could create. Many forms of infertility treatment, such as AID, and egg or embryo donation, result in a child that is genetically related to only one of the parties to the treatment: since the law recognized legal relationships of parent and child only when there was a genetic relationship, the result was that the child was the child in law of one 'parent' but not the other. While illegitimacy was important, this had significant effects on the child's status. Attempts to obviate these effects by hiding the true state of affairs were frequently criminal offences (for example, registering as father the husband of a woman who is artificially inseminated from a donor).[20] Worse (in the sense of being even more ludicrous) was the fact that the donor of the gametes, being the genetic parent, remained the parent in law and could therefore be subject to parental duties, such as the obligation of maintenance.[21]

To a certain extent, the abolition of the status of illegitimacy abolished most of the legal disadvantages that a child suffered. But, in relation to children born by means of reproductive technology, abolishing that status did not solve all the problems, since a child's relationship to its parents was still determined genetically (certainly the case in relation to the father, with whom most of the difficulties arose). Now, even while recommending the change of law that led to the abolition of the status of illegitimacy, it was recognized by the Law Commission that maintaining the emphasis on the genetic link could lead to anomalies, in particular with regard to the AID child. Although such a child would no longer be stigmatized as illegitimate he or she in fact remained in exactly the same legal position as before: the child's father was the donor, and not the husband of the mother. The father–child relationship was now to be as if it were legitimate, but it was still determined genetically, and the rights and obligations on either side arose when the genetic link was proved. The husband of the wife remained a stranger to the child, in the sense of having no rights over the child, even though he accepted the child into his family, paid for its upkeep, and acted in all important senses as the child's father.[22]

The Scottish statute that abolished the status of illegitimacy[23] made no special provision for this sort of situation;[24] but the equivalent English statute, passed a year later, did make express provision for the child born as a result of AID. Section 27 of the Family Law Reform Act 1987 provided that the husband of the AID child should be regarded in law as the father of the child, provided that he consented to being so regarded. Any parental rights and obligations of the donor were, in that case, extinguished. The result of this was that, if AID were provided to a married woman with the consent of the husband, then for all purposes of law the husband would become the father. Although this certainly reflected the aims of the procedure, it was limited in a number of important ways. First, it concerned only AID, and it is of course possible for a woman to become pregnant with a child who is not genetically related to her husband by other means — such as, for example, embryo transfer (or indeed sexual intercourse with a stranger). Yet even if the husband consented to this, he did not become legal father. Secondly, the Act created a father–child relationship only within the context of marriage. This was an important limitation. It followed that, when AID was provided to an unmarried woman because her cohabitee was sterile, the fact that the cohabitee consented was irrelevant and did not create any relationship between him and the child. The child's father remained to be determined by the genetic link (that is, the father was the donor of the sperm).

The Warnock Committee, which reported a few years before the passing of the 1987 Act, had recommended[25] that the AID child be regarded as the child of the husband if the husband consented. When the Human Fertilization and Embryology Act 1990 was passed, this recommendation, already enacted for England, was re-enacted for that jurisdiction, and enacted for the first time for Scotland.[26] Importantly, it also extended the rule to other forms of infertility treatment and, equally significantly, it extended the provision to cover unmarried couples. Section 28(3) of the 1990 Act provides that where an embryo or sperm and eggs are placed in a woman, or she is artificially inseminated, and this is done 'in the course of treatment services provided for her and a man together' and the man has no genetic link with the child,[27] then that man, and no other man, shall be deemed to be the father of the child for all purposes of the law. This extension to unmarried couples did not appear in the Bill as it was originally presented, but the feeling was clear that, when cohabiting couples are accepted onto infertility programmes, their needs and expectations are the same as those of married couples. This removes one of the great anomalies created by the 1987 Act described above, and is symbolically highly significant. Not only does it remove a difference between a child born to a married couple and one born to an unmarried couple, but it indicates the law's willingness to accept the provision of infertility treatment to the unmarried. This is a matter which will be returned to below.

A child's position in law is determined by its relationship both to its father and to its mother. The problems in establishing parentage have traditionally been with the father, and this has been reflected in the discussion above. But the newer developments in infertility treatment also raise problems in relation to the mother, since it is now possible that the woman to whom the child is born is different from the woman whose egg was used to provide the genetic material.[28] It could be said that the law traditionally regarded the carrying mother as the mother of the child,[29] but really one cannot draw conclusions either way, because, since the law had no need to distinguish the genetic mother from the carrying mother, in reality it never did. The removal of the status of illegitimacy was not the impetus to law reform here – rather it was the realization that, for the first time, two women could both have justifiable claims to be the mother of the same child.

There had been much academic discussion of the question,[30] and indeed, in other jurisdictions, judicial discussion. Thus, in the American case of *Calvert* v. *Johnstone*[31] a woman who had carried an embryo which had no genetic link to her and refused to give up the child on birth, was ordered by the court to do so on the ground that the absence of a genetic link meant that she had no parental rights or responsibilities in relation to the child. However, in the UK, when the Warnock Committee considered the matter,[32] the majority did not like the analogy with establishing paternity, which is usually determined by establishing a genetic link, and preferred to draw an analogy with sperm donation, which they had previously suggested should be dealt with by severing completely all legal links between the donor and the child.[33] These proposals were accepted, and given effect to in the Human Fertilization and Embryology Act 1990, s. 27 of which provides as follows:

> The woman who is carrying or has carried a child as a result of the placing in her of an embryo or of sperm and eggs, and no other woman, is to be treated as the mother of the child.

The result is that the carrying mother, and only the carrying mother, is to be treated in law for all purposes as the child's mother.

There is no doubt that this provision reflects a deep-seated belief that the woman who experiences the pains and pleasures of pregnancy and childbirth, and who contributes her body for nine months to the life-creating process, has the overwhelming claim to be regarded by the law as the mother. The provision also simplifies matters, of course, which is a perfectly sufficient justification for law reform. The counter argument – that it denies the significance of the genetic link – ignores the fact that the female contribution to life-creation is twofold – genetic and gestative; it ignores the fact that the genetic link has lost some of its significance even in relation to paternity;[34] and it ignores the fact that the whole policy of the 1990 Act is to reflect the reality that, with artificial techniques of reproduction, the social element of parenting is far more important to the individual than is the solely genetic element.

SURROGACY

In the sixteenth chapter of the Book of Genesis in the Old Testament, the story is told of Abraham and his wife Sarah, who had no children because Sarah was past child-bearing age. Sarah told Abraham to lie with her Egyptian slave-girl, Hagar, so that they could found a family through her. Hagar conceived, although Abraham and Sarah rejected the child that was subsequently born because Sarah, with truly biblical disregard for the laws of nature and the facts of life, suddenly became pregnant herself, with a child to be called Isaac.[35]

This story is of course very ancient, but it is in essence a form of what today would be termed a surrogacy arrangement. There are various different forms of surrogacy arrangements, including those involving egg donation and embryo transfer, but the basic idea in all is the same: a woman wishes to be a mother to a child, but cannot for some reason carry and give birth (or does not wish to), and therefore it is arranged that another woman will perform that function, the original woman herself taking over the care of the child on its birth. These are dangerous arrangements because of the risk of something going wrong, as seen in the story recited above; but the story also illustrates that the problems are by no means new.

At common law, a surrogacy arrangement that involved the woman who gives birth to a child surrendering that child to another would not be criminal, but nor would it be enforceable. It had been held in England that an agreement to surrender a child would not be enforced against a mother who changed her mind,[36] and almost certainly, if the agreement were carried out, the law would not pay any regard to it (with the result that the 'real' mother remained mother for the purposes of the law).[37] In Scotland, where the concept of fostering of children has a much longer history than in England, the agreement was probably not legally binding in the sense that the offices of the law could not force the mother to hand over the child as she had previously agreed to do, because that would interfere with her personal liberty, but it may well have been legally recognized in the sense that parental rights and duties could be transferred from the mother (if willing to effect the transfer) to the woman who was to look after the child.[38]

The legal difficulties in the practice of surrogacy are legion. They concern legality, enforceability, status, succession, custody rights, restitution of money paid, to name only the most obvious and immediate. These problems are made doubly difficult when surrogacy is combined with the process of egg or embryo transfer.[39] These and other difficulties had been recognized by legal writers long before the Warnock Committee was set up, and the problems and potential solutions had been well aired. The Warnock Committee examined the issue itself, although it did not reach a unanimous conclusion. The majority wanted to criminalize the setting up, or operating of, surrogacy agencies whether profitmaking or not,[40] while a minority saw some place for state-controlled surrogacy.[41] However, for extraneous reasons shortly to be described, the issue of commercial surrogacy was dealt with by legislation before the different views could be fully canvassed and analysed.

There really is no evidence to suggest that surrogacy was a particularly common method of alleviating the suffering caused by childlessness. Doubtless it did occur, but this would have normally been in unusual and very private situations, without strangers being involved – as, for example, in a woman agreeing to carry a child for her infertile sister.[42] If a stranger were involved, it would usually have been a doctor who arranged for the woman to become pregnant by means of artificial insemination. The idea of the pregnant woman being paid for her services, beyond expenses, was probably seldom considered, because of the very privacy of the agreement.

However as the problem of childlessness became less hidden, and society came to accept that it might be right to try to solve that problem, it also became apparent that the suffering caused might encourage people to pay large sums of money for any solution.[43] This had been seen previously in relation to adoption when it was realized early on that people who could not adopt a child through normal means would be willing to pay large sums to bypass the system. Monetary payments for adoption have long been illegal[44] due to the risk that undesirable parties might be able to adopt just because they could afford to pay large sums of money. When surrogacy came to the fore, the analogy with adoption and 'child-selling' had too great a grip on the public imagination for it to be ignored.

There are, in the United States, well known commercial organizations which make their profits by bringing together couples who cannot have children and women willing to act as surrogates.[45] There were also isolated examples in the United Kingdom of surrogacy arrangements being entered into which involved the exchange of money. This was the case in *A v. C*[46] where a couple paid a prostitute to become pregnant with the husband's sperm. The issue went to court after the birth, when the carrying mother changed her mind and refused to part with the child (the father claimed access but was denied this). The rather unfortunate circumstances of this case seemed to give credence to the view that surrogacy is more a method of prostitution than a compassionate attempt to alleviate suffering. As with prostitution, the potential exploitation need not all be one way.

The public fears, combined with the legal difficulties, should have rendered public consultation all the more important. However, events overtook the normal course of progress, and it was deemed impossible to provide the time needed for public consultation and proper consideration of the various options available for dealing with surrogacy.

On 4 January 1985 Mrs Kim Cotton gave birth to a child in a London hospital. This child had been conceived by her with the sperm of an American man who, with his wife's agreement, had arranged for Mrs Cotton to give up the child on its birth. Fulfilling her side of the bargain, Mrs Cotton left the child at the hospital, and the father was allowed to take the child with him back to the United States. The court, which had been asked to ward the child,[47] sanctioned his action. There was a public outcry at the fact not that Mrs Cotton had abandoned the child she had just given birth to, but that she had been paid a substantial sum of money for so doing. At about the same time, it became known that a number of organizations in the United States had commenced 'recruiting drives' for potential surrogates in the UK.[48] Society baulked at the thought of surrogacy becoming a means of making money, and as a result of the moral panic, fanned by a press that knows a good-selling story when it sees one, the British government rushed through Parliament, without allowing any amendments, the Surrogacy Arrangements Act 1985 which came into force on 16 July 1985.[49] In Freeman's words:

> It is unashamedly a stop-gap measure and there is no doubt that the Government was panicked into legislative action by a vociferous media and populist demand. The 'grasping' agency and the 'rent-a-womb' mothers became folk-devils overnight and this Act was the result of the moral panic reaction to them. The Act was rushed through with all demands for clarification resisted on the grounds that no delay could be brooked.[50]

The statute renders criminal any act designed to establish a surrogacy arrangement if that arrangement is made on a commercial basis, by which is meant if money or money's worth is passed as a consequence.[51] A person or an organization can be guilty of this new offence. Advertising in connection with surrogacy, commercial or otherwise, is also made a criminal offence.

However, the Act has only limited application, being expressly designed to catch the agencies who make a profit by bringing together infertile couples with women willing to act as surrogate mothers. Merely to enter into a surrogacy arrangement is not a criminal act. The infertile couple and the surrogate mother do not commit any offence if they enter into a private arrangement, even when money passes. It is only organizations who attempt to bring them together, or who advertise, that can be penalized by the terms of the Act.

The speed and urgency with which the 1985 Act was passed can clearly be seen. The issue of enforceability of the contract was expressly avoided, with s.1(9) weakly providing that the offence was committed 'whether or not' the arrangement itself was enforceable. The government felt obliged to act quickly to outlaw commercial organizations, even if this meant postponing consideration of all the other connected legal points. The 1985 Act was later amended by the Human Fertilization and Embryology Act which, by s. 36(1), made clear that surrogacy arrangements are unenforceable in law.

This history illustrates the way that law reform all too often takes place in the United Kingdom.[52] The issue was admittedly awkward – the Warnock Committee could not agree on it – and, for this reason, all the more care should have been taken in the law reforms that followed. But because of the obvious panic, public outrage and the villifying press campaign the government felt obliged to act quickly, not so much to solve the legal problems as to salve the public conscience. The difficulty with this sort of knee-jerk law reform is that, all too often, the solving of the problem as perceived by the media fails to solve all the potential legal problems; but worse still, the impression is given that all the problems are indeed solved. This is not the case. The statute today makes criminal commercial organizations making money by bringing together surrogates and those who want their help, and it makes any surrogacy arrangement unenforceable. But a whole series of other problems arising from surrogacy are simply ignored, such as the right of the father to access[53]; the position of the child if both parties reject it on birth (for example, if it is handicapped); the control of the surrogate during the pregnancy; restitution of any money paid as a result of the unenforceable contract; and the legality and ethics of surrogacy 'for convenience'.[54] All these issues are left to be dealt with by traditional concepts of law (so that, for example, during the pregnancy the surrogate is the only one who can decide to have an abortion).[55] At the end of the day, apart from the commercial ban and the clarification that in both Scots and English law the agreement is unenforceable, the law in relation to surrogacy is much as it was before the Warnock Committee sat.[56]

Section 30 of the Human Fertilization and Embryology Act 1990, though not expressly dealing with surrogacy, is designed to provide a means whereby morally acceptable surrogacy arrangements can be given legal recognition. That section provides that a married couple, at least one of whom is genetically related to a child which is carried by a woman other than the wife, can apply to the court for an order that they both be treated in law as the parents. This is effectively a shorthand adoption. The consent of all the parties is needed. This provision does not make the arrangement enforceable, but it is recognition by the law that these arrangements do exist and that the law should reflect the social reality of who will actually be looking after the child.

EMBRYO RESEARCH

It is possible to question whether there would have been a Warnock Committee and a Human Fertilization and Embryology Act at all had it not been for the development of the ability to perform research on human embryos, arising from the availability of live *in vitro* embryos obtained in the course of infertility treatment. AID has been practised throughout the twentieth century; surrogacy has been practised since biblical times.[57] Yet the law was content simply to apply its traditional concepts of parenthood, status, child law and medical law to these procedures. In one sense the development of *in vitro* fertilization was simply an extension of AID. A donated ovum has a moral status directly comparable with that of donated sperm, the moral difference lying not in the nature of the donation nor even in the aims for which the donation was given. However, a new moral environment is entered into when the donations are used to create an embryo over which the creator has some physical control and which is created not for its own good but for the good of the woman into whom the embryo is intended to be implanted. Once researchers realized that a woman's chances of conceiving a single child would be greater if more than one embryo were created, developments quickly took place. For instance, the 'spare' embryo was found to have its uses. Examination of, and research upon, the 'spare' embryo were perceived as being invaluable in increasing knowledge about the reproductive process, so giving *in vitro* fertilization itself a better chance of success. Furthermore, increased knowledge about the very early (that is, pre-implantation) embryo promised to provide knowledge that would allow the development of new and better contraceptives.[58] Also, as the genetic structure of the human being became better understood, so it was possible to identify many defective genes that cause much suffering: if the embryo is outside the woman's body, one of its cells can be removed, examined and then the decision can be taken whether or not to implant the embryo according to whether it possesses the deleterious gene. Non-implantation, of course, means that the embryo eventually does not continue in existence, or to put it another way, it 'dies'.

All of this has become possible in recent years, and, because an entity with full genetic human identity is being used, a moral status, different from, for example, independent gametes, is conferred upon that entity. It may be perceived that to allow research on such entities is to allow research on human beings, and to allow their destruction for the good of others. If five embryos are created so that a woman can give birth to one child, the other four are being used as means to her ends.[59] If an embryo is found to possess a deleterious gene and is not implanted, it is not being cured, it is being destroyed. It was these sorts of fears, whether well founded or not, that led directly to the setting up of the Warnock Committee.

It is the issue of embryo research from which all else follows. The Warnock Committee clearly regarded this issue as central. Lady Warnock, in *A Question of Life*,[60] said this: 'All the other issues we had to consider seemed relatively trivial compared with this one,'[61] Parliament agreed. The proposals on embryo research were described as 'the crucial issue',[62] the 'moral heart of the Bill'[63] and 'the pivotal question'.[64] Ultimately, the issue condensed into the question of whether a human person, entitled to all the protections of the law, was created at the moment of fertilization, or at some later stage. The Roman Catholic Church and various 'Pro-Life' organizations took the view that the morally significant point was fertilization. Many scientists took the view that an entity of two, four or eight cells could not rationally be regarded as a full human being and should not therefore be given all the law's protections.

Yet in a sense – a sense that was not only ignored but denied – that issue was decided long ago. An unborn child can lawfully be aborted[65] and therefore clearly does not have the legal protection, nor even the moral respect, that a born human person has. To argue that entities should be fully protected, even before implantation, is therefore at best inconsistent and at worst nonsense.[66]

But there seemed to have been a strong gut reaction against this conclusion, however much logic drives us to it. The embryo in the test tube is felt to be different from the embryo in its mother (from whom it has little real protection). That difference seems to lie in the appearance in the picture of a third party – that is, the doctor or scientist, who has control over the embryo. There is something very different between a mother's decision to empty her own womb (which remains part of her own body) and a scientist's actions in destroying something which in no sense is 'his'. Research and destruction of an embryo by a third party to its creation (however essential, practically speaking, that third party was) therefore demanded serious and effective control, if it were to be permitted at all.

All these arguments, and others, were put forward in the public and Parliamentary debates. The Warnock Committee could not agree, a majority being in favour of controlled research,[67] a minority accepting this only if the embryos were truly 'spare' and had not been created for the purposes of research,[68] and a different minority wishing research on embryos to be banned completely.[69] The government was so determined to demonstrate its neutrality on the issue (or possibly so determined not to lose a significant number of votes) that, when the Human Fertilization and Embryology Bill was presented, it was drafted in a unique fashion – there were two clauses, one permitting research (subject to controls) and one forbidding it (almost) completely. The acceptance of one clause was to act as the automatic rejection of the other. In the end, with the government's neutrality unimpaired, the vote was in favour of controlled research. That control is to be provided by the statutory licensing authority, which is to be known as the Human Fertilization and Embryology Authority (for brevity referred to hereinafter as the Licensing Authority).

Much of the 1990 Act is taken up with the establishing and running of the Licensing Authority. Its function is to oversee embryo research and infertility treatment in the United Kingdom, to grant licences to those working in the field, to withhold or revoke licences from those who act in such a way as infringes the standards the Authority wishes to uphold, and to publish[70] reports on its activities. Licences can be granted subject to conditions imposed by the Licensing Authority; and criminal offences are committed by anyone carrying out any of the controlled activities without a licence, or against any of the conditions thereby imposed. Importantly, the '14-day rule' suggested by the Warnock Committee has been accepted,[71] and the Licensing Authority is barred from allowing any research or destruction of an embryo created *in vitro* to take place after 14 days from the completion of the process of fertilization (which is defined as the appearance of a two-cell zygote).[72] In effect, if an embryo exists at that stage it must either be implanted into a woman for gestation or immediately be destroyed. Research before 14 days will be permitted only if it is 'necessary' to use a human embryo for the proposed research.[73]

It is clear that the '14-day rule' was one of the most difficult conclusions to reach, and one of the most difficult to convey to opponents. An immense amount of soul-searching went on, in the Warnock Committee itself and in the Parliamentary debates both on the White Paper and on the Bill that became the 1990 Act.[74] Finally, the preponderant scientific view was accepted that, on the appearance of the primitive streak (which normally occurs at around 14 days), it is no longer possible to say that human individuality has certainly not developed. In the debates, the fear of using human beings as research tools was real, and indeed dominant. But the benefits, both to the infertile individual, and to scientific knowledge in general, of allowing such research were so great – and promise to be even more impressive – that MPs accepted that a balance had to be struck. This balance was struck in favour of research because, fundamentally, a majority, both in society and in Parliament, simply did not believe that the very early embryo had a level of humanity that demanded protection.

ISSUES STILL UNRESOLVED

Although it is one of the most comprehensive statutes dealing with human reproduction in the world, the Human Fertilization and Embryology Act 1990 by no means gives the answer to all of the legal problems which arise out of human reproduction. For one thing, there are other statutes (already discussed) covering issues considered by the Warnock Committee.[75] But, more importantly, there are other issues that have not been considered, but which do affect an individual's freedom to become a parent. The 1990 Act deals almost exclusively with the new reproductive techniques designed to alleviate the suffering of the infertile. However, an individual's freedom to reproduce is also affected by the availability of methods of preventing reproduction. There is still doubt about the legality of some forms of post-coital contraception.[76] There is still doubt about the ethics and legality of using foetal material obtained by abortion for the treatment of various diseases.

Even within the limited parameters of infertility treatment certain important issues are not covered by the current legislation. Foremost amongst these is the issue of allocation of resources.[77] In a society that cannot afford to pay for all medical treatment or procedures that are needed or wanted, it is inevitable that choices have to be made concerning upon which areas the available money is to be spent, and also concerning to whom the money is to be individually allocated. A health authority or health board must decide whether to allocate part of its budget to infertility treatment or, say, provision of better facilities for the long-term senile. And a consultant who runs an infertility programme must decide whether to allocate her or his limited time and resources to attempts to provide Mrs X with a child rather than Miss Y. Decisions of this nature are almost impossible to challenge.[78] The 1990 Act provides no guidance, except to delegate a certain power to the Licensing Authority. Indeed, as was made clear in the White Paper,[79] 'the Government does not intend to specify in legislation the detailed criteria which should be applied in granting licences'. Once more we see government protecting its own position of studied neutrality, and expressly leaving criteria to be adopted to the decision of the Licensing Authority. That Authority has the right to grant licences subject to conditions.[80] Now it is possible that one such condition may relate, for example, to the patient's marital status; but there is no indication that this is the type of condition that is intended. And, indeed, since the other parts of the Act presuppose treatment being given to unmarried couples (see above) it is submitted that it would be improper for the Authority to impose any such conditions. It follows that it is left up to the individual doctor to decide whether to limit access to the married, or to exclude, say, lesbians from AID treatment, or to exclude from IVF treatment those who have previously had an abortion.

The result of course is that different centres will adopt different policies (just as they do in their interpretation of the terms of the Abortion Act). There is nothing new about this. Individual surgeons have long had their own views on who should receive, for example, sterilization operations or vasectomies. There is no law to say that a man of 22 who has had no children may not be sterilized, but it would be difficult to find a surgeon in the UK who would be willing to perform the operation on such a patient (at least within the NHS). These policy decisions, like those involving access to IVF, are effectively unchallengeable.[81] Section 13(5) of the Act provides that no treatment services may be provided 'unless account has been taken of the welfare of any child who may be born as a result of that treatment', but it is difficult to visualize the legal consequences of a failure on the part of the doctor to do so.

The issue of resource allocation was hardly mentioned in the Warnock Report, and although it received more attention in the parliamentary debates on the 1990 Act, that Act itself gives little guidance on the issue. Yet, in a very real sense, this issue is as important as any other. A person who wishes to receive infertility treatment may do so only when she or he has found a doctor willing and able to provide the treatment, and there is no effective means by which an unwilling doctor can be forced to provide the treatment to a certain individual. Had Parliament been willing to confront this issue it would of course have raised all sorts of new arguments against infertility treatment (such as, for example, that deliberately creating one-parent families disrupts the structure of society); and one is left with the strong suspicion that the avoidance of the issue was little more than a public relations exercise. Throughout the public and Parliamentary debates, and indeed in the Warnock Report,[82] infertility treatment was projected as a means of alleviating the suffering of a traditional heterosexual couple. The lesbian[83] and any other single woman who wishes to become a mother without the sexual endeavours of a man were ignored,[84] and never legislated for, apparently for fear that this might prejudice people against infertility treatment. Consequently, as stated above, it is left to the individual doctor, and practice will inevitably vary across the country.[85] One way of avoiding great diversity would be for the Licensing Authority to make it a condition of its licence that no such undesirable policy limitation is adopted by the licence-holder. But whether it is willing to adopt this directive stance – which many doctors would see as infringing their own discretion – is something that only time will tell.

A further type of issue that remains unresolved concerns a number of legalistic points, such as the status of embryos that are allowed to survive after 14 days, in contravention of the licence. The statute provides that this is a criminal offence, but it says nothing about the embryo itself. Likewise, succession and property rights are not dealt with exhaustively. It is provided that an embryo cannot later claim a succession from its father who died before its implantation,[86] but that is all. Issues such as the perpetuity periods in trusts are not mentioned, nor is the issue of ownership dealt with. It is impossible to own a living human person (and therefore impossible to sell one) and there is no doubt that an embryo in the womb would come within the category of existing things that cannot be sold. But what about the embryo outside the womb — especially the 'spare' embryo? Who owns (in the legal, proprietorial sense) gametes? Can they be sold, or left by will, or subject to a trust or a security? It is unclear how ownership falls to be determined, or even if it is possible. This reflects a similar confusion in the Warnock Report itself. Paragraph 10.11 recommends that legislation should enact that there be no right of ownership in the human embryo, whilst para. 13.13 recommends that sale or purchase of gametes or embryos should be permitted only under licence. But it is legally incompetent to buy and sell that which cannot be owned, because sale is the transfer of ownership. Again, these issues remain unresolved.

In fact, the 1990 Act has as its major aim the control of medical science. It was the fear of the maverick scientist and the confusion concerning the moral status of embryos available for research that led to the setting up of the Warnock Committee. And it was to assuage that fear, rather than to solve the potential legal difficulties, that the Act was passed. The Act deals directly with only a few of the pressing legalistic problems. It is an Act of medical control rather than legal solution, and many of the major legal issues remain in serious doubt.

NOTES

1 There is, in Great Britain, no constitutionally recognized right of privacy such as there is in the US (see *Griswold* v. *Connecticut* 381 US 479, 14 L. Ed. 2d 510 (1965)) but there is no doubt that privacy is recognized in the negative sense described in the text.

2 It might be argued that the true social engineering involved here was not directed towards the personal relationship but rather towards the proprietory relationship, the aim being to protect 'legitimate' inheritances. That, however, is another issue.

3 Marriage Act 1949 (England) and Marriage (Sc) Act 1977, both amended by the Marriage (Prohibited Degrees of Relationship) Act 1986.

4 Sexual Offences Act 1956, ss.10 and 11 (England); Sexual Offences (Sc) Act 1976, s.2A.

5   See Abortion Act 1967, s.1, as amended most notably by the Human Fertilization and Embryology Act 1990.

6   'The policy of the state, as I see it, is to provide the widest freedom of choice. It makes available to the public the means of planning their families or planning to have no family. If plans go awry, it provides for the possibility of abortion. But there is no pressure on couples either to have children or not to have children or to have only a limited number of children', per Pain J. in *Thake* v. *Maurice* [1985] 2 WLR 215, p. 230.

7   Cf. the US Supreme Court case of *Griswold* v. *Connecticut* 381 US 479, 14 L. Ed. 2d 510 (1965).

8   Again from the US, see *Eisenstadt* v. *Baird* 405 US 438, 31 L. Ed. 2d 349 (1972).

9   Though admittedly for technical reasons: see *Bradlaugh & Besant* v. *the Queen* LR 3 QBD 607 (1877).

10 The nearest an English court approached it was in Denning LJ's intemperate remarks relating to sterilization in *Bravery* v. *Bravery* [1954] 3 All ER 59, which were expressly disavowed by his two judicial brethren.

11 For a comprehensive discussion of the legal problems arising from most, if not all, of the different methods, see Cusine, D. J. (1988), *New Reproductive Techniques: a legal perspective*, Aldershot: Dartmouth.

12 See, for example, Cusine, D. J. (1977), 'Artificial Insemination with the husband's semen after death', *Journal of Medicial Ethics*, **3**, p. 163 and (1978), 'Womb leasing: some legal implications', *New Law Journal*, **128**, p. 824.

13 Cmnd 9314 (1984).

14 *Legislation on Human Infertility Services and Embryo Research: A Consultation Paper*, Cm. 46 (1986).

15 *Human Fertilisation and Embryology: A Framework for Legislation*, Cm. 259 (1987).

16 It should be pointed out that the abortion rules are not directly discussed here, not because they are not one of the most important issues in reproductive choice, but because to examine them properly would take a whole chapter or indeed a whole book. See Keown, J. (1988), *Abortion, Doctors and the Law*, Cambridge: Cambridge University Press.

17 This is not of course wholly accurate as a definition since children born outside wedlock might sometimes be regarded as legitimate.

18 See the dicta quoted in note 6 above.

19 See Law Com. no. 74, 'Illegitimacy' (1979) and Scot. Law Com. no. 62 'Illegitimacy' (1983).

20 It is interesting to note that in the Second Reading in the House of Lords of the Bill that became the Human Fertilization and Embryology Act 1990, Baroness Hooper, concluding for the government, gave a figure of one in 20 of the population having a genetic father different from that named in their birth certificate (*HL Deb.*, vol. 513, col. 1112).

21 Of course, due to the secrecy of donations practised by those who collected the sperm it was well nigh impossible to establish who the donor was. In recent years, however, this might not have been so difficult, because the development of DNA profiling makes it possible positively to identify a man as the genetic father of a child.

22 In such a situation in Scotland the husband could be legally liable for some of the obligations of parenthood, such as aliment (Family Law (Sc) Act 1985, s.1(1)(d)) but would have none of the legal rights (such as title to claim custody or succession).

23 This terminology is, in fact, not wholly accurate since there remains residual consequences of legitimacy, but these are unlikely to be important here.

24 Law Reform (Parent and Child (Sc) Act 1986, s.1(1).
25 Para. 4.17.
26 1990 Act, s.28.
27 Section 28(3)(b).
28 See the discussion of all the different possibilities by Cusine, 'Womb Leasing', op. cit., note 12 above.
29 So, for example, the wording of the Births and Deaths Registration Act 1953 (England) and the Registration of Births Deaths and Marriages (Sc) Act 1965 imply that the woman who gives birth has to register the child as hers.
30 See, for example, Cusine, *New Reproductive Techniques*, op. cit., note 11 above; pp. 59–73; Rosettenstein, D. R. (1981), 'Defining a parent: the new biology and rebirth of the *filius nullius*', *New Law Journal*, **131**, p. 1095; McKenzie, D. (1986), 'Who are a child's parents?', *SLT (News)*, p. 303.
31 22 October 1990.
32 Paras 6.6–6.8.
33 Ibid., at para. 4.22. The Law Commission had also previously suggested that this was the more apt analogy: see Law Com. 74, para. 109 (1979).
34 See the provisions discussed above whereby a man can become father (in law) simply by consenting to infertility treatment of a woman.
35 This is not the only biblical example of such an arrangement, suggesting that amongst early civilizations the use of slaves as surrogates was not uncommon.
36 See *Humphries* v. *Polak* [1901] 2 KB 385; *A* v. *C* (1978) 8 *Fam. Law 170*, (1984), *Fam. Law*, **14**, p. 241.
37 See *Humphreys* v. *Polak* [1901] 2 KB 385, in which it was held that a mother could not give up her right of custody, because that right was conferred only to allow her to fulfil her parental duties.
38 See *Kerrigan* v. *Hall* (1901) 4F 10.
39 On the myriad legal difficulties that can arise out of a surrogacy contract in a legal system that recognizes its validity, see Rothenberg, K. L. (1988), 'Baby M, the surrogacy contract and the health care professional: some unanswered questions', *16 Law, Medicine and Health Care*, p. 113.
40 Para. 8.18.
41 Expression of Dissent 'A'.
42 See the news report of such a case in *The Times*, 29 April 1983.
43 See *A* v. *C*, note 36 above cited, in which the infertile couple were willing to pay their life savings, their car and their house to obtain the child they had contracted for.
44 See now s.57(1) of the Adoption Act 1976 (England) and s.51(1) of the Adoption (Sc) Act 1978.
45 See Parker, D. (1984), 'Surrogate mothering: an overview', *Family Law*, **14**, p. 140; Singer, P. and Wells, D. (1984), *The Reproductive Revolution*, Oxford: Oxford University Press, ch. 4.
46 (1978) *Family Law*, **8**, p. 170 (1984), *Family Law*, **14**, p. 241.
47 *Re C. (A Minor) (Ward: Surrogacy)* (1985) Family Law, **15**, p. 191.
48 See, for example, the news reports in the *Guardian*, 18 October 1982 and 27 April 1983.
49 The Secretary of State for Social Services admitted while moving the Second Reading that it was the Cotton case that persuaded the government that legislation was urgently required: see HC Deb., vol. 76, col. 23.
50 Current Law Annotations: Surrogacy Arrangements Act 1985, c. 49.
51 Sections 1(8) and 2(3).
52 It is by no means difficult to find other examples of ill-thought-out panic measures. See, for example, the Human Tissue Transplants Act 1989, passed

as a result of public outrage at the 'sale' of kidneys from nationals of Third World countries to private patients in Britain; the Local Government Act 1988, s.28 of which prohibits local authorities from 'promoting homosexuality' (whatever – if anything – that means) passed as a result of Conservative backbench outrage that books giving positive images of homosexuality were found in school staffrooms. Further back, the same phenomenon can be seen with the Prevention of Terrorism (Temporary Provisions) Act 1976 and the Official Secrets Act 1911.

53 Cf. *A* v. *C*, note 36 above, cited in which access was denied.
54 This last-mentioned was regarded as 'totally unacceptable' by the Warnock Committee: para. 8.17.
55 This would seem to follow from *Paton* v. *British Pregnancy Advisory Service* [1978] 2 All ER 987, *C* v. *S* [1987] 2 WLR 1108, and from s.27 of the Human Fertilization and Embryology Act 1990.
56 For a lucid criticism of the 1985 Act, see Sloman, S. (1985), 'The Surrogacy Arrangements Act 1985', *Law Journal*, **135**, p. 978.
57 For an interesting history of various forms of infertility treatment, see Cusine, *New Reproductive Techniques*, op. cit., note 11 above, ch. 3.
58 Or at least contragestives, that is, methods of preventing fertilized eggs from implanting: see Norrie, K. (1991), *Family Planning Practice and the Law*, Aldershot: Dartmouth, ch. 4.
59 This point, amongst others, is discussed by Davies, J. (1984), 'Fabricated man: the dilemma posed by artificial reproductive techniques', *NILQ*, **35**, p. 354.
60 Warnock, Mary (1985), *A Question of Life*, Oxford: Blackwell, p. xvi.
61 Although it is interesting to note that surrogacy has given rise to vastly more literature in the academic press.
62 Lord Ennals at *HL Deb.*, vol. 153, col. 1012.
63 Archbishop of York, ibid., at col. 1019.
64 Lord Ashmore, ibid., at col. 1048.
65 Abortion Act 1967, as amended by the 1990 Act.
66 As Lady Warnock herself pointed out in the House of Lords, the pre-Act position was that an embryo *in vitro* had no rights in law whatsoever nor any protection: *HL Deb.*, vol. 513, col. 1035.
67 Para. 11.18.
68 Expression of Dissent 'C'.
69 Expression of Dissent 'B'.
70 Annually: see s.7.
71 1990 Act, s.3(3) and (4).
72 Section 1. Certain other activities cannot be licensed, such as placing non-human embryos and gametes in a woman (s.3(2)), placing a human embryo in an animal (s.3(3)(b)) and cloning by nucleus substitution (s.3(3)(d)).
73 Sched. 2, para. 3(6).
74 Indeed there were various attempts in Parliament prior to 1990 to ban embryo research: see the Unborn Children (Protection) Bills, presented on 18 January 1985, again on 21 October 1985, and again on 28 October 1987. Only the first-mentioned (sponsored by Mr Enoch Powell, MP) reached the Second Reading.
75 See, for example, the Surrogacy Arrangements Act 1985 and the Family Law Reform Act 1987.
76 See Norrie, *Family Planning Practice and the Law*, op. cit., at pp. 48–59.
77 See Wiewiorka, P. (1991), 'The Human Fertilisation and Embryology Act 1990', *SLT (News)*, p. 65.
78 See *R* v. *Central Birmingham Health Authority ex p. Collier* (unrep) 6 January

1988; *R* v. *Secretary of State for Social Services, ex. p. Walker* (unrep) 26 November 1987; and *R* v. *Ethical Committee of St Mary's Hospital, ex. p. Harriott* (1988), *Family Law*, p. 165.

79 Para. 22.

80 Section 12.

81 See the *Harriott* case, cited above, note 78, in which a woman challenged the decision of a consultant obstetrician to refuse to accept the plaintiff onto her IVF programme within the NHS. She failed on the ground that this decision was, on the facts of this case, 'clearly reasonable'. To be challengeable by way of judicial review the plaintiff would have to show that the decision had some 'public' element to it, which will be almost impossible.

82 See, for example, para. 2.6.

83 See Kottow, S. (1984), 'The right to lesbian parenthood', *Journal of Medical Ethics*, **10**, p. 54.

84 Although the unmarried *couple* are recognized in the provisions concerning the child's status: see s.28(3), discussed above.

85 There is clear disapproval by some doctors of providing infertility treatment to the unmarried: see, for example, Snowdon, D., Snowdon, E. (1985), 'A personal response to the Warnock Report', *British Journal of Family Planning*, **11**, p. 23. It has been reported that in the United States 90% of doctors would be unwilling to provide AID to an unmarried woman: (1985) *Harvard Law Review*, **98**, 669, p. 670. However, the UK Government presently has no plans to introduce legislation limiting the doctor's discretion: see the statement of the Health Minister, Virginia Bottomley, reported in *The Times*, 12 March 1991 (made in response to public disquiet at the revelation that AID was being provided to single women and 'virgins' (a clear euphemism for 'lesbians') by the British Pregnancy Advisory Service).

86 1990 Act, s.28(6).

8 United States: Surrogacy*

R. ALTA CHARO

Bill Stern:	I don't want to see you hurt. I don't want to see my daughter hurt. I really. . . .
Mary Beth Whitehead:	*My* daughter too, why don't you quit doing that, Bill, Okay?
Bill Stern:	Okay, Okay, all right. . . .
Mary Beth Whitehead:	It's *our* daughter. Why don't you say it? *Our* daughter.
Bill Stern:	All right, *our* daughter. Okay, Mary Beth, *our* daughter.
Mary Beth Whitehead:	That's right.[1]

Rarely does a telephone conversation so effectively capture the essence of a dilemma. Yet these few lines of a conversation between Bill Stern, genetic father, and Mary Beth Whitehead, fugitive 'surrogate' mother of the now-famous 'Baby M', demonstrate the essential problem of surrogate parenting. Surrogacy contracts do not ask women to give over their 'services'; they ask women to give over their babies. Surrogacy asks all the rest of us to choose one of two paths – a contractual view of human relations, in which we are all reasonable people, all rational consumers, or a more holistic view, in which human relations are determined by chance, biology, emotion, circumstance, and yes, to some extent, volition.

The first path has the attraction of simplicity, a certain philosophical neatness. It is the same view that opposes the National Organ Transplantation Act's prohibition on organ sales as an undue interference with the freedom of contract and the right to make a voluntary, informed decision concerning one's own best interests. But it flies in the face of American legal tradition of the twentieth

*This chapter is adapted from Charo (1988),'Legislative approaches to surrogate motherhood', *Law, Medicine and Health Care*, **16(1–2)**, pp. 96–112 and contains material from Charo (1989), 'Book review: NYS Task Force Report on surrogate parenting', (1989), *Journal of Legal Medicine*, 10(1), pp. 251–60, as well as new material.

223

century, in which legal realism,[2] and now critical legal studies,[3] strive to infuse case law with a greater sense of the larger political and economic realities that drive people into the often preposterous situations from which courts are called to drag them out.

By the beginning of 1988, nearly 600 babies had been born through surrogate mothering arrangements. Although there have been a number of lawsuits concerning custody or challenging adoption laws that appear to prohibit payments to surrogates, the majority of surrogacy arrangements proceed without judicial involvement. Nevertheless, surrogate mothering has engendered considerable activity in state legislatures, as well as two bills in Congress to ban the practice (HR 2433 and HR 3264) and hearings by the House Committee on Energy and Commerce and the Subcommittee on Transportation, Tourism, and Hazardous Wastes. More recently, the Congressional Office of Technology Assessment (OTA) released a report, *Infertility: Medical and Social Choices*.[4] That report included the results of a survey of surrogate-mother matching services active in the United States in late 1987 (see Table 8.1).

This chapter describes the status of surrogate mothering in American society, courts, and legislatures, drawing on the data collected in the 1988 OTA survey. By examining editorials, columns, and letters to the editor published in major American newspapers at the time of the famous 'Baby M' trial, it presents one of the underlying themes of the surrogacy debate — the definition and deification of motherhood. The chapter concludes with the suggestion that, while surrogacy arrangements ought not to be criminalized, they should not be enforceable either. Further, it suggests that payment beyond the actual and reasonable exepnses associated with surrogacy ought to be prohibited, along with the professional services of surrogate and matching services. Finally, to protect the reproductive autonomy of all women, it proposes that the federal government should recognize that there is nothing 'surrogate' about surrogate mothering, and should enact legislation to define 'mother' as a woman who carries a child to term, regardless of the source of the egg and sperm or her intentions with regard to custody.

THE STRUCTURE OF SURROGACY ARRANGEMENTS

Who Hires a Surrogate Mother?

The overwhelming majority of those seeking surrogates are white, married couples in their late thirties or early forties, although agencies reported agreeing to hire a surrogate mother for five unmarried couples and nine single men, according to the OTA survey.[5] The

Table 8.1 Demographic Surveys of Surrogate Mothers

	OTA	Linkins	Hanifin	Parker 1	Parker 2	Franks
Sample size	> 334[a]	34	89	30	125	10
Average age	27	28	28	25	25	26
Marital status						
Married	60%	73%	80%	87%	53%	50%
Single	40%[b]	18%	14%	10%	19%	40%
Divorced	—	9%	5%	3%	22%	10%
Unknown	—	—	—	—	6%	—
No. of children	N/A	1.8	2.0	1.9	1.4	1–3
Race/ethnicity						
White non-Hispanic	88%	N/A	85%	100%	100%	N/A
Hispanic	2%	N/A	14%	—	—	N/A
Black non-Hispanic	< 1%	N/A	< 1%	—	—	N/A
Asian	2%	N/A	< 1%	—	—	N/A
Other	8%[c]	N/A	< 1%	—	—	N/A
Religion						
Protestant	67%	N/A	74%	53%	55%	N/A
Catholic	28%	N/A	25%	47%	40%	N/A
Jewish	3%	N/A	< 1%	—	1%	N/A
Other	2%	N/A	< 1%	—	4%	N/A
Household income						
< $15,000	13%	N/A	N/A	N/A	N/A	N/A
$15,000–$30,000	53%	N/A	N/A	N/A	N/A	N/A
$30,000–$50,000	30%	N/A	N/A	N/A	N/A	N/A
> $50,000	4%	N/A	N/A	N/A	N/A	N/A
Average	N/A	$25,000	N/A	N/A	N/A	N/A
Range	N/A	$12K–$68K	N/A	N/A	$6K–$55K	(modest to moderate)
Education						
Some high school	61%[d]	12%	—	20%	18%[e]	—
High school graduate	—	38%	52%	53%	54%[e]	(average for sample)
Some college	35%[d]	47%	24%	27%	26%[e]	—
College graduate	—	3%[f]	24%[f]	—	2%[e]	—
Some graduate school	4%[d]	—	—	—	—	—
Previously relinquished child by:						
Surrogacy	7%	N/A	N/A	N/A	N/A	N/A
Adoption	7%	N/A	1%	10%	9%	N/A
Abortion	18%	N/A	37%	23%	26%	N/A
Are themselves adopted	12%	N/A	1%	1%	1%	N/A

Notes
a. Data supplied by matching agencies, not by surrogates themselves.
b. Includes divorced.
c. May include Hispanics.
d. Includes graduates.
e. Includes only fifty women in sample.
f. Includes category 'some graduate school'.
'N/A' means 'not applicable' or 'not available'.

Sources:
Franks, D. D. (1981), 'Psychiatric evaluation of women in a surrogate mother program', *American Journal of Psychiatry*, **138** pp. 1378–79.
Hanifin, H. (1987), *The Surrogate Mother: An Exploratory Study*, Chicago: University Microfilms International; Hanifin, H. (1987), 'Surrogate parenting: reassessing human bonding', paper presented at the American Psychological Association Convention, New York, August.
Linkins, K., Daniels, H. and Richards, E. (1988), Boston, Mass.: McLean Hospital, 8 January.
Office of Technology Assessment, US Congress, 1988.
Parker, P. J. (1983), 'Motivations of Surrogate Mothers: Initial Findings', *American Journal of Psychiatry*, **140**, pp. 117–18.
Parker, P. J. (1984), 'The psychology of the surrogate mother: a newly updated report of a longitudinal pilot study', paper presented at the American Orthopsychiatric Association General Meeting, Toronto, 9 April.

number of homosexual individuals or couples who seek to hire a surrogate mother is consistently reported as no more than 1 per cent, but three agencies have sought surrogates for a homosexual male couple, and one for a homosexual female couple. Approximately 25 per cent are Catholic, a similar proportion are Jewish, and approximately 42 per cent are Protestant. On average, agencies report that about 25 per cent of the couples are already raising a child. In one 1988 development, a family with several boys hired a surrogate in the hopes of obtaining a girl. When she conceived fraternal twins, one a boy and one a girl, the intended rearing parents accepted the girl but placed the boy in a foster home, from which his biological mother retrieved him.[6]

Those seeking to hire a surrogate mother are generally well off and well educated. Agencies reported that approximately 64 per cent of their clients have a household income over $50,000 with an additional 28 per cent earning $30,000 to $50,000 per year. Overall, the services reported that at least 37 per cent of their clients are college-educated, while another 54 per cent have attended graduate school.[7]

Who Becomes a Surrogate Mother?

Agencies report that the women waiting to be hired as surrogate mothers are generally non-Hispanic Protestant whites, twenty-six to twenty-eight years of age. Approximately 60 per cent are married (see Table 8.1). Most have had a prior pregnancy, and approximately 20 per cent have had either a prior miscarriage or an abortion. Generally fewer than 10 per cent have previously relinquished a child through adoption, and fewer than 7 per cent have been surrogates before.[8] One psychiatrist suggests that some surrogates offer this service as part of their personal effort to overcome the memory of a prior loss of a child or their own placement for adoption.[9] No study has yet confirmed this suspicion, however.

Surrogate mothers are less educated and less financially secure than those who hire them. Fewer than 35 per cent of those waiting to be hired as surrogates had ever attended college, and only 4 per cent had attended any graduate school. Thirty per cent earn from $30,000 to $50,000 per year, but two-thirds (66 per cent) earn less than $30,000.

Fees

As reported to the OTA, the most common fee for a surrogate mother is $10,000 plus expenses for life insurance, maternity clothes, required transportation to the matching centre or physician, necessary laboratory tests, and the delivery. That figure has not changed since 1984, although two agencies reported a fee of $12,000 and three stated that each fee is negotiated individually.[10] In addition, fees are paid to the commercial broker (commonly $3,000 to $7,000, but ranging up to $12,000); the physicians (from $2,000 to $3,000) and psychiatrists (from $60 to $150 per hour); and the attorneys (up to $5,000). The total cost of all these fees and expenses can be roughly $30,000 to $50,000, meaning that about $1 of every $4 actually goes to the surrogate mother herself.

At least 36 states make it illegal to induce parents to part with offspring or to pay money beyond medical, legal, and certain other expenses for a parent to give a child up for adoption. All the states, whether by statute or judicial decision, prohibit baby-selling.[11] Whether these laws apply to surrogate transactions depends upon judicial decisions in each state, as well as upon interpretations of state and federal constitutional protections of the right to procreate (see below). The preconception agreement lacks the coercive pressures of unwanted pregnancy or recent childbirth that are at the root of many prohibitions on baby-selling.[12] Further, the baby is given over to another genetic parent, who is thereby buying exclusivity of custody, rather than the actual baby. Some contracts are written to pay the mother a monthly fee, rather than a lump sum upon relinquishment of the child, perhaps to enhance the impression that it is her services that are being bought, not the baby.[13]

On the other hand, a miscarriage or stillbirth often results in only a nominal fee being paid, ranging from nothing to $3,000.[14] At least two centres reduce or eliminate the fee if the surrogate is found to have behaved in a way that resulted in a health-impaired child. Finally, the hiring couple generally will pay no fee unless the mother will relinquish the child at birth.[15] The Kansas Attorney-General, considering this point, concluded, '[W]e cannot escape the fact that custody of the minor child is decided as a contractual matter' involving the exchange of funds, and thus violating public policy that 'children are not chattels and therefore may not be the subject of a contract or a gift'.[16]

If state laws prohibiting monetary inducements to adoption are applicable to paid surrogacy, they make payment of money to surrogates illegal baby-selling. This was the conclusion of courts in Indiana,[17] Michigan,[18] and New Jersey.[19] In contrast, courts in New York[20] and Kentucky[21] have held that their baby-selling prohibitions do not specifically address the situation created by surrogate motherhood, and that therefore payments are allowable until the state legislature decides otherwise.[22] Only Louisiana's and Nevada's legislatures have acted on this point. In 1987, amendments to Nevada's adoption law exempted 'lawful' surrogacy contracts from the provisions of the statute prohibiting payment to a mother beyond her expenses.[23] Louisiana, on the other hand, found such contracts to be prohibited baby-selling, and made the arrangements void from their inception, as did legislatures in Indiana, Kentucky, Michigan, Nebraska and Utah.

Limitations on Behaviour or Medical Treatment During Pregnancy

Surrogacy contracts typically prohibit the mother from smoking, drinking alcohol, and taking illegal drugs. She must also agree to abide by her physician's orders,[24] which may oblige her to undergo amniocentesis, electronic foetal monitoring, or a Caesarean delivery. Two-thirds of the agency contracts allow the client some control over whether the surrogate mother will undergo chorionic villi sampling, amniocentesis, or abortion, as well as the type of prenatal care she will receive.[25]

A practical problem with provisions such as these is the difficulty of enforcement. It is hardly feasible to follow a woman around to observe or control her behaviour. Suits for breach of contract would also be of limited use: it is unlikely that any minor breach of these behavioural restrictions will lead to an identifiable health problem in a child, leaving it unclear how to assess damages. Even liquidated damages cannot be used, unless the figure set for the damages bears some reasonable relationship to the harm caused by the breach. Thus, both pre-natal efforts to enforce the behavioural lifestyle restrictions or postnatal attempts to collect damages for their breach are difficult propositions.

Another enforcement mechanism is specific performance. However, that remedy could unconstitutionally interfere with individual rights to privacy, personal autonomy, and bodily integrity. Behavioural and medical restrictions in the contract may give the client more control over the surrogate mother's pregnancy, as it gives the client a basis upon which to seek an injunction to force her to comply or to seek damages should she refuse to comply. Yet principles of personal autonomy would probably prevent the enforcement of any requirement to undergo amniocentesis or abortion, and many proposed state laws would prohibit enforcement of such clauses. Once involved, however, courts might seek to require certain treatments on the basis of a non-contractual duty to the foetus.

A pregnant woman may possibly have a non-contractual duty to prevent harm to her foetus,[26] regardless of whether she intends to raise the child. This is a controversial and developing area of law, and a number of commentators have expressed concern that the identification of such a duty might unconstitutionally limit women's bodily autonomy.[27] A few courts have held that women may have an obligation not only to refrain from harmful behaviour — such as taking drugs — but also to take affirmative steps to prevent harm, such as undergoing Caesarean sections.[28]

Surrogacy arrangements could affect the development of this evolving area of law because the pregnant woman is often unrelated to the intended rearing parents of the child. The couple generally invest a great deal of time and money in trying to ensure that they will raise the child she bears. They have no recourse other than legal methods to try and control her behaviour. A client might use the contractual arrangement with the birth mother and the evidence of intent to rear the child to argue that he and his partner have standing to seek an injunction ordering the mother to undergo a medical procedure such as a Caesarean section. This is particularly important in light of the controversy surrounding the use of court orders to force women to undergo Caesarean sections because their physicians or husbands disagree with the decision to forego the procedure.[29] How the courts might react in the contractual surrogacy situation, however, is difficult to predict, as is the extent to which judicial decisions would be taken to apply equally to women who intend to raise the children they bear.

The Surrogate Mother's Rights to the Child

Surrogate contracts typically require the mother immediately to relinquish custody of the newborn baby. (Only three agencies do not use this provision, each reporting that it would appear to be unenforceable under their state law.) She is then required to sign papers terminating her parental rights.

The central issue in surrogacy is whether a contract can determine custody and parental rights when the surrogate mother refuses to relinquish either. Courts and attorney-general opinions have consistently stated in dicta that a surrogate mother has the same rights to her child as does a mother who conceived with the intention of keeping her baby, and that the best interests of the child would dictate the court's decision regarding custody.[30] The courts reasoned that a surrogate motherhood contract, while not void from inception, is nevertheless voidable. This means that, if all parties agree to abide by the contract terms, and the intended rearing parents are not found to be manifestly unfit, then a court will enter the necessary paternity orders and approve the various attorney's fees agreed upon.[31] If, on the other hand, the surrogate mother changes her mind about giving up her parental rights within the statutory time period provided by the applicable state law, then '[s]he has forfeited her rights to whatever fees the contract provided, but both the mother, child and biological father now have the statutory rights and obligations as exist in the absence of contract'.[32]

ENFORCEABILITY OF SURROGACY CONTRACTS

Until the *Baby M*[33] and *Yates* v. *Huber*[34] cases, no custody dispute ever made it to trial in the United States. In both of these 1988 decisions, however, surrogate motherhood contracts were voided and held irrelevant to determining custody of a child wanted by both the surrogate mother and the genetic father. The New Jersey decision is particularly important because that state's nationally influential Supreme Court held that commercial surrogacy contracts are void (and possibly criminal), not merely voidable. Finding the contract void has several important consequences. First, as noted above, it removes an important basis upon which a court could order a surrogate mother to relinquish a child to the genetic father pending resolution of a custody dispute. Second, it eliminates the contractual authority of a genetic father to control the behaviour of a surrogate mother during pregnancy or to specify the conditions of her prenatal care and delivery. Finally, it makes a surrogacy contract unenforceable, so that courts would not be allowed to order even monetary damages for its breach. This complete lack of enforceability could be a tremendous deterrent to the further popularization of surrogate motherhood, although it should be noted that similar unenforceability with regard to prenatal independent adoptions has not eliminated that practice. Discussing the analogy of commercial surrogacy to prohibited baby-selling, the New Jersey Supreme Court acknowledged that the surrogate consents to adoption before conceiving the child, and therefore does not act under the duress of an unintended pregnancy.[35] Nevertheless, it stated:

> The natural mother is irrevocably committed before she knows the strength of her bond with her child. She never makes a totally voluntary, informed decision, for quite clearly any decision prior to the baby's birth is, in the most important sense, uninformed, and any decision after that, compelled by a pre-existing contractual commitment, the threat of a lawsuit, and the inducement of $10,000 payment, is less than totally voluntary.

The idea of informed consent to engage in a surrogacy arrangement is made even more problematic in transnational surrogacy arrangements, where language barriers, absence of legal counsel, and immigration considerations may affect the transaction. For example, one surrogacy contract between an American couple and a Mexican cousin has resulted in a custody dispute complicated by allegations of misunderstanding and violations of immigration law. The surrogate understood that she was to undergo *in vivo* fertilization and embryo transfer, a commitment of several weeks. The couple asserts, however, that the handwritten contract and oral understandings always contemplated a full-term pregnancy, with the child relinquished to the genetic father and his wife at birth. In exchange, the couple was to provide clothing, medical care, food, and assistance in obtaining a visa for permanent residency in the United States.[36] The arrangement was complicated by the fact that it included providing housing in the United States for the Mexican mother, in violation of immigration regulations.

One proposed solution to the problem of ensuring informed and voluntary consent would require that surrogacy contracts be reviewed in a court before being signed by all parties. As described below, several state Bills, as well as recommendations by advisory bodies in the Netherlands and Ontario, Canada, have suggested that the contract be enforceable if a court has fully satisfied itself that it is not overreaching and that the parties are fully aware of the meaning of their promises. However, the problem of the inherent coercion created by economic need resulted in the Dutch proposal being limited to non-commercial arrangements, with commercial surrogacy still disapproved.

To date, only Indiana, Kentucky, Louisiana, Michigan, Nebraska and Utah have passed legislation specifically addressing enforceability. The Kentucky, Louisiana, Michigan, Nebraska and Utah statutes void all surrogacy contracts involving 'compensation' or 'consideration'. As the term 'consideration' is not always defined, it remains somewhat unclear whether payment of a surrogate's actual and reasonable expenses would void a contract. Indiana's statute voids all surrogacy contracts, regardless of payment.

Nevada's legislation, which exempted 'lawful' surrogacy from baby-selling prohibitions, does not speak to enforceability. Nevada law still invalidates a mother's consent to relinquish a child for adoption if made less than 48 hours after birth. It is not clear whether a surrogacy contract that commits the mother to relinquish the child is in and of itself a violation of the law, making the contract 'unlawful' and therefore outside the provisions of this amendment. Further, the statute is not clear on how the courts should balance the competing provisions of the contract terms and the statutory 48 hour cooling-off period, should there be a dispute. Although the intent of the amendment clearly seems to be to exempt surrogacy from the prohibitions on baby-selling, it is not clear whether the amendment is also intended to render surrogacy agreements fully enforceable.

SURROGACY: WHY ALL THE FUSS?

Surrogacy has captured the American imagination in a way unmatched by any other bioethics issue except abortion. Why?

The first, and most obvious, answer has to do with the technological unsophistication of the arrangement. Unlike *in vitro* fertilization, it involves no surgery, no elaborate equipment, no statistically nuanced discussion of success rates. Second, it involves no abstract questions of morality — whether embryos are alive, whether genetic manipulation is inherently bad, or whether conception in a dish is more or less natural than conception in a fallopian tube. Rather, surrogacy poses very stark questions that can be answered by reference to values we all possess, if not share. What business is it of the government to tell me (or them, or her) what to do? Why shouldn't a promise be a promise? Why shouldn't I make money the way I want to? What makes a good mother? What makes a real mother? And, most accessible of all, because it permits binary choices whose rightness and wrongness can be checked against the judicial outcome in the case, who gets to keep the baby?

But surrogacy captured America in 1987 and 1988 for more than its accessibility for debate over dinner tables. And although many commentators have focused on the potential of surrogacy for the creation of a class of professional breeders, the truly shocking aspect of the arrangement is hardly its class biases. After all, such economic inequities have long led some parents to sacrifice time with their children, their health, and even their lives due to economic necessity.

What appears to have truly caught the American imagination during the *Baby M* trial was the fact that surrogacy forces us to confront our most basic confusions concerning maternal instinct and the appropriate role of women in modern society. The *Baby M* case was quite cathartic in that it gave the American public a chance to vent its ambivalence about the women's liberation movement under the guise of bemoaning the unintended consequences of taking feminist analysis to its seemingly logical conclusion. In sum, Americans have been fascinated with surrogacy because it has let each and every one of us express our strong opinions on the meaning of motherhood, and has let many of us express our hostility at the changes forced upon us by the feminist movement.

First, it allowed numerous commentators to assert that feminism requires the adoption of a libertarian philosophy, and to note gleefully the disjunction between feminist principles of self-determination and feminist political strategies of communal action for the communal good. Then other commentators 'rescued' feminism from this dilemma by asserting the sanctity of maternal instinct. But many took this opportunity to comment that if feminists had not abandoned this notion of biological determinism to begin with there would be no welfare mothers or pornography, let alone surrogacy, to worry about today.

This approach at least put an end to surrogacy as a commercial enterprise. It did not, however, protect the rights of surrogates to retain custody of their infants. Ironically, whether one argued that women were coldly calculating individuals capable of choosing to relinquish a child for payment or that women are too trapped by their hormones and emotions to make free and voluntary decisions, the arguments could be used to undercut a surrogate's fitness for parenthood and her chances of retaining custody.

Surrogacy arrangements begin with a woman agreeing to become pregnant for a fee, and agreeing even before conception that she will relinquish the child at birth. Some members of the public, subscribing to a sort of free-market theory of human relations, balance this seemingly bizarre behaviour against the other interests present:

> [Childless couples], even though they are in a very small minority in this country at present, have a real human need, and they are willing to put up their own money to pay for it. On the other side are consenting surrogate mothers who would like the income, and who feel that the money amply compensates them for their labor. And let us not forget Baby M herself — she has come into the world because of surrogacy. . . .[I]f she [the surrogate] chooses to give up the baby. . . her choice is certainly as well informed as that of parents who give up their infant child for adoption. This result [losing the child] preserves the rights of consenting adults. . .[37]

This portrayal of surrogacy presents women as 'consenting adults'. Denying them the 'right' to become surrogate mothers implicitly denies them an important aspect of personhood — that is, autonomy. As men have this right and routinely risk their safety or self-respect in dangerous or demeaning employment, it is sexist paternalism to protect women from the potentially devastating choice of being a surrogate.

Arguing the case for the right to make a surrogacy contract, one commentator stated:

> The basic moral case for contract law, and indeed for capitalism itself, rests on the voluntary nature of exchange. . . .[N]o one is forcing women to do this, and no one who wants to deny them the opportunity is offering them an alternative source of funds. This, once again, is the powerful logic of capitalism. And, once again,

almost all surrogate mothers are apparently quite pleased with the arrangement.[38]

This, of course, is the same logic that underlay the series of substantive due process decisions in the 1930s that the Supreme Court used to dismantle worker health and safety legislation. Still, it is a portrayal of women that, taken at its most flattering, grants them the right and duty to be fully competent adults who are in control of their lives and their choices.

Juxtaposed with this rational view of the universe was the frequent recourse to the argument of maternal instinct. The *Wall Street Journal*, normally the bastion of the market approach to life, somewhat sympathetically characterized the events in the *Baby M* case:

> All went well until the moment Baby M was born. Mrs. Whitehead says at this point, 'It overwhelmed me. I had no control. I had to keep her.'[39]

Similarly, the New Jersey Supreme Court, while reinstating Whitehead's legal status as mother of the child and invalidating the surrogacy contract, stated:

> She was guilty of breach of contract, and she did break a very important promise, but we think it is expecting something well beyond normal human capabilities to suggest that this mother should have parted with her newly born infant without a struggle. Other than survival, what stronger force is there?[40]

Professional commentators and many members of the public characterized the two views as presenting a stark choice, with women either rational beings with decision-making power or emotional beings with irresistible impulses and emotions, at least when it comes to babies:

> Wait a minute. In the beginning, feminism said biology was not destiny. Feminism argued that women had the right to control their bodies, to have children or not, to have abortions or not, to have surrogate children or not.
>
> Now, it seems, that commitment is wavering. Feminists have rediscovered the biological imperative. Feminists, who have labored long and hard to re-educate society about what is and is not biologically determined, have succumbed to the tyranny of the womb. Feminists, who argue that biology is secondary when it comes to abortion, are now saying that biology is all when it comes to surrogate mothering.[41]

This was the public challenge to feminism. The attorney for the Sterns used it in his closing arguments, when he told the judge that invalidating the contract would be 'unfairly paternalistic' and 'an insult to the female population of this country',[42] and its implications are already the subject of journalistic musings. 'Beware the double edged sword,' one person wrote in a letter to the editor. 'If a contract with a woman can be invalidated *solely* because of her sex and hormones, the apparent feminist angle, does that standard apply only to childbirth?'[43]

Charles Krauthammer, in a *Washington Post* editorial, characterized the *Baby M* case as a 'perverse triumph of feminist ideology'. First, having fought for, and won, the right to control their bodies and to abort their foetuses, how can they be denied the right to grow a foetus for payment? Second, feminist success in defeating the idea that fathers can, and should, be active parents has undercut the previously held notions of inherent female superiority in parenting – a superiority that gave women an edge in custody disputes over infants. For surrogacy arrangements, this has particularly trouble-some results. 'Take away the idea of biological supremacy of the mother', he writes, 'and the class supremacy of the father will allow him to win nine times out of ten.'[44]

In discussing this perverse result of the feminist movement, both Krauthammer and other commentators linked the struggle to free women of stereotypes to the general disintegration of family vaues and morality in America.

> Public policy in the U.S. for a good many years now has been aimed perhaps unconsciously at trivializing a basic natural force – procrea-tion. Sexual acts become nothing more than a means of gratification in the popular culture. Abortion becomes a 'right' in public debate. Public support for unwed mothers becomes an entitlement defended by a large welfare bureaucracy. And now we have lawyers earning very large incomes by arranging contracts between childless couples and young women who are willing to be impregnated with the husband's sperm, bear children, and collect a fee for their services.
>
> Those in our society who raise objections to all of these practices are brushed off by sophisticates as prudes or reactionaries. While the sophisticates have held sway for years now, we detect, not least in the soul searching over the Baby M case, a rising level of concern among reasonable people over some of the outcomes and abandon-ing traditional ideas about sex and procreation.[45]

Thus, the policies that have been developed to protect women who terminate their pregnancies or carry them to term outside the protections of marriage were characterized as an abandonment of traditional ideas about sex and procreation, directly leading to unap-petizing life choices, such as surrogacy. Others noted that it is the feminist sexual freedom that led to an epidemic of sexually transmitted diseases that, over the new extended premarital sexually active years, resulted in increased infertility. And it was asserted that the feminist-inspired right to abortion and feminist-sought financial support for single mothers led to a dearth of adoptable healthy white babies. Thus, feminism was blamed for increasing infertility, inhibiting adoption, and creating a decadent moral climate that would tolerate outrageous solutions such as commercial surrogacy.

Krauthammer, in the above-mentioned column, links this to other 'unintended consequences' of the feminist movement:

> [T]he Baby M case is a caution. This is not the first time that feminist victories have come back to haunt. In the early days, the women's movement was instrumental in advancing the cause of freedom of sexual self-expression. Now, twenty years later, many feminists are fighting the plague of pornography, which thrived in the more tolerant moral and legal climate they helped to create. The women's movement is not the first liberation movement to be dismayed by the fruits of its own successes.[46]

Of course, one could argue that the question was not whether women can make informed choices or enforceable contracts. Rather, it is whether some subjects are simply not appropriate for contract law. How is one to make sense, for example, of the contract clause requiring Whitehead to 'in the best interests of the child, not form or attempt to form a parent–child relationship with the fetus'? How can one not form a relationship with one's own body?

Nonetheless, American debate seemed far more focused on this seeming dichotomy between women as autonomous decision-makers versus women as irrational, vulnerable victims. Ironically, to succeed on both maternity and custody, the Sterns' attorney had to argue both. As columnist, Ellen Goodman, wrote:

> In the contract debate, the Sterns' lawyer wants to prove that Mary Beth Whitehead was competent, cool, strong enough to make a rational decision. In the custody debate, he wants to prove that she is too emotional, unstable and unfit to be the better parent of the child.[47]

In fact, either characterization makes the surrogate appear an unpalatable mother and affects her chances of retaining custody. Cool and competent, she loses public sympathy because only an unnatural woman would relinquish her child, and the subject of the same sort of anger directed at women who choose to abort their foetuses. 'Would that Mary Beth Whitehead Gould were as truly loving a mother as her biblical predecessor' wrote one person who insinuated that Whitehead ought to relinquish the child rather tear her in two over a debate on who is the real mother.[48]

In the event, the New Jersey court recognized this as such a threat to a surrogate's ultimate chances on custody that it specifically directed the lower court to make its custody ruling without penalizing her 'one iota for the surrogacy contract. Mrs. Whitehead, as the legal mother, is entitled to have her own interest in visitation considered.'[49]

Conversely, presenting her as emotionally overwhelmed by childbirth and loss led to a number of inane findings by psychiatrists. She was unstable because she dyed her hair. The lower court characterized her as dominating the family and her husband, implicitly finding that such behaviour is inappropriate for a woman. She had her daughter on brief supervised visits during which she hugged the child too often, gave her water before she was thirsty and, all in all, seemed too enmeshed with the child. The conclusion was not that this was a woman who behaved within the normal range associated with motherhood. Nor was it concluded that she was abnormally emotional with the child due to the stress of separation and the artificiality of the infrequent visits. Rather, it was concluded that this was evidence of instability, just as her attempt to breach the contract showed an inability to make a decision. Wanting to retain custody was characterized as an inability to separate her needs from those of the child. Was this reasonable, or was it punishment for having the audacity to choose to be a surrogate, and the further audacity to change her mind? In her provocative 1988 article 'On being the object of property', Patricia Williams suggests that Whitehead's greatest sin was disobedience:

Contract law reduces life to fairy tale. The four corners of the agreement become parent. Performance is the equivalent of obedience to the parent. Obedience is duly passive. Passivity is valued as good contract-socialized behavior; activity is caged in retrospective hypotheses about states of mind at the magic moment of contracting. Individuals are judged by the contract unfolding rather than by actors acting autonomously. Nonperformance is disobedience, disobedience is active; activity becomes evil in contrast to the childlike passivity of contract conformity.

One of the most powerful examples of all this is the case of Mary Beth Whitehead, mother of Sara — of so-called Baby M. Ms. Whitehead became a vividly original actor *after* the creation of her contract with William Stern; unfortunately for her, there can be no greater civil sin. It was in this upside-down context, in the picaresque unboundedness of breachor, that her energetic grief became hysteria and her passionate creativity was funnelled, whorled, and reconstructed as highly impermissible. Mary Beth Whitehead thus emerged as the evil stepsister who deserved nothing.[50]

The terms of the *Baby M* contract only highlight the problem.

Limiting her 'right' to form an attachment with the foetus growing inside her, limiting her 'right' to experience her own pregnancy, reduces the surrogate to an 'ARV' — an alternative reproductive vehicle — as it was termed by the lower court in the *Baby M* case.

> [I]f the womb is a rented fetal container, the personhood of the woman renting it is of no significance. So if suddenly the fetal container (a.k.a. mother) starts acting like a person — 'Oh God, what have I done' — she is acting incongruously. Thus the natural bonding between mother and child is made to seem like the mother's caprice and seemed irresponsible in light of her contract.[51]

What is the result of this public disapproval of women, whether active or passive, autonomous or enslaved to biology? If actively in control of their lives, competently agreeing to birth a child for pay, they are unnatural women who cannot possibly stand on equal footing with their more tender-hearted sisters when it comes to custody. Result: no child. If appropriately passive, then they become bound by the four corners of the contracts they sign. Result: no child. And if they once again assert control, and dispute the contracts with lies, threats, flight, and any other tool available, then they are characterized as disobedient, unstable, and unfit. Result: once again, no child.

So surrogates are unsympathetic characters in America, no matter how many columns and letters to the editor decried the *Baby M* decisions. But how about the other women — the relatively hidden infertile women who are hiring these surrogates?

> Elizabeth Stern is a woman. I wonder what feminists have to say to her. In some media accounts, she is an aging careerist, a pediatrician who dared to postpone childbearing. In others, she is a selfish hypochondriac with a 'mild case' of multiple sclerosis, who wouldn't risk pregnancy when it was easy enough to hire someone else to do the work. Sometimes, she is referred to simply as the wife of the father, Bill Stern. Always, she is the other woman, a non-person. And I wonder if that isn't after all because she did not bear a child, society's most ancient definition of womanhood.[52]

Neither Mary Beth Whitehead nor Elizabeth Stern can come out winners. Women are

> . . . faulted by both political leaders and by some segments of society for working, for working too much, for going back to work too early, for caring too much about their work. . . They are charged with something close to neglect for availing themselves of childcare . . .[53]

So, how could someone like Mary Beth Whitehead care for her

children without being a bad mother — a mother who abandons them for the workforce? Only by working at home, as a surrogate. But, of course, surrogates are bad, too. And how could Elizabeth Stern, whose career and late decision to have a family interfered with the chances of a successful adoption, gather sympathy for her desire to have a family and to satisfy her husband's desire to have a genetic as well as emotional link to the next generation? She, too, is a highly unsympathetic character. There appears to be no single way to escape the public anger at modern mothering.

Thus it would seem that frustration at the new patterns of family life, at the choices women make, and at the changes they have wrought in motherhood underlie much of the fascination with surrogacy, as well as the

> . . . bizarre anti-surrogacy consensus . . . between liberals and feminists siding with Mrs. Mary Beth Whitehead on sex and class grounds, and social conservatives upset at the general implications of messing around with procreation. . .[and] those who see this as part of a general trend they don't care for involving working women, divorce, abortion, untraditional families, welfare, and so on.[54]

The reaction to this public debate has been legislative debate. At first, before the *Baby M* case, most Bills proposed to legitimize surrogacy as a 'business arrangement' to which the 'rights of motherhood do not apply'[55] or, at most, to regulate the procedure heavily, with the emphasis on psychological screening to weed out women likely to renege on the deal. Legislation introduced after the *Baby M* case has generally invalidated surrogacy contracts.

SURROGACY ARRANGEMENTS: MODELS OF STATE POLICY

Legislation related to surrogate motherhood has been introduced in over half the state legislatures since 1980;[56] many of these bills are still pending. Only nine states have passed legislation. Their approaches have differed: Arkansas endorsed surrogacy, Kansas simply exempted surrogacy from prohibitions on adoption-agency advertising, and Nevada exempted it from its prohibition on baby-selling. Kentucky, Louisiana, Michigan, Nebraska and Utah, on the other hand, voided commercial surrogacy contracts, and Indiana voided all surrogacy contracts. The approaches taken by state legislatures may be broadly grouped into five categories: static, private ordering, inducement, regulatory, and punitive.[57]

The Static Approach

The static approach is basically one of inaction, an effort to maintain the status quo. To date, it has had mixed results. Several courts have so far declined to find that surrogates lose their rights of motherhood by virtue of their preconception agreement to relinquish parental rights. But most courts have at the same time agreed to enforce the paternity and fee-payment provisions of these contracts, at least when all parties to the agreement still desire its enforcement. In other words, although these courts have found surrogate agreements to be voidable, they generally have not found them to be void. A notable exception is the New Jersey Supreme Court, which held that these agreements are void.[58]

This socially and psychologically conservative approach seeks to minimize the impact of noncoital reproductive techniques upon the structure and relationships of the traditional family, mainly by refusing to recognize new parental configurations. 'The family unit has been under severe attack from almost every element of our modern commercial society, yet it continues as the bed-rock of the world as we know it. Any practice which threatens the stability of the family unit is a direct threat to society's stability,' stated the dissenting justice in *Surrogate Parenting Association, Inc.*, the 1986 case finding that paid surrogate matching services are permissible under Kentucky law. This attitude is typical of the static approach, which aims to support traditional family configurations.

One legislative method for furthering this viewpoint would be to define 'mother' as the woman who either gives birth to a child or who obtains a child through a legal adoption proceeding. Such a definition could guarantee surrogate mothers control of their pregnancy and at least those rights held by all mothers with respect to their children. However, given the economic and educational disparity between surrogates and those who hire them, merely having equal footing will not ensure that surrogates who wish to retain custody of their children will have success at least half the time. For example, Mary Beth Whitehead did not win exclusive or primary custody of 'Baby M', and Laurie Yates (of the *Yates* v. *Huber* case) relinquished custody of her twins to their biological father rather than proceed with a custody trial after the surrogacy agreement had been declared void. Ms Yates and her husband were both unemployed, and despite the fact that the children had lived with them in the seven months since their birth, the Yates' success in a custody trial was far from assured.

Thus, although the static approach will undoubtedly slow the growth of surrogate motherhood as an industry, it will not eliminate it entirely. The expansion of these services since 1980, in the absence of judicial or legislative guidelines, demonstrates that this arrangement can be used when all parties abide by their original intentions. There can be some problems with the use of state laws and courts to manage birth certificate recordations and paternity orders. It is primarily when the parties change their minds, however, that state action becomes important and that the absence of governmental guidelines becomes an active barrier to the successful conclusion of the arrangement.

The Private Ordering Approach

The private ordering approach holds that government's primary role is to facilitate individual arrangements, and thus would compel recognition and enforcement of any conception and parenting agreement freely formed among consenting adults. Such an approach could accommodate commercializing the services of surrogate mothers.[59] Private ordering is, of course, subject to some limited constraints, such as those offering special protection to vulnerable parties in the transaction. Children are traditionally viewed as such vulnerable parties, and thus judicial intervention to ensure that custody is awarded to a fit parent would be consistent even with this approach of limited governmental intervention.

Examples of such private-ordering philosophy can be found in several of the Bills introduced in state legislatures, such as the Nevada amendment that exempts surrogacy from prohibitions on baby-selling. Proposed legislation in Oregon would also follow this model, and another Oregon proposal goes further to specifically legalize paid and unpaid surrogacy, while providing for breach of contract. An early Rhode Island Bill also aimed to make surrogacy contracts enforceable, stating that surrogate motherhood 'is to be viewed as a business venture' and that the 'rights of motherhood' do not apply to the surrogate mother.[60]

Without addressing the question of the enforceability of surrogacy contracts, an amendment to an Arkansas artificial-insemination statute explicitly contemplates surrogate arrangements. With respect to unmarried women at least, it allows an exception to the presumption that the woman who bears a child is its legal mother. The amendment states that, in the case of surrogate motherhood, the child 'shall be that of the woman intended to be the mother'. The statute does not address questions of evidence, such as the kind of agreement necessary to demonstrate who was intended to be the mother or the enforceability of these arrangements. Nevertheless, it is the first statute in the United States of its kind. A Wisconsin Bill calling for a presumption that the intended social parents are in fact more fit to raise the child also exemplifies the private ordering approach, but with some protection for the vulnerable child. Further, the Bill attempts to ensure that, if all the adult parties refuse custody, an adoptive home will be found for the child.

Consistent with the private ordering approach are state law provisions to ensure the informed and voluntary consent of all parties. A number of Bills require that the surrogate and the intended rearing parents be represented by attorneys; many further specify that the parties be represented by separate counsel. Bills in at least five states require that the intended rearing parents review the results of medical, psychological, and genetic examinations of the surrogate mother before agreeing to hire her. Bills in Michigan and the District of Columbia propose that at least 30 days pass between the time that the contract is signed and the first insemination, to allow a cooling-off period.[61] It is unclear if such provisions could meet all the objections of the New Jersey Supreme Court, but the *Baby M* decision did say that state legislatures could legalize and regulate surrogacy, within constitutional limits.[62]

The private ordering approach can be inadequate if parties fail to agree to a contract that spells out all contingencies and their outcomes. For example, a contract might fail to specify a remedy if one or both of the intended social parents were to die, leaving it unclear whether the surrogate mother or the state is responsible for the child. Contracts may also fail to specify the medical tests to be performed during pregnancy, remedies for failure to abide by lifestyle restrictions, or the lines of authority for emergency medical decisions concerning the health of the newborn. In the absence of state guidelines that create presumptive responses to these situations, private contracts may lead to disagreement and confusion. Courts attempting to enforce contracts and carry out the parties' intentions could find it necessary to decide on matters not explicitly contemplated under the contract, making even these arrangements unclear as to their outcome and highly variable from state to state.

The Inducement Approach

The inducement approach offers individuals an exchange. If the contracting parties agree to follow prescribed practices — such as judicial review of the contract, adherence to a model set of terms and conditions, or use of a licensed surrogate matching service — the state will facilitate legal recognition of the child born by the arrangement.[63] For example, a Missouri bill introduced in 1987 would require that judges approve surrogate contracts before insemination takes place. In exchange, the Bill would automatically terminate the rights of the surrogate mother, thereby offering the intended rearing parents the certainty that they will be able to gain custody of the child. The penalty for failure to follow these practices might be that the contract is unenforceable under state law or that adoption proceedings are ineligible for expedited treatment. Of course, penalties that harm a baby's psychological, physical, or even legal well-being would probably be unacceptable. A preliminary draft by the National Conference of Commissioners on Uniform State Laws took a similar approach.[64] A 1986 report by the independent Health Council of the Netherlands also endorsed this approach,[65] although only for non-commercial contracts and only with the proviso that a surrogate have three months following birth to change her mind about relinquishing custody. Commercial contracts were disapproved in the report.

Another form of this approach is to induce use of a particular approved procedure or agency by offering some governmental assurance of its quality. Thus, for example, government could license particular adoption agencies to operate as surrogate matching services. As a condition of licensing, the agency could agree to certain conditions, such as use of a standard contract or psychological screening of participants. The state would also ensure that the personnel of the agency meet certain minimum criteria, such as years in practice or professional training. Although there would be no penalty for failure to use the service, many participants would probably be interested in assuring themselves that the surrogates they hire have been screened for drug or alcohol abuse, that the persons for whom they bear children have been interviewed to identify the kind of home they plan to provide for the child, or that the contract they sign has been reviewed for fairness, completeness, and enforceability.

Any inducement approach that relies at least partly upon licensing surrogate matching agencies permits the government to prevent abuses without necessarily limiting the freedom of individuals who wish to pursue these agreements. For example, licensing could specify permissible and impermissible ways of recruiting surrogates and infertile couples, standardize the medical testing and screening of the participants and their gametes, require monitoring of the health of the baby, or set standard fees and expenses. To allow poorer couples access to surrogacy, licensing could provide sliding fee scales and agency-financing. Inducement or regulatory approaches may also, however, enable the government to specify who will be permitted to take advantage of the agencies. Agencies might, for example, be limited to serving married couples, thereby leaving unmarried couples, homosexual couples, and single persons without access to the advantageous state-approved method of surrogate adoption. Any such limitations would be subject to constitutional review, particularly to the extent that they are viewed as state interference in the right to privacy with regard to procreative decisions.

The Regulatory Approach

State regulation can also be used to create an exclusive mechanism by which an activity may be carried out. A number of proposals have been made to regulate surrogacy. Bills in Florida, Illinois, New Jersey, and South Carolina, for example, would permit only married couples to hire a surrogate. Bills in at least eight states would further specify that surrogates can be used only for medical reasons, such as inability to conceive or to carry a pregnancy to term.[66] A South Carolina Bill would require extensive investigation of the intended parents' home, as is generally done prior to adoption. Bills also propose standards for potential surrogate mothers, such as excluding women who have never had children before.

Besides regulating who may participate in surrogacy arrangements, a number of bills specify that the surrogate and at times the intended parents undergo psychological screening or counselling, and bills would require the biological mother and father to be tested for sexually transmitted diseases. This latter point takes on particular importance after the report that one surrogate who was not stringently screened before she became pregnant bore a child who was seropositive for the human immunodeficiency virus. The biological father and his wife rejected the child.[67] Regulations have also been proposed in South Carolina to require the surrogate mother to follow physician's orders during pregnancy, to adhere to a particular prenatal care schedule, and to forgo abortion unless medically indicated.

Regulations have also been proposed to limit compensation to the surrogate mother, or to set forth pro rata schedules of fees in the event of abortion, miscarriage, or stillbirth. Some proposals have also been made to maintain state records of surrogacy arrangements and, in a few cases, to provide the child, at age eighteen, with information about his or her conception. State proposals have split on whether to allow the surrogate a period after birth in which to change her mind about relinquishing custody and on whether the remedy should she do so would be monetary damages or specific enforcement of the contract's custody provisions.[68]

The Punitive Approach

The punitive approach is hostile to surrogacy arrangements. To put an end to them, it prohibits the practice, or at least its commercial forms. An alternative mechanism is to make the contracts unenforceable.

Punitive measures may be directed at a variety of parties. Civil and criminal sanctions could attach to the professional matching services, to the physicians and attorneys who are involved in the arrangements, or to the surrogates or couples themselves.[69] Nevada's legislature, for example, is to consider a bill making surrogate matching a felony punishable by up to six years in prison. A Michigan Bill also treats surrogate matching as a felony, making the penalties particularly stiff for any person who matches a couple to a surrogate who is not of legal age. The Bill would make the participation by the surrogate and the genetic father a felony as well. However, the fact that surrogacy does not require the services of a physician or an attorney, and therefore is not easy to detect, means that prohibitive approaches are unlikely completely to eliminate surrogate arrangements, although they may drive them underground.

The United Kingdom's 1985 Surrogacy Arrangements Act bans commercial surrogacy, although without criminal penalty. The Spanish report, however, recommended criminal penalties for both commercial and non-commercial surrogacy.[70] The Surrogacy Arrangements Act in the United Kingdom, as well as regulations in France[71] and court decisions in the Federal Republic of Germany,[72] also outlaw the operation of surrogate matching services in those countries. In fact, with the exception of reports recommending limited approval of supervised, non-commercial surrogacy contracts in the Netherlands and in Ontario, Canada, every nation that has examined surrogacy arrangements has taken a punitive approach and concluded that they should be at the least unenforceable and at the most criminal.[73] The recommendations of the two approving reports have not yet been implemented, although they are under review in Canada.[74]

In the United States, the idea of prohibiting all forms of surrogacy, including those involving no compensation beyond direct expenses, raises the question of interference with the right to procreate. Such a prohibition would seem to interfere more with the ability of a couple to raise a genetically related child than with an individual's right to have a child, however. Limitations on surrogacy do not prevent the man from procreating (albeit outside marriage), nor do they affect his wife's inability to procreate. Rather, they interfere with their ability, as a couple, to raise a child genetically related to at least one of them.

As such, prohibitions on surrogacy may invite judicial challenge but would probably be upheld.

The courts in *Doe* v. *Kelly*[75] and *Baby M*[76] characterized surrogacy as an effort to use contract law to further the statutory right to change the legal status of a chid via adoption, rather than as an effort to exercise the right to procreate *per se*:

> The right to procreate very simply is the right to have natural children, whether through sexual intercourse or artificial insemination. It is no more than that. Mr. Stern has not been deprived of that right. Through artificial insemination of Mrs. Whitehead, Baby M is his child. The custody, care, companionship, and nurturing that follow birth are not parts of the right to procreation; they are rights that may also be constitutionally protected, but that involve many considerations other than the right of procreation.[77]

The question can be recast as: Is there a constitutional right to have custody of a biologically related child? No such right has been identified in the past:

> There is nothing in our culture or society that even begins to suggest a fundamental right on the part of the father to the custody of the child as part of his right to procreate when opposed by the claim of the mother to the same child.[78]

Thus, prohibitions on surrogacy pose a somewhat attenuated threat to the right to procreate.

Short of prohibiting surrogacy, a state could take a punitive approach by making surrogacy contracts unenforceable. Thus, for example, a Bill could prohibit payment of fees to surrogates, by stating that commercial surrogacy contracts are void and therefore unenforceable. This was the approach taken in the Kentucky, Louisiana and Nebraska laws. Proposals in Alabama, Minnesota and New York take this same approach. Proposals in Connecticut, Illinois, North Carolina, and Rhode Island would void even non-commercial contracts, an approach adopted into law in 1988 by Indiana. Voiding these contracts means that, should the surrogate change her mind about relinquishing the child, she will stand on at least equal footing with the genetic father when she seeks permanent custody. In some states, if the surrogate is married, her husband will be presumed by law to be the child's father, leaving the genetic father with a difficult task should he seek custody of the baby.

A number of countries have taken this approach. Legislation, court cases, or regulations in South Australia and Victoria, Australia,[79] the Federal Republic of Germany,[80] France,[81] Israel,[82] Norway,[83] South Africa[84] and the United Kingdom[85] state that surrogacy contracts, whether commercial or non-commercial, are unenforceable. Other countries, such as Spain[86] and Sweden,[87] have issued Parliamentary reports recommending that these nations enact similar legislation, as has the Council of Europe's Ad Hoc Committee of Experts on Progress in the Biomedical Sciences (CAHBI). Quebec's Council on the Status of Women[88] has also been highly critical of surrogacy.[89] Even if there were a constitutional right preventing states from prohibiting or criminalizing surrogacy, they could still refuse to enforce the contractual agreements. Although failure to enforce the agreements may constitute a significant interference with an extended interpretation of procreative freedom,[90] such unenforceability of prebirth adoption agreements has not prevented couples from using the technique for private adoption. Failure to enforce surrogacy contracts is not a sufficiently direct interference with the right to procreate or even with the privilege to adopt to be outside the limits of governmental authority.

Even if states were obliged to enforce the agreements, they would not necessarily be required to order the mother to relinquish custody of the child and to terminate her parental rights. Imposing monetary damages for breach of contract could be considered a sufficiently strong mechanism for ensuring the general regularity of these arrangements, and should meet any test of a state's obligation to facilitate the use of social arrangements for the formation of families. To announce a constitutional right to contractually obtain custody of a child would deprive the surrogate mother of the same constitutional right to custody. 'It would be to assert that the constitutional right of procreation includes within it a constitutionally protected contractual right to destroy someone else's right of procreation,' said the New Jersey Supreme Court.[91]

THE DEFINITION OF MOTHERHOOD: MODELS FOR POLICY

For many years, a woman who bore a child was clearly the mother of that child: *mater est quam gestatio demonstrat*.[92] This relationship is no longer unequivocal. The possibility of embryo transfer or egg donation separates biological motherhood into genetic and gestational components. It opens the door to fresh legal consideration of the definitive aspect of motherhood – whether genetics, gestation, or intention – that entitles a particular woman to *a priori* rights to a child. 'I always considered myself her aunt,' said Linda Kirkman, gestational mother of a baby conceived with a sister's egg and destined to live with the infertile sister and her husband.[93] By contrast, Carol Chan, who donated eggs so that her sister Susie could bear and raise a child, said 'I could never regard the twins as anything but my nephews.'[94] The two births occurred in Melbourne within weeks of each other.

The dilemma of gestational surrogates, those who are not genetically linked to the foetuses they carry and deliver, most clearly poses the question of whether a genetic or gestational relationship, in and of itself, ought to determine maternal parentage and legal rights. The determination of their rights will in turn affect the definition of the rights of mothers who conceive with the intention to relinquish custody. Ultimately, it might affect determination of the rights of those women now offering naturally conceived children up for adoption.

The question of legal maternity and surrogacy has been addressed by law in only two states. Arkansas Statute s.34–721, touching on birth certificates, declares:

> For birth registration purposes, in cases of surrogate mothers, the woman giving birth shall be presumed to be the natural mother and shall be listed as such on the certificate of birth, but a substituted certificate of birth can be issued upon orders of a court of competent jurisdiction.

Thus, in Arkansas, a court order is needed to issue a birth certificate with the name of a woman other than the one giving birth. Whether a court would issue such an order based upon genetic maternity or contractual intent to take custody is not clear.

Another approach is to mimic the law of paternity, by providing that genetic parentage is definitive. This would mean that a genetic mother could apply to a court for a prebirth ruling that she is the legal mother of a child being carried to term by another. Such a ruling has been issued at least twice,[95] although in those cases the orders were made with the consent of all the parties involved and in furtherance of their stated intentions. A similar request was made in 1987 by a Massachusetts couple who had a Virginia woman carry their genetic child to term and relinquish the infant at birth.[96] The very need to resort to a court order, however, implies a *de facto* presumption that the birth mother is the child's legal mother. In many ways this is analogous to the determination of paternity, in which a presumption exists that the husband of a pregnant woman is the father of her child, with the presumption rebuttable by evidence that another man is the genetic father.

Recent regulations issued by the Israeli Health Ministry follow this sort of genetic model of maternity.[97] A woman who accepts a donated ovum but gives birth herself must nonetheless formally adopt the child she bore. Although the regulations forbid all forms of surrogacy, thereby making them irrelevant to the question of legal rights for surrogate gestational mothers, they do reflect the Ministry of Health's intention to consider genetic connections to be determinative of parentage, pending a legal change of status.

Another approach is to enforce the surrogacy agreements, regardless of the various genetic, gestational and intended social arrangements. In the case of gestational surrogacy, this would grant the parental rights of motherhood to a genetic mother who intends to rear a child brought to term by another. Such an approach was taken for the first time when the Wayne County Circuit Court in Michigan issued an interim order declaring a gamete donor couple to be the biological parents of a foetus being carried to term by a woman hired to be the gestational mother. The judge also held that the interim order would be made final after tests confirmed both maternity and paternity.[98] Upon the child's birth, the court entered an order that the names of the ovum and sperm donors be listed on the birth certificate, rather than that of the woman who gave birth. The gestational mother was termed by the court a 'human incubator'.[99]

One state law attempts to define motherhood in terms of contractually stated intentions for all surrogacy arrangements, not merely those involving ovum transfer. Arkansas Statute s. 34–721(B) states:

A child born by means of artificial insemination to a woman who is unmarried at the time of the birth of the child, shall be for all legal purposes the child of the woman giving birth, except in the case of a surrogate mother, in which event the child shall be that of the woman intended to be the mother.

This provision avoids the complications of adoption by declaring the intended rearing mother to be the child's legal parent, without the usual elaborate procedures for home review.[100] Thus, if all parties agree to fulfil the contract terms, the surrogate mother's rights would be cut off in favour of those of the intended rearing mother, without the need to get a court order or approval. (The birth certificate however, would still identify the birth mother as the presumed mother, pending a judicial order for change).

The statute is unclear, however, on certain points. First, by its terms it applies only to unmarried women, leaving open the question of the child's legal parentage if the surrogate is married. (In 1987 a Bill to extend the provision to married women was passed by the Arkansas legislature but vetoed by the governor.) Section 34–721(A) of the statute states without reservation that a child born by artificial insemination to a married woman is presumed to be her husband's child. Second, the statute concerns 'presumptions' of legal parenthood. Unless clearly stated otherwise, presumptions are generally rebuttable. The statute does not address the problem of a surrogate mother changing her mind and deciding to retain parental rights, and it is unclear whether this statute would automatically cut off her rights should she choose to rebut the presumption. Artificial insemination statutes are similarly written in terms of 'presumption of paternity', and those presumptions are rebuttable under certain circumstances – for example, if the husband can show that he did not consent to the insemination. The Arkansas law does not specify the reasons for which a surrogate mother can rebut the presumption of maternity.

A third approach is to consider the woman who bears the child as the legal mother, with any further changes in parental rights to be made as per agreement or, in the event of a dispute, as per court order. Such an approach implicitly asserts the primacy of the nine-month pregnancy experience as the key factor in designating a 'mother'. The approach has simplicity as one advantage. For example, hospital officials would always know at the time of birth the identity of the legal mother. This is also the approach taken in the Arkansas statute discussed previously, which addressed the use of birth certificates in the context of surrogate mother agreements.

The United Kingdom,[101] South Africa[102] and Bulgaria[103] have explicitly adopted this approach, with legislation stating that the woman who gives birth is to be considered the mother of a child. In West Germany, an advisory Federal-State Parliamentary Working Group[104] and the national medical association[105] have recommended similar legislation, as has CAHBI.[106] The Swiss Academy of Medicine, and the Swiss public through referendum, expressed general hostility to the idea of using *in vitro* fertilization or embryo transfer in conjunction with surrogacy.[107]

One unusual gestational-surrogacy case involving a model of maternity has drawn international attention to South Africa. In 1987 a 48-year-old grandmother bore triplets conceived *in vitro* from her daughter's ova and her son-in-law's sperm.[108] Experts disagreed on the legal status of the children, but tended to find that the daughter might have to adopt the children to protect her rights.[109] Nevertheless, the Department of Home Affairs registered the babies as children of their genetic parents. Had they been born after 14 October 1987, when the Children's Status Act came into operation, such registration would have been impossible. They would then have been deemed by law as the children of their birth mother.[110]

SUGGESTIONS FOR FEDERAL ACTION

Surrogacy arrangements are based upon principles of contract and family law, and therefore fall largely within the traditional domain of state legislative activity. As surrogacy is an interstate business,

Congress has the power under the Interstate Commerce Clause to enact regulatory legislation. Just as it does with interstate adoption activity, however, Congress may choose to leave this area primarily to state and local oversight. State legislators have not moved to coordinate their efforts as yet, with the exception of certain committees of the National Conference of Commissioners on Uniform State Laws and of the American Bar Association.

Absent federal direction, surrogate motherhood is likely to be the subject of extensive state legislative debate and action over the next few years. Statutes, when enacted, are likely to vary considerably, ranging from complete bans to only minimal oversight of contractual arrangements. This period of state legislative activity may be a useful experiment toward finding a workable legislative scheme for either banning or promoting the practice. But lengthy and complicated custody battles could ensue if courts must first decide choice-of-law questions. The problem can become particularly acute if the choice between using one state's law rather than another's could essentially decide the case. Lengthy custody suits are troubling because it becomes progressively more difficult to remove the child from his or her initial home, regardless of the merits of the case. Numerous custody battles may exact a heavy toll on the families and children involved.

Congress ought to step into this arena to accomplish four goals: to reduce the demand for surrogacy, to harmonize the state and transnational laws that govern the arrangement, to ban commercial surrogacy, and to define the legal uses of the term 'mother', in order to protect the rights of all pregnant women.

Reduce the Demand for Surrogacy

To avoid the need for state and federal involvement, Congress should focus on preventing infertility and on facilitating adoption for those who are already infertile.

Reducing infertility is an exceedingly difficult task, but some progress might be achieved through more research, education, and data collection on the prevention of sexually transmitted disease.[111] Congress could also help by facilitating the integration of employment, career development, and reproduction, so that couples might be better able to have children during their peak fertility years.

Another path would be to facilitate adoption. The Adoption Assistance and Child Welfare Act of 1980, the Title IV funding of child welfare (including foster care) and adoption assistance under that Act, and the 1978 Child Abuse Prevention and Treatment and Adoption Reform Act have produced results worthy of Congress's consideration. These programmes have been used to develop a limited national database of adoptable children for use by couples seeking private adoption, as well as to remove barriers to the adoption of children with physical or mental handicaps, older children, or children of a different race. Much better use could be made of a national clearinghouse for adoptable children to make adoption a more manageable and successful, even if time-consuming, effort. Finally, Congress should improve the opportunities for domestic and international adoption, by offering couples the same economic benefits to finance this choice as they would receive in conjunction with childbirth (for example, maternity and paternity leave) and by simplifying the search for adoptable babies.

Facilitate Harmonization of State Laws

To forestall fragmentation of state laws, Congress should at least exercise oversight of trends in those laws, in order to ascertain whether federal action is necessary. Topics of interest could include state legislation and case law on resolution of custody disputes; development of standard contract provisions, including provisions relating to a surrogate's choice of diet, medical care, and pregnancy continuance; fee structures; and protection for offspring in the event of the death or disability of an adult participant.

Further to this end, Congress could facilitate the development of state laws on surrogate motherhood. Congress could authorize the use of challenge grants to encourage states to explore approaches to surrogate motherhood. Funds could be used to finance studies of proposed legislation; to begin pilot projects for licensing of professional surrogate matching services or review of surrogate contracts; to determine the need for home studies of couples seeking a surrogate mother; or to carry out research concerning the psychological impact of surrogacy arrangements on a child, any siblings, and the adult participants.

Congress could also facilitate joint efforts by states to develop a uniform approach to surrogate motherhood. It could pass a joint resolution, for example, calling on the states to adopt one of the model laws developed by various professional groups, such as the American Bar Association and the National Conference of Commissioners on Uniform State Laws. Congress could also draft such a model law itself, to be published in the *Federal Register*, as was done in a 1981 effort to harmonize state laws on the adoption of children with special needs.

Although joint resolutions and model legislation are not binding upon the states, they could be used to express the sense of Congress concerning the use of surrogate motherhood. Congress could also encourage states to develop interstate compacts in order to avoid difficult choice-of-law problems in the event of a custody dispute surrounding an interstate arrangement and to harmonize regulations concerning surrogate-mother matching and child placement. The Interstate Compact on Placement of Children provides a precedent for the use of such compacts in the area of family law, with respect, in that case, to placing children in foster care or adopting homes.

A particularly useful provision that Congress should encourage states to adopt would be to prohibit specific performance of lifestyle and medical care restrictions or of custody provisions. Thus, while allowing states to differ on whether surrogacy contracts should be criminal, void, voidable, or enforceable with monetary damages, uniformity on prohibiting specific performance would protect the personal autonomy of surrogate mothers and prevent child custody from being determined wholly or in great part by contractual terms.

Of course, any regulatory option is quite unworkable. It inevitably places the state in the business of assessing who may enter into a surrogacy contract and which of its terms may be enforced, whether by damages or injunctions. Can a gay couple hire a surrogate? What about those who are poor, or who have criminal records? What psychological tests must a woman pass to demonstrate minimum competence to carry out pregnancy for payment? Is she to be tested for her health or for her likelihood to stick to a promise? No matter how it is fashioned, regulation of surrogacy arrangements puts the state in the business of determining fitness for pregnancy and parenthood. Many would regard such a cure as being worse than the disease.

Regardless of its stance on state regulation of surrogacy, Congress should encourage states to follow the lead of the New York State Task Force on Life and the Law, and to adopt rebuttable presumptions that surrogates can retain custody of disputed children.[112] Declaring surrogacy contracts unenforceable does not avoid this issue, and the Task Force faces the reality that custody disputes between surrogates and intended fathers are likely to be unbalanced affairs. Money, education and, presumably, legal expertise are likely to be on the father's side. Simply leaving surrogate mothers with the same rights as intended fathers to fight for custody may do them little good, since determinations as to the child's 'best interest' are almost certain to be influenced by the obvious disparities of socioeconomic advantage – as, for example, with Mary Beth Whitehead[113] and Laurie Yates.[114] Although neither of these women was held bound by her surrogacy contract, both lost custody of their children anyway. No matter what the decisions and statutes say, it is hard to ignore the fact that a father's custody case includes such advantages as the prospect of private schooling or summer camps. And so, in a chapter devoted to nothing but this point, the Task Force describes its thinking concerning presumptions of custody in disputed surrogacy cases.

The Task Force's proposed 'Surrogate Parenting Act' states in s. 4(a) that, in the event of a custody dispute, the court should 'award custody to the birth mother unless it finds, based on clear and convincing evidence, that the child's best interests would be served by awarding custody to the genetic father, genetic mother, or both'. This is, of course, a most controversial provision. It echoes the old custody traditions, in which mothers got custody of toddlers and fathers got custody only of childen old enough to need an education.

The Task Force's approach offers women an apparent edge when it comes to obtaining custody, but even feminists may find this troubling. American feminists have traditionally favoured equality in process over equality in outcome, because to give women special preferences might invite giving them special burdens not shared by men as well. Further, it attempts to correct only for surrogacy what is acknowledged as a systemic problem – the very difficult question of whether and how to consider financial advantages when making custody awards.

The Task Force argues convincingly, however, that surrogacy poses a special case in which class differences will be the norm, in which neither parent will have an established relationship with the child for the court to evaluate, and in which the fact that the surrogate entered the arrangement intending to relinquish the child may well prejudice her case. Given these factors, the best way to even the contest is to weight it in favour of the disadvantaged party. This was a courageous decision by the Task Force based on a sensitivity to the world beyond theory and principle, and it should be followed.

Another topic for forceful Congressional action is requiring that surrogacy brokers, if permitted to continue doing business, be licensed by their state. In lieu of federal licensing legislation or regulations, Congress could exercise its power to attach conditions to the receipt of federal funds to require states at least to license professional surrogate matching services, if they are not already outlawed in that state. For example, conditions could be attached to federal funding for Aid to Families with Dependent Children, family planning agencies, or adoption assistance programmes. Some of these programmes are heavily dependent on federal funding, and many states would probably feel compelled to pass the necessary legislation.

Another area of federal activity should focus on facilitating international agreements concerning transnational surrogacy arrangements. Already, in the brief history of commercialized surrogate motherhood, women of other countries have contracted with American women to act as surrogates, and vice versa. This may become more common in the future. Gestational surrogacy may also become more common. Affluent couples, for example, could hire women from developing nations, for whom a fee of far less than $10,000 would still constitute a considerable sum.

To ensure that there is no confusion concerning the rights of these women, and to avoid conflicts of national law concerning maternity and child custody in the event of a dispute, Congress could work to facilitate international cooperation and agreement on transnational surrogacy arrangements. This could be accomplished by submitting proposals to amend one of the existing child welfare agreements (for example, the Hague Convention on International Parental Kidnapping), in order to state clearly who — at least initially — shall be considered the mother and the father of a child, and who shall have initial rights to physical custody.

Ban Commercial Surrogacy

Congress should enact legislation to ban for-profit surrogate motherhood, leaving individuals able to engage in the practice as long as no money changed hands beyond actual expenses. Such a ban would probably have the effect of drastically reducing the scope of the practice. Alternatively, Congress could outlaw commercial intermediaries while leaving individuals free to make their own arrangements even if they involve payments to the surrogate. This too would probably reduce the scope of the practice.

The purpose of such a ban would be to ensure that children are not simply offered to the highest bidder. Parents cannot at this time sell their parental rights to strangers or to each other, even when they are estranged or divorced. Surrogacy should provide no exception to this rule. Further, the commercialization of pregnancy and childbirth creates a dangerous temptation to resort to courts to determine the limits of pregnant women's control over their own bodies, because the people waiting to take the baby home have nothing other than a commercial relationship with the woman to whom they have entrusted the gestation of this child. To prevent a dispute over a surrogate's refusal of foetal monitoring from becoming the test case for all women refusing foetal monitoring, it is probably best to remove commercial relationships from the delivery room.

At the same time, allowing individuals to pursue their own private, contractually unenforceable arrangements reduces the degree of possible interference with the right to procreate and form a family, as well as demonstrating respect for the ability of competent adults to make informed and voluntary choices. Further, it does not foreclose surrogacy entirely to those interested infertile couples with a willing friend or relative. In addition, criminalizing such private activities is unlikely to end surrogacy, but would merely drive it entirely underground.

A ban on commercialized surrogacy, however, would not only be consistent with the spirit behind the prohibitions on baby-selling in place in every state, but would also bring the United States in line with the unmistakable majority of other nations that have considered this issue. It would also prevent the United States from continuing to grow as a surrogacy haven, to which foreign couples come to arrange for a baby. One Michigan broker has made a number of such arrangements, and it may be only time before this practice leads to a painful transnational custody dispute.

Even if the states and the federal government could not ban all forms of surrogacy, they could prohibit its commercialization, based on the need to avoid encouraging individuals to view embryos, mothers, and babies, as articles of commerce.[115] While commercialized surrogacy finally acknowledges the economic value of women's reproductive capabilities — that is that 'labour' is labour — it also makes biological mothers into 'workers on a baby assembly line, as they try to convert their one economic asset — fertility — into cash for their other children'.[116] Other sales of the body, whether in prostitution, peonage, or slavery, are prohibited under law when there is broad social agreement that the sale violates basic principles of personhood. Unfortunately, surrogacy has a strong potential for leading to a view of women as childbearers for hire and of babies as articles of commerce.[117] As a commercial ban interferes only with an asserted right to pay for surrogacy, not with the right to procreate, and as women's self-reported motivations for becoming surrogates usually include non-commercial considerations, such as a desire to help other people,[118] a commercial ban should be upheld as a rational expression of state interest that does not unduly interfere with the right to procreate. This conclusion is shared by at least two state courts.[119]

Commercialized reproduction might also lead to the exploitation of certain women. Because of the considerable difference in average income and education between surrogates and those who hire them, some argue that there is an inherent element of coercion in surrogacy arrangements, even if the surrogate is free of the pressure of an unwanted pregnancy at the time she agrees to enter into the contract. A woman faced with an inability to feed her existing children may find herself making a choice that is, albeit autonomous, not genuinely free. Another consideration, beyond economic need, is that surrogacy may be the most efficient way for women with children to supplement the family income without having to leave home. With this consideration, commercial surrogacy may be viewed as a sinister relief from the situational coercion created by the widespread preference for in-home parental care of small children coupled with the small proportion of fathers willing to take on that responsibility. The New Jersey Supreme Court, while recognizing that surrogates consent to the arrangement before conception, nevertheless equated surrogacy with traditional baby-selling:

> The essential evil is the same, taking advantage of a woman's circumstances (unwanted pregnancy or the need for money) in order to take away her child, the difference being one of degree.[120]

While American society has long tolerated the idea that economic need and limited opportunity may lead people to give their children up for adoption or to relatives, and to work under unpleasant and even somewhat hazardous conditions, there has been little tolerance for the idea that such circumstances can be alleviated through the sale of children.

Of course, even as statements of 'rational' state interest, arguments based on protecting public morality are generally weak, if only because the harms to society are usually speculative and attenuated. In this case, however, the state rationale is further supported by a history of prohibitions against buying adoptable babies, because it degrades human life and puts children at risk of being placed in inappropriate homes simply because the occupants were able to outbid a competing set of aspiring parents. The New Jersey Supreme Court's *Baby M* decision considered this a crucial point:

> There is not the slightest suggestion that any inquiry will be made at any time to determine the fitness of the Sterns as custodial parents, of Mrs. Stern as an adoptive parent, their superiority to Mrs. Whitehead, or the effect on the child of not living with her natural mother. This is the sale of a child, or, at the very least, the sale of a mother's right to her child, the only mitigating factor being that one of the purchasers is the father. . . . In surrogacy, the highest bidders will presumably become the adoptive parents regardless of suitability, so long as payment of money is permitted.[121]

Undoubtedly the ban on baby-selling in ordinary adoption makes it more difficult for some couples to raise a family, but the limitation has been tolerated in light of the need to protect the interests of the available children. Despite the fact that childlessness is an unhappy afflication for many, there has never been a recognized right to obtain custody of a child.

One leading proponent for the constitutional protection of commercial surrogacy has speculated that prohibitions on private, paid adoptions might indeed be affected if the courts were to find that there is a right to contract for reproductive services and custody of a child:

> Recognition of such a [surrogacy] contract right also raises the question of why contracts to adopt children made before or after conception but before birth would not be valid, nor why parties should not be free after birth to make private contracts for adoption directly with women who want to relinquish their children. The logic. . .is that *persons, at least if married, have a right to acquire a child for rearing purposes,* and may resort to the medical or social means necessary to do so. Although IVF and its variations preserve a genetic or gestational link with one of the rearing parents, the right at issue may not be so easily confined. It may be that the law of adoption needs to be rethought in light of the right to contract for noncoital reproductive assistance.[122]

Traditionally, prohibitions on paying for adoptable babies are based on a collective judgement that certain things simply should not be bought and sold. Prohibitions against buying human organs have been based on the same reasoning;[123] and no successful challenge has ever been mounted to the fact that this interferes with the rights of individuals willing to purchase organs without which they might die. The New Jersey Supreme Court, considering this point in the *Baby M* case, stated:

> There are, in a civilized society, some things that money cannot buy. In America, we decided long ago that merely because conduct purchased by money was 'voluntary' did not mean that it was good or beyond regulation and prohibition. Employers can no longer buy labor at the lowest price they can bargain for, even though that labor is 'voluntary', or buy women's labor for less money than paid to men for the same job, or purchase the agreement of children to perform oppressive labor, or purchase the agreement of workers to subject themselves to unsafe or unhealthful working conditions. There are, in short, values that society deems more important than granting to wealth whatever it can buy, be it labor, love, or life.[124]

Even if surrogacy fees purchased 'services' rather than a baby, the overall transaction is one that has the potential to submerge biological ties and children's interests beneath monetary and contractual considerations. 'The profit motive predominates, permeates, and ultimately governs the transaction,' said the New Jersey Supreme Court. State regulations forbidding parents to buy and sell custody rights to each other have long been recognized as constitutional.

Overall, commercialization of familial rights and duties is one area in which courts have consistently upheld the constitutionality of legislation based both on protecting the interests of the children involved and more generally on protecting society's morals.

Define the Term 'Mother'

Finally, regardless of what else is left to state courts and legislatures, Congress should choose to set forth a national definition of the term 'mother' for the purposes of all federal legislation, international agreements, and other areas under federal jurisdiction. Congress could enact a provision such as that in the United Kingdom, which defines a child's 'mother' as the woman who was pregnant and gave birth.

While it could serve at times to defeat the interests of one or more interested persons, one advantage of this last choice is that it makes it easy to determine a child's mother. Hospitals, immigration services, and others would not need to enquire further into the circumstances surrounding the conception of a child in order to determine maternity. Pregnancy and childbirth would speak for itself. Legal maternity could change, as it does now, with formal adoption.

As discussed above, the most important reason for this action is to protect the reproductive autonomy of pregnant women. Even if commercial surrogacy continues, and other parties have a legally cognizable interest in the child being carried by a woman, her undisputed legal status as mother of the child she carries may help to protect her from any efforts by the intended rearing parents to force her to undergo any treatment or delivery method she wishes to refuse.

SUMMARY AND CONCLUSIONS

The legal status of surrogate arrangements is still unclear. Despite activity in over half the state legislatures, only seven have enacted legislation either facilitating or inhibiting the arrangement. Kentucky, Louisiana and Nebraska have voided commercial surrogacy contracts, and Indiana has voided all contracts regardless of payment. On the other hand, Arkansas has begun to regularize the legal parentage of the child. Nevada has exempted surrogacy contracts from its prohibition against baby-selling, and Kansas from its prohibition on adoption-agency advertising. With the exception of two advisory reports offering cautious approval of non-commercial forms of surrogacy, every other nation examining this issue has concluded that surrogacy arrangements are unenforceable and, at times, criminal. Several countries have implemented these findings in legislation, regulations, or judicial decisions.

State court decisions are sparse, but consistently find surrogacy contracts unenforceable in the event of a custody dispute, although the decisions do split on whether the contracts necessarily violate state adoption law. The 1988 *Baby M* case held that commercial surrogacy contracts are completely void and possibly criminal. This decision, coming from the highest court in that state, may well be influential in other state courts. Every judicial decision and legislative action by other nations examining this issue has resulted in making contracts unenforceable. Nevertheless, absent federal legislation or a federal judicial decision identifying constitutional limitations on state regulation in this field, state courts and legislators are likely to continue to come to different conclusions about whether these arrangements can or should be enforced, regulated, or banned.

The federal government ought to step into this arena to reduce the need to resort to surrogacy, to encourage states to harmonize their local laws on this topic and to prohibit specific enforcement of surrogacy contracts, to clarify procedures in the event of a transnational surrogacy dispute, to ban commercialized forms of surrogacy, and to define the legal meaning of the word 'mother'. Most importantly, it needs to protect all women, but especially surrogates, from the public antipathy towards those modern mothers who break the mould.

AN AMERICAN POSTSCRIPT

Mommies Dearest

Who's going to tell women that they may have to adopt their own children these days? It's true. A California appellate court just held that a woman giving birth may be nothing more than a glorified wet nurse, and the child's real mother is the woman whose egg was used for the conception. This all may come as a real surprise to the growing number of women who are selling their eggs to ovum donation programs in Southern California, as well as to the women using those donor eggs because they can't ovulate or carry a serious genetic disorder. After in vitro fertilization, they have the embryos implanted in their wombs, and spend nine months waiting for the big day. Naturally (to coin a phrase), such a woman would expect to return home after delivery with her baby. *Her* baby.

But not in California. There, in a mirror image situation, a woman named Crispina C. had usable ova but no uterus. So she had one of her eggs fertilized with her husband's semen and hired a second woman, Anna J., to carry the pregnancy to term. When a dispute broke out after birth, California trial and appellate courts both concluded that the woman who gave birth was merely a 'foster parent' for the 'natural' mother whose egg had been used.

Undoubtedly the California judges' opinions on the definition of motherhood were influenced by the pre-conception intentions of the parties: all agreed that the gestational mother would relinquish the child to the genetic mother. What then, will they do when a genetic mother who sold her eggs asks for some legal status with regard to the child? Will the gestational mother suddenly become the 'natural' mother?

Perhaps the definition of 'natural' mother depends not upon nature but upon who plans to take the baby home. Consider two stories from Australia. In the first, Linda K. agreed to gestate and give birth to a child conceived with her infertile sister's egg. As she relinquished the child she'd borne to the infertile sister, she denied feeling as if she was giving up her own baby girl: 'I always considered myself her aunt.' By contrast, Carol C. donated eggs to her infertile sister so the sister could gestate and bear children. Reflecting on her relationship with the resulting children, who were her genetic offspring, she said 'I could never regard the twins as anything but my nephews.' The two births occurred in Melborne within weeks of each other.

But if the definition of the natural mother depends entirely upon the intention to take care of the resulting child, then another California court decision, in the *Moschetta* case, makes no sense. The Moschettas hired a woman to act as a 'surrogate' mother because Mrs. Moschetta was infertile. The 'surrogate' was impregnated with Mr. Moschetta's semen, and relinquished the child at birth to the hiring couple. Mrs. Moschetta cared for the baby at home for seven months, until the day Mr. Moschetta walked out on the marriage, taking the baby with him. In a three-way custody battle between Mr. Moschetta, Mrs. Moschetta, and the 'surrogate', the California court promptly threw out the application of the one parent who had actually taken care of the child, day in and day out, for over half a year. Mrs. Moschetta, the court explained, was not the child's natural or (yet) adoptive parent, and therefore had no rights at all.

So it is clear that here in America we are intent upon identifying the single, 'natural' parent who gets first crack at keeping the baby. A majority of American courts, newspapers, and academic commentators have already adopted the term 'natural' or 'biological' mother to mean 'genetic' mother. They write of conflicts between genetic and gestational mothers as that of 'nature versus nurture,' as if nine months of pregnancy isn't biological, isn't natural, but is some kind of extended babysitting job.

Perhaps it shouldn't surprise us that so many confuse genetic links with biological links. After all, most of these judges and commentators are men whose only possible biological links *are* genetic. They'll never have 'morning' sickness in the afternoon or swollen ankles in the eighth month because there's a baby in the belly. They'll never worry before drinking a second cup of coffee, lest it affect a developing fetus.

In a woman's world, pregnancy is indisputably a biological fusing of fetal and maternal bodies, health, and well-being. In a man's world, biology begins and ends with the DNA chains that link one generation to another. This rush to impose a male definition on a uniquely female biological experience is almost a bad feminist joke.

And it might be a joke if the consequences for women weren't so frightening. Sticks and stones can break our bones and names *can* harm us. When Mary Beth Whitehead, a genetic *and* gestational parent, was called a 'surrogate' instead of a 'mother', the infamous *Baby M* case was already halfway decided, regardless of whether a pre-conception parenting contract should be enforceable. In the words of courts and commentators, a pregnant woman may be no more than a walking womb, a human incubator working on behalf of a future child. A month before the birth, one Michigan court declared that 'plaintiff Mary Smith is the mother of the child to be born to defendant Jane Jones on or about July 1987'. Imagine: you can be pregnant and already a legal stranger to the unborn child within you.

This country has seen prosecutors, hospital lawyers, and judges use court orders to stop pregnant women from smoking or to force them to undergo caesarean sections – all on behalf of a diffuse 'societal interest' in the as-yet-unborn child. Think what could happen when it's not strangers but the 'natural' and 'legal' parents of an unborn child still in another's womb who are trying to ensure the gestational mother, this 'foster parent,' does everything the way they would have done it. Will a pregnant woman's sense of fused biological well-being stand any chance against a legal property interest that others have in the fetus still within her body?

California's *Anna J.* decision that a gestational mother is no more than a foster parent to her own child is almost without precedent in the world. Only Israel, bound by unique aspects of religious identity law, has adopted a genetic definition of motherhood. Every other country that has examined the problem – including the United Kingdom, Germany, Switzerland, Bulgaria, and even South Africa with its race-conscious legal structure − has concluded that the woman who gives birth is the child's mother.

It is a conclusion that is essential if women are to maintain any degree of control over their own bodies during pregnancy. Anything less makes them ever more subject to the whims and coercive power of those deemed to have a superior interest in the child being carried. If, as the trial court judge in the *Anna J.* case asserted, it would be 'crazy making' to recognize the reality of two natural mothers, then for the sake of womens rights and bodily integrity the one who is chosen ought to be the one who has given birth.

But in fact, there is a better solution. Let's toss out legal fictions and recognize in court what has already happened in the physical world. Some children have three biological parents, not two. Some children have two biological mothers, not one. Acknowledging that *two* women are biologically related to the same child, that *both* women are 'natural' mothers, does not necessarily determine which will have superior claims to raise the child. As every divorced parent in America knows, biology alone does not dictate custody.

Perhaps it is time to take an even greater leap in family law. All biological relationships − genetic and gestational − are irrevocable. They cannot be undone by signing a contract or adoption papers. The thousands of children who have wondered about the biological parents who gave them up for adoption or the sperm donors used to conceive them already know this.

At the same time, the voluntary social responsibilities we take on when we adopt children are equally permanent, and no less profound. That is why so many adopted children, though they may wonder about their biological parents, take no action to find them. Forced by society to choose among various adults, these adopted children understand that the most important parent is the one who tries to stay around.

Why not give these children a break? Once a parent enters into a child's life, whether by virtue of genes, gestation, or declaration, there is an unbreakable bond of psychology and history between the two. Crispina C., Anna J., Mrs. Moschetta, and Mary Beth Whitehead are *all* mothers to their children. Even for those whose parents are absent due to contract, abandonment, or involuntary events there is a mutual tie of emotion, of wondering how the other is doing, and of moral responsibility. While courts and legislatures may see the need to determine who has a primary role in raising the child, there is no need to cut these other people out entirely. Indeed, from the child's point of view, it is simply wrong to do so. It has been said that you can never be too rich or too fit. Shall we add, perhaps, that you can never have too many parents to love you?

NOTES

1   Transcripts of taped conversation of Mary Beth Whitehead and William Stern, 15 July 1986, when Mrs Whitehead called Mr Stern from the Florida home in which she was hiding with 'Baby M' while evading a court order to return custody of the child to Mr Stern, *Associated Press*, 5 February 1987.

2   Fried, C. (1988), 'The Jurisprudential Responses to Legal Realism', *Cornell Law Review*, **73**, p. 331; Posner, R. A. (1987), 'Legal Formalism, Legal Realism, and the Interpretation of Statutes and the Constitution', *Case W. Res.*, **37**, p. 179.

3   Unger, R. Ma. (1983), 'The Critical Legal Studies Movement', *Harvard Law Review*, **96**, p. 561; Tushnet, M. (1991), 'Critical Legal Studies: A Political History', *Yale Law Journal*, **100**, p. 1515.

4   US Congress, Office of Technology Assessment, (1988), *Infertility: Medical and Social Choices*, OTA-BA-358, Washington, DC.: US Government Printing Office.

5   Ibid.

6   'Surrogate mother troubled by lack of regulation of contracts', *Associated Press*, 23 April 1988.

7   OTA, *Infertility*, op. cit., note 4 above.

8   Ibid.

9   Assoc. Press, op. cit., note 6 above; Parker, P. J. (1983), 'Motivation of surrogate mothers: initial findings', *American Journal of Psychiatry and Law*, **140**, pp. 1–4; Parker, P. J. (1984), 'Surrogate motherhood, psychiatric screening and informed consent, baby selling, and public policy', *Bulletin of the American Academy of Psychiatry and Law*, **12**, pp. 21–39.

10 Andrews, L. B. (1984), 'The stork market: the law of the new reproduction technologies', *American Bar Association Journal*, **70**, pp. 50–6; Dickens, B. (1985), 'Surrogate motherhood: legal and legislative issues', in A. Milunsky and G. J. Annas (eds), *Genetics and the Law III*, New York: Plenum Press; OTA, *Infertility*, op. cit., note 4 above.

11 OTA, *Infertility*, op. cit., note 4 above.

12 Katz, A. (1986), 'Surrogate motherhood and the baby selling laws', *Columbia Journal of Law and Social Problems*, **20**, pp. 1–53.

13 Dickens, B., University of Toronto, Faculty of Law, personal communication, 12 October 1987.

14 Gladwell, M. and Sharpe, R. (1987), 'Baby M winner', *The New Republic*, 16 Feb., pp. 15–18; OTA, *Infertility*, op. cit., note 4 above.

15 OTA, *Infertility*, op. cit., note 4 above.

16 Kansas Attorney General Opinion No. 82–150, 1982.

17 *Miroff* v. *Surrogate Mother*, Marion Superior Court, Probate Division, Marion County, Indiana (October 1986).

18 *Doe* v. *Kelly*, 307 NW 2d 438, 106 Mich. App. 169 (1981); 122 Mich. App. 506, 333 NW 2d 90 (1983).

19 *In the Matter of Baby M*, 525 A.2d 1128, 217 NJ Super. 313 (Superior Ct. Chancery Division 1987), reversed on appeal, 537, A2d 1227, 109 NJ 396 (NJ S. Ct. 1988).

20 *In the Matter of Adoption of Baby Girl L.J.*, 505 NYS 2d 813, 132 Misc.2d 172) (Surr. Ct. Nassau Cty. 1986).

21 *Surrogate Parenting Associates* v. *Commonwealth of Kentucky, ex rel Armstrong*, 704, SW2d 209 (1986).

22 *Baby Girl L.J.*, cited above, note 20; *Surrogate Parenting Assoc.*, cited above, note 21.

23 Nevada Revised Statutes, ch. 127.

24 Andrews, 'Stork market', note 10; Brophy, K. M. (1982), 'A surrogate mother contract to bear a child', *University of Louisville Journal of Family Law*, **20**, pp. 263–91; OTA, *Infertility*, op. cit., note 4 above.

25 OTA, *Infertility*, op. cit., note 4 above.

26 Robertson, J. A. and Schulman, J. (1987), 'Pregnancy and prenatal harm to offspring: the case of mothers with PKU', *Hastings Center Report*, **17**, (4), pp. 23–8.

27 Dworkin, R. B. (1986), 'The new genetics', in J. Childress *et al.* (eds), *Biolaw*, Frederick, Md.: University Publishers of America; Gallagher, J. 'The fetus and the law – whose life is it anyway?', *Ms. Magazine*, November); Gallagher, J. 'Prenatal invasions & interventions: what's wrong with fetal rights?', *Harvard Women's Law Journal*, **10**, pp. 9–58; Johnsen, D. E. (1986), 'The creation of fetal rights: conflicts with women's constitutional rights to liberty, privacy and equality', *Yale Law Journal*, **85**, pp. 599–625; Johnsen, D. E. (1987), 'A new threat to pregnant women's authority', *Hastings Center Report*, **17**,(4), pp. 33–8.

28 Rhoden, N. (1986), 'The judge in the delivery room: the emergence of court-ordered cesareans', *California Law Review*, **74**, pp. 1951–2030.

29 Kolder, V. E. B., Gallagher, J. and Parsons, M. T. (1987), 'Court ordered obstetrical interventions', *New England Journal of Medicine*, **316**, pp. 1192–6.

30 *Baby Girl L.J.*, cited above, note 22; Kansas Atty General, cited above, note 16; Louisiana Attorney General Opinion No. 83–869, 1983; *Miroff*, cited above, note 17; Ohio Attorney General Opinion No. 83–001, 1983; *Surrogate Parenting Assoc.*, cited above, note 21.

31 *Baby Girl L.J.*, cited above, note 22.

32 *Surrogate Parenting Assoc.*, cited above, note 21.

33 *Baby M*, cited above, note 19.

34 *Yates* v. *Huber*, as reported by Associated Press, 2, 3, and 10 Sept., 1987; 22 January and 14 April 1988.

35 Katz, op. cit., note 12 above.

36 *Haro* v. *Munoz*, as reported by Associated Press, 10 June and 29 November 1987; US Congress, House Committee on Energy and Commerce, Subcommittee on Transportation, Tourism, and Hazardous Wastes, Hearings on HR 2433 ('The Anti-Surrogacy Act of 1987'), 16 October 1987.

37 D'Amato, A. (1988) Letter to the Editor, *New York Times*, 18 February, p. 26, col. 4.

38 Kinsley, M. (1987), 'Baby M and the moral logic of capitalism', *Wall Street Journal*, 16 June, p. 31, col. 3.

39 Review and Outlook, 'Whose Baby M?', *Wall Street Journal*, 22 January 1987, p. 30, col. 1.

40 *In the Matter of Baby M*, cited above, note 19.

41 Leavy, J. (1987), 'My baby and Baby M: as an adopting mother, my heart is with Elizabeth Stern', *Washington Post*, 22 March, p. C5, col. 4.

42 Goodman, E. (1987), 'Baby M: the right to give away your rights?' *Washington Post*, 24 March, p. A19, col. 1.

43 Hartman, T. (1987), Letter to the Editor, *Washington Post*, 18 March, p. 20. col. 4 (emphasis in the original).

44 Krauthammer, C. (1987), 'The Baby M verdict: a triumph of feminist ideology', *Washington Post*, 3 April, p. A22, col. 3.

45 Review and Outlook, 'Beyond Baby M', *Wall Street Journal*, 2 April 1987, p.28, col.1.
46 Krauthammer, 'The Baby M verdict', op. cit., note 44 above.
47 Goodman, 'Baby M', op. cit., note 42 above.
48 Faulkner, S. (1988), Letter to the Editor, *New York Times*, 18 February, p. 26, col. 6.
49 *In the Matter of Baby M*, cited above, note 19.
50 Williams, P. (1988), 'On being the object of property', *Signs: Journal of Women in Culture and Society*, **14(11)**, pp. 5–24.
51 Will, G. (1987), 'The "natural" mother', *Washington Post*, 22 January, A21, col. 1.
52 Leavey, 'My baby and Baby M', op. cit., note 41 above.
53 Cohen, R. (1987), 'Could any parent pass the Baby M test?', *Washington Post*, 13 March, p. A27, col. 5.
54 Kinsley, 'Baby M and the moral logic', op. cit., note 38 above.
55 Katz, 'Surrogate Motherhood', op. cit., note 12 above.
56 American College of Obstetricians and Gynecologists, Governmental Affairs Division, personal communication, 23 November 1987; Andrews, L. B. (1987), 'The aftermath of Baby M: proposed state laws on surrogate motherhood', *Hastings Center Report*, **17(5)**, pp. 31–40; Jaeger, A. and Andrews, L., American Bar Foundation. personal communication, 24 November 1987; Katz, op. cit., note 12 above; National Committee for Adoption, personal communication, 13 October 1987; Pierce, W. (1985), 'Survey of state activity regarding surrogate motherhood', *Family Law Reporter*, **11**, p. 3001.
57 Dickens, 'Surrogate Motherhood', op. cit., note 10 above. Wadlington, W. (1983), 'Artificial conception: the challenge for family law', *Virginia Law Review*, **69**, pp. 465–514.
58 *Baby M*, cited, note 19 above.
59 Dickens, 'Surrogate motherhood', op. cit., note 10 above.
60 HB No. 83H-6132, 1983.
61 Andrews, 'Aftermath', cited above, note 56.
62 *Baby M*, cited above, note 19.
63 Dickens, 'Surrogate motherhood', op. cit., note 10 above.
64 Robinson, R. C., Chair, National Conference of Commissioners on Uniform State Laws, Committee on the Status of Children, Portland, Maine, personal communication, 17 October 1987.
65 de Wachter, M. and de Wert, G. (1987), 'In the Netherlands, tolerance and debate', *Hastings Center Report*, **17**, Supp. pp. 15–16.
66 Andrews, 'Aftermath', op. cit., note 61 above.
67 Frederick, W. R. *et al.* (1987), 'HIV testing on surrogate mothers', *New England Journal of Medicine*, **317**, pp. 1251–2.
68 Andrews, 'Aftermath', op. cit., note 61 above.; Katz, op. cit., note 12 above.
69 Dickens, 'Surrogate motherhood', op. cit., note 10 above.
70 Spain, Congreso de los Diputados, Comisión Especial de Estudio de la Fecondación 'in Vitro' y la Inseminación Artificial Humanas (Special Commission for the Study of Human in Vitro Fertilization and Artificial Insemination), (1986), 'Informe', *Boletin Oficial de las Cortes Generales*, **166**, 21 April,   AD 38–1.
71 Cohen, J. Chief of Obstetrics and Gynecology Clinic, Hospital of Sèvres, Paris, France, personal communication, 21 October 1987.
72 'Court orders U.S. agency promoting surrogate motherhood to close', *Associated Press* (1988), 1 January; Wagner, W., Medical Director, Duphar Pharma, Hannover, Federal Republic of Germany, 30 October 1987.

73 OTA, *Infertility*, op. cit., note 4 above.
74 Whitman, G. J., Counsellor for Scientific and Technological Affairs, Embassy of the United States of America, Rome, Italy, personal communication, 7 October 1987. See also Chapter 3.
75 *Doe v. Kelly*, cited, note 18 above.
76 *Baby M*, cited, note 19 above.
77 Ibid.
78 Ibid.
79 Infertility Medical Procedures Act, Nos. 10122–71, 1984.
80 Deutscher Juristenag (German Law Association) (1986), 'Beschluesse: Die kuenstliche Befruchtung Beim Menschen/Recht auf den Eigenen Tod', *Deutsches Artzeblatt*, **83**, pp. 3273–6; Federal Republic of Germany, Bund-Länder Arbeitsgruppe (1987), *Zwischenbericht: Fortpflan-zungsmedizin*, Bonn; Federal Republic of Germany, Bundestag, Enquete-Kommission (1987), *Chancen und Risiken der Gentechnologie*, Bonn; Wolf-Michael Catenhausen, Hanna Neumeister; Hirsch, G. E., Doctor of Jurisprudence, Augsburg, West Germany, 11 January 1988; Kottow, M. H., Stuttgart, Federal Republic of Germany, personal communication, 10 October 1987; Sass, H. M. (1987), 'Moral dilemmas in perinatal medicine and the quest for large scale embryo research: a discussion of recent guidelines in the Federal Republic of Germany', *Journal of Medicine and Philosophy*, **12**, pp. 279–90.
81 Cohen, cited, note 71 above; Comité Consultatif National d'Ethique pour les Sciences de la Vie et de la Santé (1986), *Journées Annuelles d'Ethique, Sommaire*, Paris and Lyons; Comité Consultatif National d'Ethique pour les Sciences de la Vie et de la Santé (1987), *Lettre d'Information*, no. 9, Paris.
82 'Israel outlaws practice of surrogate motherhood', *American Medical News*, 12 June 1987, p. 23, as cited in Childress *et al.*, *Biolaw*, op. cit., note 27 above.
83 Act No. 68 of 12 June 1987.
84 Battersby, J. D. (1987), 'Woman pregnant with daughter's triplets', *New York Times*, 9 April, p. 1; Bell, H. A., Office of Science and Technology Policy, Embassy of South Africa, Washington, DC, personal communications, 7 April 1988.
85 United Kingdom, Department of Health and Social Security (1986), *Legislation on Human Infertility Services and Embryo Research: A Consultation Paper*, London: HMSO.
86 Congreso de los Diputados, op. cit., note 70 above.
87 Sweden, Ministry of Justice, Insemination Committee (1985), *Barn Genom Befrunktning Utanfor Kroppenmm*, Stockholm: Liber Allmnna Frlaget.
88 Byk, C. (1987), 'The Developments in the Council of Europe on Reproductive Medicine', paper submitted to the Colloquium of the United Kingdom National Committee of Comparative Law, Cambridge, England, 15–17 September (1987), reprinted in Byk, C., 'Eléments de Droit Comparé Relatifs à la Procréation Artificielle Humaine', in C. Byk (ed.), *Procréation Artificielle: Analyse de l'Etat d'une Reflexion Juridique*, Paris: Ministère de la Justice; Council of Europe, Ad Hoc Committee of Experts on Progress in the Biomedical Sciences (CAHBI) (1986), 'Provisional principles on the techniques of human artificial procreation and certain procedures carried out on embryos in connection with those techniques', Secretariat memorandum, prepared by the Directorate of Legal Affairs.
89 Québec, Conseil du Statut de la Femme (1985), *Nouvelles Technologies de la Reproduction: Questions Soulevées dans la Littérature Générale*, Québec: Gouvernement du Québec, September; Québec,. Conseil du Statut de la Femme (1986) *Nouvelles Technologies de la Reproduction: Analyses et Questionnements*

Féministes, Québec: Gouvernement du Québec, March; Québec, Conseil du Statut de la Femme (1986), *Nouvelles Technologies de la Reproduction: Etudes des Principales Législations et Recommendations*; Québec, Conseil du Statut de la Femme (1986), *Nouvelles Technologies de la Reproduction: Pratiques Cliniques et Expérimentales au Québec*, Québec: Gouvernement du Québec, January.

90   Robertson, J. A. (1983), 'Procreative liberty and the control of conception, pregnancy, and childbirth', *Virginia Law Review*, **69**, pp. 405–64.

91   *Baby M*, cited, note 19 above.

92   Mason, J. K. and MacCall-Smith, R. A. (1987), *Law and Medical Ethics*, (2nd edn) London: Butterworths.

93   Dixon, R. (1988), 'Sisters tell of planning their special baby', *The Age*, Melbourne, 9 June, p. 3.

94   Brennan, B. F. (1988), 'A Sister's Priceless Gift – Twins', *Australian Women's Weekly*, **56**, May, pp. 14–15.

95   *Smith v. Jones*, CF 025653 (Los Angeles Superior Court, 1987); *Smith & Smith v. Jones & Jones*, 85-532014 DZ, Detroit, 3d Dist. 15 March 1986, as reported in Childress *et al.*, *Biolaw*, op. cit., note 27 above.

96   *Doe v. Roe*, Fairfax County (VA) Circuit Court (Chancery No. 103–147), as reported by Associated Press, 16 August 1987, and 12 January 1988.

97   Israel, Ministry of Health, Public Health (Extra-corporeal Fertilization) Regulations of 1987 (unofficial translation by A. Shapira, Tel Aviv University Law School, 1987).

98   King, P. (1984), 'ReproductiveTechnologies', in Childress *et al.*, *Biolaw*, op. cit., note 27 above.

99   *Smith & Smith*, cited, note 95 above.

100 National Committee for Adoption (1985), *Adoption Factbook: United States Data, Issues, Regulations and Resources*, Washington, DC.

101 UK DHSS, op. cit., note 85 above.

102 Bell, cited, note 84 above.

103 Byk, C. and Galpin-Jacquot, S. (1986), *Etat Comparatif des Règles et Juridiques Relatives à la Procréation Artificielle*, Paris: Ministère de la Justice, Ministère de la Santé et de la Famille.

104 Federal Republic of Germany, *Zwischenbericht*, op. cit., note 80 above.

105 Federal Republic of Germany, Bundesministerium für Justiz and Bundesministerium für Forschung und Technologie (1985), *In Vitro Fertilisation, Genomanalyse und Gentherapie*, Munich

106 Byk, 'Developments', op. cit., note 88 above; Council of Europe, op. cit., note 88 above.

107 Campana, A. Servicio di Endocrinologia Ginecologica, Ospedale Distrettuale di Locarno, Switzerland, personal communication, 18 November 1987; Questions Familiales éditorial/sommaire 'Commission d'experts pour les questions de technologie génétique chez l'homme', Bern: December 1986 issue); Zobrist, S.M.D., Special Assistant for International Affairs, Federal Office of Public Health, Bern, Switzerland, personal communication, 5 November 1987.

108 Erasmus, C. (1987), 'Test-tube babies common in South Africa', *Daily Nation*, Nairobi, 3 October, p. 2; Michelow, M. C. *et al.* (1988) 'Mother–daughter in vitro fertilization triplet surrogate pregnancy', *Journal of in Vitro Fertilization and Embryo Transfer*, **5(1)**, pp. 1–56.

109 OTA, *Infertility*, op. cit., note 4 above.

110 New York State Task Force on Life and the Law (1988), *Surrogate Parenting: Analysis and Recommendations for Public Policy*, New York.

111 *In the Matter of Baby M*, cited, note 19 above.

112   *Yates* v. *Huber*, cited, note 34 above.
113   *In the matter of Baby M*, 537 A. 2d 1227 (NJS Ct 1988).
114   *Yates* v. *Huber*, as reported by the Associated Press, 2, 3 and 10 September; and 22 January and 14 April 1988.
115   Radin, M. J. (1987), 'Market-Inalienability', *Harvard Law Review*, **100**, 1849–1946; Ramsey, P. (1970), *Fabricated Man: The Ethics of Genetic Control*, New Haven: Yale University Press.
116   Lamanna, M. A. (1987), 'On the baby assembly line: reproductive technology and the family', paper presented at the University of Dayton conference *Reproductive Technologies and the Catholic Tradition*, 30 October.
117   Goerlich, A. and Krannich, M. (1986), 'Summary of contributions and debates at the hearing of women on Reproductive and Genetic Engineering', *Documentation of the Feminist Hearing on Genetic Engineering and Reproductive Technologies*, 6–7 March, Brussels: Women's Bureau, European Parliament.
118   Hanifin, H. (1987), 'Surrogate parenting: reassessing human bonding', paper presented at the annual meeting of the American Psychological Association, August; Parker, 'Motivation', op. cit., note 9 above; Parker, 'Surrogate Motherhood', op. cit., note 9 above; Sutton, J., paper presented to the Pennsylvania State Legislature on behalf of the National Association of Surrogate Mothers, 1987.
119   *Doe* v. *Kelly*, cited, note 18 above; *Baby M*, cited, note 19 above.
120   *Baby M*, cited, note 19 above.
121   Ibid.
122   Robertson, J. A. (1986), 'Embryos, families and procreative liberty: the legal structure of the new reproduction', *Southern California Law Review*, **59**, pp. 939–1041 (emphasis added).
123   US Congress, Office of Technology Assessment (1987), *New Developments in Biotechnology: Ownership of Human Tissues and Cells*, OTA-BA-337, Washington, DC: US Government Printing Office.
124   *Baby M*, cited, note 19 above.

PART TWO

9 The Unscrambling of Egg Donation

MICHAEL D.A. FREEMAN

A lot of attention has been given in recent years to the legal implications of many of the activities associated with the 'reproduction revolution'.[1] In some spheres and in some parts of the world this has led to legislation.[2] Disputes have sometimes arisen, notably over surrogacy arrangements,[3] and courts have become involved, leading to the formulation of some guidelines. The question of egg donation has remained relatively immune from such thinking or lawmaking activity. This chapter looks at some of the questions this poses, at possible and optimal solutions, and asks, Why has so little attention been given to egg donation?

EGG DONATION

There are two main reasons for wishing to resort to egg donation. Most obviously, it may be a way of overcoming infertility.[4] In most cases where ovum donation is sought for this reason, the cause of non-functioning ovaries is premature ovarian failure in women between the ages of 17 and 40 (Professor W. Thomson estimates *80 per cent* of cases come into this category).[5]

Other, less common, causes are ovarian dysgenesis, bilateral oophorectomy (tumours, cancer) and, more controversially, the fact that the woman concerned is post-menopausal. Egg donation may also be used to avoid passing on a genetic defect, such as Huntingdon's Chorea.

Eggs can be obtained in a number of ways. First, they can be garnered from women on IVF programmes who produce excess eggs. This is ironic, for it is possible for the recipient to succeed at the donor's expense. Second, eggs can be obtained from women who volunteer to undergo laparoscopies or ultrasonic treatment and allow their ova to be used. There will be few true volunteers prepared to do this for altruistic reasons. It is possible that sisters or other relatives may donate in this way, but other women also may be prepared to subject themselves to this treatment for a fee, or for compensation or expenses. Sums of between £1,000 and £5,000 per ovum have been cited. In Britain no law prohibits this, but doubts have been cast on whether it should be allowed.[6] Third, it is possible that a relative (a sister, or even a mother, for example) or a friend may be prepared to come to the assistance of an infertile relative or friend. There are social and psychological pressures involved in 'transactions' of this nature, as well as legal conundrums, and the practice is controversial. The practice has been carried out at the Humana Wellington Hospital in St John's Wood in London and is deprecated by the Voluntary (now Interim) Licensing Authority, the rules of guidance of which caution against donations between sisters.[7] A fourth source of ova is from women who are undergoing voluntary sterilization or having a hysterectomy. However the average woman becomes sterile ten years before menopause, so that the donation of older women's eggs is not advisable. It is thought that women undergoing such surgery, who are asked to participate in egg donation programmes at the same time, are likely to cooperate with the doctors who make what may seem reasonable requests of them to assist other, less fortunate, women. But exactly to what extent their decision is based on 'informed consent' remains an issue. Such women are vulnerable to pressure, to hints, suggestions, encouragement. Whether the consent they give is informed and uninhibited may be doubted. The revelation, in May 1989, that clinics in Britain are waiving fees of up to £600 for private sterilizations to induce women to denote their eggs is a graphic illustration of these fees. The practice has been described as 'unacceptable' and 'unethical' and the Voluntary Licensing Authority, which envisages that legislation will make it a criminal offence,[8] has threatened to withdraw the licences of any clinic using such a practice. Nevertheless, sterilization remains an obvious source where the women themselves genuinely desire to donate ova.[9] There is a fifth way in which ova can be obtained, that is by uterine lavage or flushing; this involves the washing out of pre-embryos. In 16 American states this is regarded as coming under the umbrella of abortion.[10] There are also risks involved, including that of losing the embryo and of ectopic pregnancy. The Warnock Report rejects the procedure.[11] It cannot at present be considered as a real source for egg donation. It is thought that Parliament is likely to endorse this view.

LEGAL IMPLICATIONS

In its first annual report, the British Voluntary Licensing Authority pointed to 'obvious legal implications' in ovum donation.[12] It did not, however, specify them. The report strongly recommends urgent clarification 'before the practice becomes more widespread'.[13] In its second report, it notes that, once successful freezing techniques are established, with the possibility of egg banks and the widespread use of donated ova in IVF treatment, it will be important that 'a number of legal implications affecting children born as a result of egg or pre-embryo donation should be clarified'.[14] Four particular problems are identified: registration, legitimacy, parentage and the right to know the identity of genetic parents. THE VLA urged the Government to give consideration to these matters.

Some consideration has, of course, been given to the unravelling of the legal problems of egg donation, both in Britain and else-where.[15] At the same time opportunities were missed, an example of which was the Family Law Reform Act 1987. This Act, in providing that children born to married women as a result of AID with their husband's consent should be treated in law as legitimate, and there-fore as the children of the husband and not the donors, could have extended this principle to egg and embryo donation, but did not do so. The existing provision (in s.27) was controversial. It was said to legitimate perjury and was, accordingly, confined. The Warnock Report had recommended that the new provision should cover egg and embryo donation,[16] as well as semen donation. The force of this logic was rejected.

The first legislation in Britain to make specific reference to egg donation is the Human Fertilization and Embryology Act of 1990. In Sweden it has been banned,[17] and no other country has detailed laws as such. Previously the ILA guidelines[18] were the closest the United Kingdom came to legislation. These were, and still can be, regularly amended and updated to take account of new developments, new understanding and informed debate. With the new legislation on assisted reproduction a Statutory Licensing Authority (The Human Fertilization and Embryology Authority) has been established. But a problem which remains and is shared by other countries is the extent to which (on a matter such as egg donation) an agency such as the new Authority should be left to make its own rules or whether its guidelines should be embodied in legislation, primary or secondary. Whether the compromise effected by the new British legislation is appropriate must be considered.

Egg donation poses numerous ethical and legal problems. Should the donation be anonymous? If so, how should the anonymity be preserved? What records should be kept? Who should take responsi-bility for any such records? What is the legal status of the offspring? Should donations be offered only to married women or only to heterosexual women? If we permit donations to 'single' women, should we insist that they are truly 'single', thus countenancing the creation of another one-parent family, or do we extend donations beyond marriage to women in stable cohabitations? If so, how do we define these? The variations on this theme are legion. Should the offspring have the right to know about the circumstances of his or her birth? If so, should the information be so comprehensive as to identify the genetic mother, or non-identifying, specifying her age, culture, background, occupation, possible hair and/or eye colour, height, other physical characteristics? In Britain, controversy has not yet centred on these questions, about which there has been little discussion. Two other problem areas have, however, provoked a good deal of comment, not to say bitter dispute. Should a sister, or other close relative, be permitted to donate an egg to an infertile sister? If so, how many ova should be transferred? These questions have divided VLA, and one hospital in particular, although the other questions are at least as important and could well stimulate contro-versy in the coming years. It is as well to turn our attention to them now.

The pragmatist response might be to solve problems when they arise. Certainly this is an approach of which lawyers in particular are fond. But this presents two major drawbacks. First, courts (and therefore those whose decisions are taken in the light of what courts can be expected to do) will find themselves bound by policies and statutes adopted to resolve unrelated past problems and will, as a result, be hamstrung in their efforts to reach appropriate conclusions. As Walter Wadlington put it, in an early but authoritative article: 'Old legal categories often constrict courts confronted with problems that arise from new technology and limit their efficacy in attempting to find creative solutions.'[19] Whether a court is in fact the appropriate forum for such decision making may be questioned: judicial knowledge and understanding of biotechnology is limited. Second, there is a danger of a piecemeal, ad hoc approach, which can lead to gaps and inconsistencies, an absence of principles and of a coherent framework. Complex ethical questions, matters of public policy, are not the province of the judge.

So it is to the legislature that we must look. There are some matters upon which it must pronounce: Who is the mother? Is the child legitimate or not? Should there be a right to knowledge about parentage? To whom would the ova preserved in an egg bank belong? These are matters of public policy which call for clear and unequivocal legal answers. There are other matters, donations between sisters are a good example, which are concerns of public policy and upon which legislative guidance is imperative. The legis-lature would have the capacity to ban such donations and could do so effectively (it must be presumed that even 'rogue' clinics would not circumvent such a prohibition). But, on a matter as sensitive as this, the legislature should not act alone. The advice of a multi-disciplinary body, such as a licensing authority, should be sought. It may even be thought appropriate to delegate to such a body the power to license such donations in particular circumstances, in which case the details may best be left to the authority itself. On other matters regulation by a licensing authority may be more appropriate than legislation by a legislature: for example, the questions of what records should be kept, and who should take responsibility for them. The dividing line between the appropriate provinces of legislature and licensing authority is itself a matter of debate. Where the line should be drawn may become clearer as we proceed. The issues themselves will be discussed, the problems identified and the choice of solutions outlined.

THE BIOLOGICAL CONNECTION

There is no definitive answer to the question of who is the mother of a child born following *in vitro* fertilization with a donor ovum. Mason and McCall Smith, in their standard legal text, state that the 'genetic or biological parentage of the child will be confused but natural parentage will be acceptably clear'.[20] This is hardly helpful: the word 'natural' is highly tendentious. They say, following the Warnock view[21] and precedents in Australia (a Victorian Act of 1984[22] and one from Western Australia in 1985[23]) that the act of carrying a child to term is what constitutes true motherhood. This, of course, emphasizes the social, the psychological, the nurturing aspect of mothering over the genetic. On the other hand, if the genetic link is determinative, it would be the egg donor who would be the legal mother. British legislation (the 1990 Act) has now adopted the social, rather than the genetic, test. But the consequences of concluding that the genetic consideration should prevail are nevertheless worth considering.

Looking at this from the perspective of English law, a child would be illegitimate unless produced by a donated ovum fertilized by the ovum donor's husband's sperm, in which case the child would be the legitimate child of the donor and her husband. Second, the ovum donor alone would have parental responsibility for the child including rights and duties in respect of the child, a conclusion that would be very unrealistic. Third, it would be necessary for the gestational mother (and her husband) to adopt the child if they wanted to become true or at least legal parents. Such a transfer would require the agreement of the donor (and possibly her husband). This could be dispensed with by a court, though ironically not on the grounds of abandonment or persistent failure without reasonable cause to discharge the obligations of a parent. There could be no doubt, however, that her agreement would be readily dispensed with on the general ground that it was being withheld unreasonably, the criterion being what a reasonable mother in her position would do.[24]

Amongst other sundry consequences are the following. The child would take the donor's domicile.[25] This could have far-reaching consequences, including the implications of political status. For example, if the donor were a British citizen but the gestational mother's husband were not, the child would not acquire British citizenship at birth, even if the birth took place in the United Kingdom. The laws of succession would be affected. The ovum donor would be the only parent from the viewpoint of current child care legislation. For example, if the child came into care, she (the ovum donor) might be obligated to contribute towards the child's maintenance. Of course, this is theory: no local authority would even contemplate taking such action. But, if we are looking for arguments to support different conclusions, it is valuable to draw out the logical implications of particular answers. This is by no means an exhaustive list: there would also be implications in the fields of social security, education and undoubtedly in numerous other areas.

Common sense dictates against this way to resolve the problem. So does the analogy of the paternity question. Currently the semen donor is not regarded as the father of the child although there can be no doubt that he is the genetic father. Indeed, the case for attributing parentage to him (which we do not do) is even greater than labelling the ovum donor as the mother. Another woman has carried the child for nine months with all that this entails for herself and the child, whereas no man other than the semen donor has contributed anything (emotional and financial support of the mother apart) to the production of the child. Since the husband of the gestational mother is now treated as the father of the child, where there has been artificial insemination with the husband's consent, consistency, the need for coherence, seem to dictate that there should be a presumption in favour of regarding the gestational mother as the mother rather than so regarding the ovum donor.

In deciding eventually to designate the gestational mother as the mother, not only was the precedent of AID followed but also the method usually commended to tease out who is the mother in the situation of a surrogacy arrangement. Thus, as an example, during the passage of the Surrogacy Arrangements Act of 1985, Lord Denning moved the following amendment in the House of Lords: 'A child born to a surrogate mother in pursuance of a surrogacy agreement shall for all purposes be regarded in law as the child of that mother.'[26] This amendment was withdrawn, but it is expected to find its way into legislation in due course. Whether this is the right conclusion is outside the scope of the present discussion, though one can hardly fail to notice that the gestational mother in surrogacy (who is also the genetic mother save where the surrogacy is total and she merely leases her womb) will only become the 'social' mother in those cases where the arrangement breaks down.

Whatever conclusion we come to regarding surrogacy, a provision along the lines of Lord Denning's amendment to deal with ovum donation would have much to commend it. At the very least, there should be a presumption in favour of the donation being absolute. And, if such a presumption were to be adopted, it is difficult to think of evidence which could be adduced to rebut it.

The case for regarding the gestational mother as 'the mother' is thus substantial. Such a conclusion has now been embodied into British legislation. Section 27(1) of the 1990 Act states: 'The woman who is carrying or has carried a child as a result of the placing in her of an embryo or of sperm and eggs, and no other woman, is to be treated as the mother of the child.' Whether this extends to the case of an embryo removed by lavage has been doubted,[27] leaving yet another question to await clarification.

This leads on to the next question which centres on the birth registration of the child. Once it is decided that the gestational mother is the legal mother of the child, her husband is the father, either because his sperm fertilized the donated ovum or, if this too was donated, because of the 1987 legislation, and the names of the persons presumed in law to be the parents should be recorded in the register of births. Registration is an administrative, not a judicial, act.[28] Normally no investigation takes place into the truth of the statements made by the informant. Therefore nothing will emerge from a birth certificate to suggest to the world at large or to the child in years to come that the birth was the result of an egg donation.

Should birth records also refer to genetic parents? To insist that they should would be to impose rules on the infertile that are not imposed on anyone else. There is a conflict of interests and a conflict of values at issue here. As far as 'interests' are concerned, the gestational parents (who are also the social parents) may well wish to keep the method of their child's conception secret. It may, however, be in the interests of the child, *qua* adolescent or adult, to seek out his true origins as he searches for an identity. It is already acknowledged that some adopted children experience personality crises, and others go in search of their genetic parents. But will men donate semen or women ova if it is possible that years later they will be 'pestered' by their genetic products? Evidence from Sweden shows that following the abolition of anonymity there was initially a decline in the number of men willing to donate semen for fear that their identity might subsequently be disclosed.[29] The number of couples seeking AID and doctors prepared to continue AID practice also declined. However the decline was temporary.[30]

Which is most valuable: privacy or freedom of information? The case for emphasizing the interests of donors and therefore the value of privacy is strong. It is difficult to see what benefit can come from birth records referring to the ovum donor or even the fact that the child was born as a result of an egg donation. The social profile suggestion, found in the Warnock Report[31] and elsewhere, has little to commend it. It may provoke a curiosity which cannot readily be satiated, and this in itself may do psychological harm. An analogy is often drawn with adoption but this is misleading. The adopted child who wishes to trace his 'real' mother seeks a person who contributed to his make-up during pregnancy and often for a considerable period thereafter. There is no need for a child born as a result of an egg donation to feel rejected or to worry about acceptance.

It may be said that birth registers which make no reference to the child's true origins are 'perjuries', even if, in surrogacy cases, 'pious perjuries'. There is some truth in this, although less than is sometimes supposed. This is because, implicit in such a criticism is the view that the birth register purports to be a source of genetically accurate information. If this were so, there would be no such thing as an entry which failed to disclose the father's name. We would also have rather more qualms about accepting that husbands of married women were unquestionably the fathers of their children.[32]

The question of whether children produced as a result of egg donations are legitimate or not was discussed earlier in the context of 'who is the mother'. A few further comments on the child's status are, however, in order.

It is true to say that, in the world as a whole there has been movement in favour of removing legal disabilities from illegitimate children. Successive reforms in those countries which penalized illegitimacy have attenuated the legal disabilities attached to it. Social stigma also holds less weight. Many countries do, however, still distinguish between those children born outside marriage and those born within. In England, where the rights of the illegitimate child are close to those of his legitimate brother (though distinctions do remain), the law still imposes legal penalties on the fathers of such children. They are able to acquire parental responsibility through a court order under the Family Law Reform Act 1987, and now by agreement with the mother.[33] But without such an order or agreement they have no parental responsibility vested in them, whatever their relationship with the child. The mother too is still discriminated against, although she no longer suffers the indignities of affiliation procedure: the Family Law Reform Act 1987 abolished this. She applies for maintenance as any other mother may against the man she claims is the father.[34] She will still have to prove however that the man whom she alleges is the father is indeed the child's progenitor in order to obtain financial provision for the child. There is no such requirement in the context of marriage, where children are presumed to be those of the husband and where no proof is required.

It is therefore important how we classify the child born as a result of an egg donation. It is difficult to see what arguments can be adduced to characterize the child as illegitimate, particularly now that the child produced as a result of AID is regarded as a legitimate child. The 1987 reform can be criticized (and has been),[35] but it is the case that with both donor insemination and egg donation births the child is born within marriage. That the conception has taken place outside marriage (or introduced a third party into the process) should not be regarded as significant, given that the non-genetic parent has participated in the arrangement. It cannot be regarded as comparable to adultery.[36]

The 'biological connection' raises one final matter: the implications for marriage. All legal systems restrict marriage and, for that matter, sexual intercourse between certain persons of close kinship.[37] The restrictions, which are far from uniform, are justified on eugenic and social and moral (even religious) grounds.[38] Marriage between close blood relatives has potential disgenic effects. There must always be the remote possibility, as there is in adoption, that a child produced as a result of an egg donation will wish to marry (or may already have gone through a ceremony of marriage with) a person who is genetically a half-sibling.[39] This could come about as a result of a woman donating a number of ova (perhaps at the time of sterilization), or as a result of the product of a single donation marrying a child of hers produced in the normal way.

Is this scenario anything more than a 'moral panic'[40] engineered by those who oppose the reproduction revolution? The potential for such a 'disaster' to occur has always existed in the context of adoption and, so far as is known, it has never happened. If it should occur in either context the English legal system (and indeed most systems) would regard the purported marriage as no marriage, that is it would be declared void.[41] This would not affect the legal status of any children born of the relationship: the marriage would almost certainly be a putative marriage and the children would accordingly be legitimate.[42] But the decree (which in England could be sought by a third party with an interest in the marriage) would be retrospective, and could wreak havoc in the area of property. Is there a solution? An exception could be created by the legislature permitting marriage for adopted or artificially conceived siblings. In the United States this would fall foul of the 'equal protection' clause in the Constitution,[43] but in England, for example, there would be no such obstacle.

Alternatively, a legislature could enforce kinship bans, but it would be realistic to do this only if persons produced as a result of an egg donation (or AID) were given full access to the details of their biological origin and this, I have argued, has in-built disadvantages. The contingency of marrying a half-sibling is so remote and the chances of not discovering it has happened until after a child with a genetic disorder is born is so unlikely that, of the two alternatives, the statutory exception, where constitutionally feasible, seems preferable.

EGG BANKS

As the Voluntary Licensing Authority acknowledged in its second Annual Report, once successful freezing techniques are established, it may be possible to set up egg banks.[44] Britain's first human egg bank has recently been set up at the Royal Free Hospital in London. In Australia three babies have been born as a result of a technique which freezes ova for later use. The implications of these, ethical as well as legal, are considerable. There has already been litigation in France, Australia and most recently the 'custody battle' in the Jones divorce in Tennessee.[45] This concerned not egg donation but the status of seven frozen embryos produced during an IVF procedure. The wife wanted them implanted in her so that she could have a child: the husband wanted them to remain in their frozen state. The trial judge ruled that the embryos were children and awarded the wife custody. The result ('crazy-making', as it has been described)[46] was reversed by the appellate court which ruled that the couple 'shared an interest in the seven fertilized ova' and concluded that they should be given 'joint control with equal voice over their disposition'. But this 'non-decision' is hardly helpful; if the couple had spoken as one voice the case would not have come to court. More disputes can be expected and will require much more rigorous reasoning than the Jones case. A large number of questions can and are likely to be raised.

Who would own the pre-embryo in the bank? Applying normal legal principles, ultimately derived from the philosophy of John Locke,[47] the answer might well be the doctors who 'created' it. But this would imply that they own potential children and, arguably, also the children born as a result of this technique. Russell Scott speculates further: 'What if the community decided to take control of all the procedures? Would we then have a state which literally owned its citizens? Would the notion of individual freedom and personal autonomy become moot?'[48]

This speculation belongs to some Huxleyian 'New World' — and it is foolhardy, rather than 'brave'. At least English law is quite clear in that it does not recognize general property rights in human bodies or tissues. Indeed, Scott himself recognises this. Control of human tissues remains with the possessor, and once tissues or organs are removed from a person, that person has no legal right of ownership, nor the right to recover them or dictate their destination. Similarly, in common law the woman and her partner (if any) whose ova are frozen (or fertilized and frozen) and stored in a bank have no rights of property over them. The IVF clinic is not under any obligation to keep ova or conceptuses for a particular couple. It could use them for research purposes (subject to any limitation imposed by law or licensing authority guideline) and it could donate them to another woman.

However, if the woman (or the couple) has made a contract with the clinic, what would be the status of such a contract? The New South Wales Law Reform Commission, in its discussion paper on *In Vitro Fertilisation*, is of the opinion that, in the event of a dispute, the courts of NSW would recognize an 'implicit agreement between the couple and the clinic that the gametes be kept for the couple's own use'.[49] It does, however, concede that this 'could not be predicted with confidence'. It is highly dubious whether an English court would imply a contract in these circumstances (nor ought it or any other court to do so).

The question ultimately is whether this is a matter best left for private ordering or one on which, as a matter of public policy, the state must be involved in a regulatory capacity. The principal arguements against private ordering are well-rehearsed, particularly in the context of the debate over surrogacy.[50] They centre on whether the market has a role to play in assisted reproduction. Is this an area where there are important interests to protect, so that it should belong to the public domain rather than be left for private autonomous decision-making? It cannot be denied that there are issues of public policy, but the existence of these may go towards the limitation of matters upon which private autonomy may prevail rather than to its total exclusion.

There is clearly also a distinction between providing for the storing of ova or gametes and egg donation. The woman (or couple) should be able to claim greater control over the storing arrangement than over the destination of the donated ovum or ova. But, even in the former case, a dispute (between the couple or one or both of them and the clinic) has more of the characteristics of a custody dispute than one concerned with determination of title. In the latter case the analogy with semen donation may be thought to warrant consideration. It has never been questioned that when a man donates semen for use in AID he does so unconditionally and, therefore, cannot assert control over its subsequent use. If this is correct (and it may be that with the advent of egg donation we may wish to reconsider something previously seen as unproblematic), should different considerations prevail with donations of ova? Should the fact that such donations are physically more difficult and dangerous and emotionally more traumatic give the donors greater property rights? I do not believe the case for distinguishing between them has been established. The case for legislation providing clinics with the power to determine questions relating to disposal of ova is thus a strong one. The maximum length of time of storage, whether or not ova may be used for research and, if so, under what circumstances, are clearly questions of public policy which must be taken by an informed legislature. They are also questions outside the remit of this article.

DONATION BETWEEN SISTERS

Thus far this chapter has assumed that there should be no limits on donation, the implicit assumption being that a woman should be entitled to donate ova to whomsoever she pleases. But, as is well-known (it having sparked considerable controversy), the question has arisen whether as a matter of policy ovum donation should be allowed between sisters or other close relatives.

In its first Annual Report the VLA emphasized that it did not advocate banning egg donation between sisters, but it thought 'the procedure should be carried out only under exceptional circumstances and only after very careful counselling of both donor and recipient'.[51] Its reason for feeling some disquiet about the practice is that the donor ceases to be anonymous in such a family arrangement. By its second Annual Report, donation between close relatives is described as 'inadvisable'.[52] It is said that it 'may not be in the best interests of the child'.

In September 1988 VLA held a joint meeting with the King's Fund Centre to look at the broader implications of egg donation and in particular to focus attention on donation between close relatives. The fourth report of the VLA (or ILA as it is thenceforward to be called) contains a summary of the discussions.[53] These were broadly opposed to the practice and the VLA accordingly considered 'the weight of the argument lay on the side of caution'.[54] The Authority's Guideline 13 (j) stating that donors should remain anonymous has been retained.

Note that the arguments against the practice underwent a subtle change from the first to the second VLA report, from the undesirability of a breach of anonymity to a 'best interests of the child' argument. The second argument, if it can be sustained, is the stronger of the two. Anonymity, although an important consideration, is not an overriding one. It is not an end in itself, nor is it an absolute value.

Some people, however, may prefer a known donor.[55] In this way, they may feel, they will get a child more like themselves. This may well be the case, particularly with members of ethnic minorities. The 'best interests of the child', though a vague and value-laden concept,[56] is one to which we still do obeisance. However, it has to be said that in the areas in which questions of a child's best interests arise (for example, a custody dispute between parents or between parents and foster parents) there *is* a child whose best interests are in question. Introducing the 'best interests' concept into the egg donation debate raises the somewhat intractable problem of whether it is in someone's best interests to be born into a particular set of circumstances.

The analogy that is often drawn between ovum donation between sisters or close relatives and the adoption of a child by a close relative is thus far from perfect. For adoption to be contemplated there must be a child and the decision to allow or not to allow adoption to take place is based on what is best for that child, who may be a few weeks, a few months or even several years old (in which case he will have a history and an identity). Thus, for example, in English adoption law the child's welfare is the 'first consideration'.[57] Clearly the older the adopted child is, the greater the chances are that he will experience an identity crisis if his aunt or grandmother becomes his mother, with concomitantly his mother becoming an aunt or sibling. This is surely what is meant by distorting real relationships, and was the target of the Houghton report in England in 1972,[58] which recommended that such adoptions should not take place. This recommendation found its way into legislation in 1975.[59]

In fact, a child born as a result of an ovum donation between sisters is, unless the sperm is also donated, genetically half of the couple's in any case and has been carried to term by the woman who is to be the social mother. She is the mother on two levels, gestational and social: her husband (or partner) is the father on all accounts. Nevertheless, a child will grow up with an aunt who is genetically his mother, and possibly with cousins who are his half-siblings. Although the same distortions occur with semen donations between brothers, there has been no call to ban or even control this. Perhaps this is not surprising, given the relative ease and privacy with which this can be carried out. But is it desirable to want to stop this practice if we could?

We can, of course, control ovum donation, provided we can

control the practices of clinics. But should we wish to do do so? This is interfering with procreative freedom[60] and it requires, as do all restrictions on liberty, a strong moral case for instigating. There have been ovum donations between sisters (they were the subject of a bitter controversy between the VLA and the Humana Wellington Hospital in London in 1987)[61] and there is no empirical evidence (at least not as yet) that they are unsuccessful.

Where, exactly, do the objections lie? To put it bluntly, the gift of an ovum is not a simple gift. It lies outside the realm of normal social intercourse. We know that the ability to give gifts in normal circumstances is demonstration of power.[62] But where the gift enables the donee to fulfil the deep desire for maternity, the power implications are even greater, for any prospects of reciprocity are missing; it is the sort of gift that cannot be returned in any way.[63] It may be argued that this is a major objection to inter-familial donations. It may also be argued that it leads to a further objection in that such a disequilibrium may disturb normal family relationships. Do family secrets distort conventional beliefs about how a family should function? These may well be valid objections. Certainly there are intuitive feelings that these disturbances may occur, though as yet there is no evidence one way or the other. Much may depend on how far the 'secret' of a child's origins is allowed to extend. But confidentiality on the part of the donor cannot be guaranteed. This is not an area where the murky waters of a breach of confidence action are likely to, or should, flow.[64] If the donor is considered in law to be, or to remain, the mother, she will, of course, technically have legal responsibilities. Whether or not this is held to be the case, she may well feel social or moral responsibilities towards the child. This may be a good thing but it may also lead to interference, jealousy, to conflict and even to rivalry. What if the donation does not turn out as anticipated and a handicapped child is born or there is an unexpected multiple birth or there are birth complications? The consequences of this for family relationships, supports and obligations may be far-reaching.

The relationship of the husband (assuming the donee is married)[65] to his wife's sister (the donor) is complex. He knows that 'his' child is genetically also that of his sister-in-law. The Victorians were anxious to distance men from their wives' sisters: legislation to allow marriage with the sister of a deceased wife was resisted for decades.[66] Perhaps they embodied 'thoughts' that lay 'too deep for tears' (in Wordsworth's memorable phrase).[67] Certainly, they feared what the same poet called 'strange fits of passion'.[68] Our awareness of sexual abuse has been heightened by the Cleveland affair.[69] It should also alert us to the possibilities of exploitation inherent in sexual relationships.[70] It is as well not to ignore these latent dangers in considering whether to allow egg donations between sisters. In addition, whatever the relationship of the husband to the sister-in-law, the child's perception of the relationship and his own cognitive and emotional understanding of his own identity may cause him concern and disturbance, and may lead to the conclusion that such a use of biotechnology is not in the child's best interests. It will be recalled that the British Voluntary Licensing Authority's main reason for urging caution (in its second report) emphasized this very consideration.

A key factor here is whether the child is told and, if so, what. As indicated earlier in this chapter, the case against divulging information appears strong when the general non-relative donation is in question. Do different considerations prevail in the context of a donation between sisters or other close relatives? Research by Dr Virginia Bolton at King's College Hospital, reported at the joint VLA/King's Fund Centre meeting in September 1988, found that, whilst a majority of those questioned were in favour of the availability of egg donations and a significant number (over a third) believed that a relative could be a donor, many of those who were not against the use of known donors were nevertheless against the donor having a continuing relationship with the child, or the child learning of the donation.[71] This reflects an ambivalence towards the known donor, which ought to be taken into account. One could argue that the child must know his 'cousin' is genetically his sister if for no other reason than that cousins may marry and siblings may not. Although marriage must be seen as a remote contingency, and therefore not a major consideration in any calculation, if donation between sisters or other close relatives is to be allowed, there should be openness and honesty. The extent of what is told, and when, must depend on individual circumstances and counselling may assist those involved. In most cases it will be better for the functioning of the family if secrets are not bottled up; in any case it is impossible to prevent someone telling and an 'unofficial leak' in anger or at the wrong time could do irreparable damage to the child. A belief that the child's welfare must be paramount dictates that, where donation between sisters or close relatives is allowed, the child should be told. Here we can draw on the accumulative wisdom of the adoption process where nowadays openness is unquestioned.

This, however, is on the assumption that we allow egg donation between close relatives. On balance the counter arguments are the weightier and at the very least extreme caution should prevail.

CONCLUSION

There is a legal minefield ready to explode under the egg donation revolution. This chapter has surveyed some, but far from all, of the questions that the development of ovum donation provokes. The issue of professional negligence (the liability of a clinic to a child born deformed as a result of negligence) is not unique to egg donation and has not been discussed. Again, it is an example of where legislation (in this case the Congenital Disabilities (Civil Liability) Act of 1976) antedates developments and not surprisingly fails to foresee them.[72] The Human Fertilization and Embryology Act 1990 has, however, attempted to tackle the question by extending the 1976 Act to cover infertility treatments.[73] But the new provision creates almost as many problems as it solves.[74] One, in particular, may be noted here. In order to commence proceedings it will often be necesarry to identify the genetic parent, in other words to trace the donor. It is clear from the Act that she herself may be liable, in addition to the treatment centre. On the application of the child the court may make an order[75] requiring the new Authority to disclose registered information such that the donor could be identified. Once again such a person becomes a 'parent'. Questions of the donor's knowledge may well be relevant, since defences in the 1976 Act apply,[76] but this would seem to be the case only if the donor is the 'mother' and the new legislation in general makes it clear that she is not. Neither has the legal status of the surplus or spare embryo been addressed. Selective foeticide is technically abortion (although not covered by the Abortion Act) but is not murder (the spare embryo is not regarded as 'life in being').[77] These questions require articles in themselves.

Enough has been written to show that the legal implications of egg donation have been neglected. The reasons for this are worth considering briefly. In part the answer lies in the rapid developments which have taken place in biotechnology. For example, human oocyte cryopreservation was not developed as a technique until 1985, a year after the Warnock Report was published. Warnock was thus able to use difficulties in egg collection and storage as a reason to make an exception to the principle of donor anonymity 'where the egg was donated by a sister or close friend'.[78] The complexity of the subject matter may also explain the lack of concern. Surrogacy, by contrast, is straightforward and readily comprehensible. A third reason may be the absence, at least until the Tennessee 'custody' battle in 1989,[79] of a *cause célèbre*. Scandal is known to be a great motivator of legislation. It causes moral panics and it hurtles legislatures into action. Surrogacy had 'Baby Cotton' in Britain and the Mary Beth Whitehead case in the USA. Disputes between the VLA and the Humana Wellington Hospital hardly merit the same attention. Hitherto, other techniques (such as surrogacy and AID) have led to disputes and to litigation. Problem cases have been tested in courts. Most of the questions considered in this chapter have not troubled the courts — as yet: this is a fourth reason why it may be that so little attention has been given to the legal issues surrounding egg donation. Finally, it may be surmised that it is confidence in the medical profession which has shielded many of the issues surrounding ovum donation from public attention and scrutiny. Should these questions now be raised, as is likely, focus on the legal problems will surely follow.

NOTES

1. Singer, P. and Wells, D. (1984), *The Reproduction Revolution: New Ways of Making Babies*, Oxford: Oxford University Press.
2. A good account is Robert H. Blank (1990), *Regulating Reproduction*, Columbia University Press. Appendix 1 is a helpful list of legislation and reports. See also Bonnicksen, A. L. (1989), *In Vitro Fertilization*, Columbia University Press.
3. See Field, M. A. (1988), *Surrogate Motherhood: The Legal and Human Issues*, Cambridge, Mass.: Harvard University Press; Chester, P. (1988), *Sacred Bond: The Legacy of Baby M*, Times Books; Morgan, D., 'Surrogacy: an Introductory Essay', in R. Lee and D. Morgan (eds) (1989), *Birthrights*, Routledge, pp. 55–84. On the case for surrogacy see Shalev, C. (1989), *Birth Power*, New Haven: Yale University Press.
4. 'The only chance of their having a child which the woman can carry to term, and which is the genetic child of her husband' per Warnock Report, *Committee of Inquiry into Human Fertilization and Embryology*, Cmnd. 9314, HMSO, 1984, para.6.5. See also Sauer, M. V. *et al.* (1990), *New England Journal of Medicine*, **323**, 1157–60.
5. As reported at joint meeting of the VLA (as it then was) and King's Fund Centre in London, September 1988.
6. See the *Observer*, 14 May 1989.
7. Guideline 13(j).
8. See *The Independent*, 19 May 1989; the *Guardian*, 19 May 1989. Corea, G. (1988), *The Mother Machine*, Women's Press, is highly dubious of supposed consent (see p. 135n.2).
9. See Kemeter, P., Feichtinger, W. and Bernat, E. 'The Willingness of Infertile Women to Donate Eggs', in W. Feichtinger and P. Kemeter (eds) (1987), *Future Aspects in Human In Vitro Fertilization*, Berlin: Springer-Verlag, pp.145–53. Though Brazier, M. (1987), *Medicine, Patients and the Law*, Harmondsworth: Penguin, regards this practice as 'of dubious legality' (p. 193). If there is true informed consent, it is difficult to see why she should think this.
10. But see Trounson, A. *et al.* (1983), 'Pregnancy established in an infertile patient after transfer of a donated embryo', *British Medical Journal*, **286**, 835. Attempts to prohibit the practice in Britain were successfully resisted (see *Hansard*, H. L., 6 February 1990, col. 805). The argument offered in favour is that it is of great importance to research into pre-implantation diagnosis.
11. Op. cit., note 4, para. 7.5. For other problems involved see Bustillo *et al.* (1984). 'Non-Surgical Ovum Transfer as a Treatment in Infertile Women' *J. Am. Med. Assoc.* **251**, 1171.

12   Voluntary Licensing Authority for Human In Vitro Fertilization and Embryology, *First Report*, 1986, VLA, London, para. 5.10.

13   Idem.

14   Voluntary Licensing Authority for Human In Vitro Fertilization and Embryology, *Second Report*, 1987, VLA, London, p.8.

15   In the Warnock Report (op. cit., note 4); a DHSS Consultation Document (*Legislation on Human Infertility Services and Embryo Research*, 1986, HMSO, London); the final report of the DHSS, *Human Fertilization and Embryology: A Framework for Legislation*, Cm. 259, HMSO, London, 1987, as well as in some academic literature (for example Frances Price, 'Establishing Guidelines: Regulation and Clinical Management of Infertility', in R. Lee and D. Morgan, *op. cit.*, note 3, pp. 37–54 (particularly pp. 46–9 and Brazier, M. (1987), *Medicine, Patients and the Law*, London: Harmondsworth, pp. 192–5).

16   Op. cit., note 4, para.6.8.

17   See Åke Saldeen, 'Sweden: Some Status Reforms', in (1990) *Journal of Family Law*, **28**, 619–21.

18   The Voluntary Licensing Authority has renamed itself the Interim Licensing Authority (see its *Fourth Report*, 1989, p. 2). The guidelines are, therefore, now those of the ILA, though most references in this article are to the VLA, where that is more apposite.

19   'Artificial conception: The challenge for Family Law' (1983), *Virginia Law Review*, **69**, 465–514, at p. 477.

20   Mason, J. K. and McCall Smith, R. A. (1987), *Law and Medical Ethics*, London: Butterworths, p. 47. But a recent 'twin' study by Thomas J. Bouchard *et al.* (1990), *Science*, **250**, (12 October), p. 223) on the importance of the genetic over the environmental may call this into question, although the authors themselves do not make major claims for their research to date.

21   Op. cit., note 4, para. 6.8.

22   Status of Children (Amendment) Act 1984 s. 10E (2).

23   Artificial Conception Act 1985 ss. 5(1), 7(1). See also NSW (Artificial Conception Act 1984); South Australia (Family Relationships Amendment Act 1984); Tasmania (Status of Children Amendment Act 1984); Northern Territory (Status of Children Amendment Act 1985); Capital Territory (Artificial Conception Ordinance 1985).

24   See *Re W* [1971] AC 682.

25   Illegitimate children take on birth the domicile of their mothers. See Dicey, A. V. and Morris, J. (1987), *The Conflict of Laws*, London: Stevens, pp. 125–8.

26   And see *Hansard*, H. L., (26 June 1986): debate on Third Reading of Surrogacy Arrangements (Amendment) Bill 1986.

27   By Jacob, J. (1990) 'Human Fertilization and Embryology Act 1990', *Current Law Statutes Annotated*, Sweet and Maxwell, p. 59.

28   See Law Commission, *Illegitimacy*, Law Com. no. 118, London: HMSO, 1982.

29   Research by Erikson (1986) referred to by Dr Bridget Mason at a Conference on 'Assisted Conception and the Law: A Medical/Legal Forum', Royal Society of Medicine, 5 June 1989. According to this it has led to more using AID facilities abroad and to more illegal activity.

30   See, further, McWhinnie, A. (1990), 'Visit To Sweden', unpublished paper, Dept. of Social Work, Dundee University.

31   Op. cit., note 4, para 4.21. See, further, Family Care (1988), *Truth and the Child*, Edinburgh, and Walby, C. and Symons, B. (1990), *Who Am I?*, British Agencies for Fostering and Adoption, ch. 5; O'Donovan, in R. Lee and D. Morgan (eds) (1989), *Birthrights*, Routledge, pp. 96–114, and Haimes, E. (1988), *Int. J. of Law and the Family*, **2**, 46–61.

32   What percentage are not cannot be known (unless there is blanket genetic finger-printing). All sorts of figures are quoted. In Birmingham in the early 1970s one piece of research suggested that the figure might be as high as *30 per cent*. The research has not been published: indeed, it is possible that it may have been suppressed.

33   See s.4 operative in 1989. With the coming into force in 1991 of the Children Act 1989 they will be able to acquire 'parental responsibility' as it will be called (see s.4 of that Act) by agreement with the mother, as well as by court order.

34   With the implementation of ss. 12 and 17 of the Family Law Reform Act 1987 (in April 1989).

35   Including from the then Chief Rabbi (Lord Jakobovits) (1984), *Human Fertilisation and Embryology – A Jewish View*, London: Office of the Chief Rabbi.

36   The question whether AID constitutes adultery was never solved in England. But it arose (*inter alia*) in Canada (*Orford* v. *Orford* (1921) 59 DLR 251) where Orde J. described it as a 'monstrous act of adultery', in Scotland (*MacLennan* v. *MacLennan* 1958 SC 105) where Lord Wheatley stated it was not adultery 'although a grave breach of the marriage contract' and at least three times in the USA (*Hoch* v. *Hoch* (1945 and unreported, *Doornbos* v. *Doornbus* 139 NW 2d 844 (1956) and *People* v. *Sorensen* 437 P. 2d. 495 (1968) (only in *Doornbos* was AID held to constitute adultery). Justice McComb observed in *Sorensen*: 'the doctor may be a woman or the husband himself may administer the insemination by a syringe [and] the donor may be a thousand miles away or may even be dead'.

37   See Mead, M. (1961), 'Some Anthropological Considerations Concerning Natural Law', *Natural Law Forum*, **6**, 51.

38   See Cretney, S. (1984), *Principles of Family Law*, Sweet and Maxwell (4th edn) pp. 48–55. See, more generally, Bettelheim, B. (1977), *The Uses of Enchantment*, New York: Vintage Books.

39   On genetic attraction see Kirsta, A. (1989), 'A Family Affair', *Guardian*, 12 December, p. 21.

40   See Cohen, S. (1972), *Folk Devils and Moral Panics*, Paladin.

41   In England see Matrimonial Causes Act 1973, s. 11.

42   Legitimacy Act 1976, s. 1.

43   The 14th Amendment.

44   See p. 8. See also the *Guardian*, 20 May 1989.

45   *Davis* v. *Davis* 15 Family Law Reporter 2097 (26 September 1989): The trial decision. The appellate decision is reported at 1990 Tenn. App LEXIS 642.

46   By Annas, G. J. (1991), *Hastings Center Report*, **21(1)**, p. 35.

47   See Drury, S. B. (1982), 'Locke and Nozick on Property', *Political Studies*, vol. 30, pp. 28–41. Nozick's position is clear: 'Whoever makes something ... having bought or contracted for all other held resources used in the process ... is entitled to it' (*Anarchy, State and Utopia*, New York: Basic Books, 1974, p. 160).

48   *The Body as Property*, Allen Lane, 1981, p. 220.

49   (1987). para. 7. 17.

50   I discuss these in 'After Warnock – Whither the Law?' (1986), *Current Legal Problems*, **39**, 33.

51   Para. 5.10.

52   Page 8.

53   Pp. 15–16.

54   Page 16.

55   Illustrated clearly in Channel Four's *Mother's Day*, transmitted on 23 March 1990. See also, as regards ethnic minorities, *Guardian*, 26 March 1990.

56   See Mnookin, R. (1975), *Law and Contemporary Problems*, **39 (3)**, 26.

57   Adoption Act 1976, s.6.

58   *Report of Department Committee on the Adoption of Children*, Cmnd 5107 (1972), London: HMSO.

59   Children Act 1975, s.10(3).

60   On which see Robertson, J. (1983), *Virginia Law Review*, **67**, 405–62 and (1986) *Southern California Law Review*, **59**, 942–1041.

61   See *The Lancet*, 1987.

62   See Mauss, M. (1954), *The Gift* (translated by I. Cussison), See also Levi-Strauss, C. (1969), *The Elementary Structures of Kinship*, London: Eyre and Spottiswoode. Gifts and the wide context of women's political inequality are discussed by Janice G. Raymond (1990) in *Hastings Center Report*, **20 (6)** 7–11.

63   See Finch, J. (1989), *Family Obligations and Social Change*, Polity Press, pp. 162–7. 'Reciprocity' in the context of egg donation was addressed by Finch at the VLA King's Fund conference. See op. cit, note 5.

64   Even after *Spycatcher*: see Jones, G., 'Breach of Confidence After Spycatcher' (1989), *Current Legal Problems*, **42**, 49.

65   Some guidance on the attitude of the English courts to an IVF clinic which limited treatment services to the married may be gleaned from *R* v. *St Mary's Hospital Manchester ex parte Harriot* [1988] 1 FLR 512. And see now Human Fertilization and Embryology Act 1990, s. 13(5) (account must be taken of the welfare of any child 'including the need of that child for a father').

66   See Turner, E. (1950), *Roads To Ruin*, London: Michael Joseph, ch. 6, and Twitchell, J. B. (1987), *Forbidden Partners*, Columbia University Press.

67   Intimations Ode.

68   In a poem of that name. See, further, Bateson, F. W. (1956), *Wordsworth: A Re-interpretation* (2nd edn), London: Longman.

69   See Freeman, M. D. A., 'Cleveland, Butler-Sloss and Beyond – How Are We To React To the Sexual Abuse of Children?' (1989), *Current Legal Problems*, **42**, 85.

70   See Ennew, J. (1986), *The Sexual Exploitation of Children*, Polity Press.

71   Perception differed between men and women, with men more reluctant to agree to the use of known donors, particularly relatives.

72   But see the case of Sandra Roberts, reported in *The Times*, 26 July 1986. Note also *B* v. *Islington Health Authority* [1991] 1 All ER 825, in which it has been held that pre-natal tortious liability to a child subsequently born alive existed prior to the 1976 Act at common law. The claim was 'contingent' and crystallized on the child's live birth.

73   See s.44.

74   See, further, Morgan, D. and Lee, R. G. (1991), *Blackstone's Guide To The Human Fertilization and Embryology Act 1990*, Blackstone, pp. 170–6.

75   See s.35.

76   In particular those in s.1(4) of the 1976 Act.

77   See Keown (1987), *New Law Journal*, **137**, pp. 1165–6.

78   Op. cit., note 4, para 6.7.

79   See op. cit., note 45.

10 Policy and Procreation: The Regulation of Reproductive Behaviour in the Third World

ANNE GRIFFITHS AND ANNE E. FINK

PROCREATION AND KINSHIP

The regulation of procreation in the Western world has in the past been concerned largely with the clarification and definition of family membership. The social value placed on biological parenthood which is embedded in Western society has clearly influenced much of that legislation in this area. There has been a presumption of biological paternity with regard to the relationship between a child and its mother's husband (*pater est quem nuptiae demonstrant*) and this principle continues to be operative, as exemplified by Scots law. However, there is always the possibility that the demonstration of alternative paternity by biological evidence can overrule the presumption.[1]

At another level, legal restriction on the immigration of 'children' of immigrants also demonstrates very clearly the importance placed on biological kinship. While other cultures define kinship in many different ways, in some cases as *all* the offspring of a couple *and* their siblings,[2] such definitions are unacceptable to British legislators. Indeed there have recently been a number of cases where families have tried to bring evidence based on newly developed genetic fingerprinting techniques in order to overrule decisions made by British immigration authorities who have assumed that the intending immigrants are defining 'children' by their own cultural norms.[3]

There has always been socially or legally defined parenthood in Western society in the form of foster and adoptive parents. While in the past such parents enjoyed unambiguous rights in relation to their children, in more recent times the emphasis on 'biological' parenthood in the Western world has led to an assertion of the 'rights' of children to access to information about their families of origin.[4] Since 1960, advances in pharmaceutical and medical technology have provided women with convenient and safe means of determining their own fertility, and these developments have raised new issues. The rights of men to decide on the outcome of the conceptions they have engendered and the right to life of the unborn child are seen, in some quarters, as conflicting with the right of the woman to make decisions on matters affecting her own body – something on which the Church, as well as the state, has had much to say.

During this past decade, medical science has made further advances, and the issues arising from the techniques employed in resolving problems of infertility have become a focus for much debate. Again, the value attached to biological parenthood is clearly central to this issue. With the development of techniques such as AID and IVF and the practice of surrogacy, we have had, in the West, to confront directly the fact that genetic and social parenting can be separated. Such activities involve three individuals: a couple who wish to have a child but are infertile and a third party who rectifies the position through the provision of semen, eggs or a womb. For the first time we are faced with the position that a woman who gives birth may not be the genetic mother of the child (*genetrix*). The reassessment of roles and obligations that such developments involve was considered in detail in the UK by the Committee of Inquiry Into Human Fertilization and Embryology (Warnock Committee)[5] whose recommendations are now the subject of legislation.[6]

Infertility is also experienced in the Third World but, in many societies in this area, biological parenthood has a less important function in defining kinship than in the West. Five different forms of parenting have been distinguished in traditional societies.[7]

1. *Biological.* Here, the parents are the *genitor* and *genetrix*.
2. *Social.* In this case, the child's parents are defined according to the rules of that society. 'Ghost marriage' among the Nuer, as described by Evans Pritchard, is one example of this sort of socially or culturally defined parenthood,[8] just as foster and adopting parents in Western cultures are distinguished as the social or legal parents.
3. *Nurturing.* In some societies, at some stages of the child's life, the biological or social parent is of less importance than is the nurturing parent. In some Muslim societies, it is the father who decides which woman will feed the child. A sum of money is set aside during the woman's pregnancy specifically to ensure payment for this service. While in most cases it is the biological mother, it can happen that another woman is chosen. The

woman who bears the child must be paid for her services just as if she were a chosen wet nurse.[9]

In some societies where wet nursing is practised, children not related biologically but nursed by the same woman are termed 'milk siblings' and, while not specifically prohibited from marriage and sexual relations, enjoy a spiritual relationship with one another similar to those who have godparents in common; and marriage in this circumstance would not be considered appropriate. Such children may also have the same obligations to their 'milk' parents as they would to their natural or social parents.[10]

It is also common practice in traditional societies for couples with many children to share their offspring with childless kin, including elderly relatives whose households have become childless or with wealthier kin who are obligated by the cultural norms of those societies to share with the biological parents the burdens incumbent on rearing children. Responsibility for the upbringing of children varies widely throughout the traditional societies of the Third World. In parts of Africa, the mother's brother plays a far more important role than does her husband or the biological father of the child.[11]

4. *Education*. Yet another form of parenting which has been distinguished is that of the parent/educator. Whereas in the developed world a wide variety of institutions such as schools, colleges and universities train young people in the skills and occupations which they will require in order to survive in their society, in the underdeveloped areas of the world these skills are imparted either by the parents or by other adults who have been selected by the parents to train their child.[12]

    Apprenticeship in Great Britain and Europe from medieval times until the late nineteenth century might have been similarly characterized, the apprenticed child retaining an obligation for life to his or her master or mistress.[13]

5. *Sponsorship*. The fifth form of parenting has been termed 'sponsorship' and may be spiritual, as is the case in godparenthood; or social, political and economic, as is common in many societies in Central and South America where the *Compadrazgo* or godparenthood combines elements of all four.[14]

With so many different strategies available for the formation of kinship relations, the problems of infertility, as experienced in the Western cultures, assume far less importance in most parts of the Third World. In those societies, however, where a woman's marital status depends on her providing her husband with a child, infertility may assume an even greater significance.

FERTILITY AND POPULATION CONTROL

In other areas of the world the problem is not so much individual infertility but, rather, problems arising from diminishing populations due to the rapid decline in birthrates after the Second World War. The socialist countries of Central and Eastern Europe had adopted pro-natalist policies which maintain both fertility and population growth at high levels. They have fostered legislation against abortion, sterilization and the production, importation and distribution of contraceptive devices as well as the provision of financial incentives to women to reproduce. In the 1960s a number of countries tightened up their abortion laws. Romania, for example, prohibited induced abortion in 1966.[15] Since 1962 abortion laws in Czechoslovakia have become more restrictive; permission not only involves medical approval but also requires the consent of the local abortion commission. Since the 1970s these commissions have been officially urged to limit the number of applications that they will accept. A further disincentive is provided by the fact that the service is no longer free.[16]

Such measures have been complemented by attempts at the positive reinforcement of fertility. These include the introduction of maternity allowances, preferential tax rates and housing benefits for those with large families. In these countries population problems are considered part of a broader socioeconomic context.

In contrast, the overriding concern of Third World policymakers is overpopulation. At the 1984 Mexico City International Conference on Population, 147 governments expressed their support for voluntary programmes to help their citizens control their fertility. There is an explicit recognition that policies, laws and programmes which influence fertility are an integral part of efforts to promote social and economic development.[17] However, not all countries with high fertility rates necessarily perceive increases in population as a problem for development. This issue has aroused strong feelings in the past, with some countries taking the view that population control is an example of a capitalist-inspired conspiracy – an imperialist intervention. At the World Population Conference in Bucharest in 1974 a number of countries contested the view that overpopulation was the cause of underdevelopment and argued instead that what was required was a restructuring of the world economy. Roman Catholic countries, such as Argentina, formed an alliance with the Eastern bloc communist and African nations to oppose the Draft World Population Plan aimed at reducing fertility rates, submitted to the conference, in favour of a much broader perspective involving the transformation of international economic relations and the redistribution of resources and power between the industrial nations and the developing nations of the Third World. This arguing for a restructuring of the international system meant that the political nature of population control was directly confronted and the conference became polarized between those countries, such as Algeria, which advocated such an approach and those, such as the United States, which were vehemently opposed.[18]

There is also considerable divergence between the perceptions of governments, international aid agencies and individual citizens in those countries where overpopulation is claimed to be inhibiting development. For subsistence-farming families, eking out a precarious existence in the Third World countries whose governments cannot provide economic security for old age or disability, the need for children to provide such security is obvious. Studies of individuals' perceived needs reveal that in India, for example, rural couples report the need to have at least six children if they are to be secure in their old age. Such couples argued that at least four adult children were needed to ensure that the burden of caring for the parents should not be too onerous. Given the prevailing child mortality rates when this study was conducted, this common wisdom was not unrealistic.[19]

The perception of an ideal finite number of children per family is one which sits strangely in many societies. Where children are seen as a measure of male sexual potency, as is the case in parts of rural Mexico, a woman who tries to limit her childbearing may find herself deserted in favour of another woman who is willing to bear children.[20] In urban areas of Central and South America and in the Caribbean, many women survive economically only by making a 'career' of motherhood. In these societies where relationships are often very short-term, unskilled job opportunities are scarce and literacy levels low, women have little alternative. The only way in which they can ensure economic support is by bearing a child. Financial provision is made by a series of men, each one staying while his child is in its infancy. Where social service provision does exist in these areas it reinforces and enhances this pattern of dependency by offering support dependent upon, and proportionate to, the number of dependent children.[21]

The number of children born in any society will reflect not only individuals' perceived economic needs and desires but also the social and cultural norms of that society. If male children are valued, whether it is in order to provide for the needs of elderly parents, to perpetuate the family line or to ensure adherence to the rituals of ancestor worship, the completed family numbers will reflect this preference; the pattern will be similar if female children are valued for any particular social or economic reason. In those societies where bride-price and dowries accompany marriage it may be necessary for couples to ensure even numbers of male and female children in order to be able to afford to fund their marriages. Legislating against such customs in order to control fertility appears to have had little success.[22]

Policies, laws and programmes aimed at regulating reproductive behaviour in the Third World are wide-ranging and have included legalizing the distribution of contraceptives as in the Cameroons, Mali and Mexico; widening the categories of workers who are allowed to supply contraceptive devices as in Barbados, India and Sri Lanka; easing import requirements as in Bangladesh and Egypt; allowing increased public information and advertising of contraceptives as in Brazil and Haiti; and providing services and/or education for young people as in Costa Rica and the Philippines.[23]

Many countries have established national population policymaking or coordinating mechanisms at a high governmental level to ensure that policies are implemented. There is great diversity worldwide in the form that these mechanisms take, but at least three distinct types of administrative body can be identified — technical units, interministerial and family planning coordinating councils. In many Asian countries, small technical units are placed at a high level of government to ensure that demographic considerations are included in development planning. In Latin American and African countries, however, interministerial councils are more popular because policies are often still in the process of formulation. The function of these councils is to develop, monitor and, in some cases, coordinate population policies. Countries such as Indonesia and Mexico have favoured family planning coordinating councils which have a role in coordinating funding and even implementing the government's family planning programme.[24]

National policies aimed at controlling population growth encourage the proliferation of family planning programmes. These programmes may form part of a government's national health service or, alternatively, be administered by private organizations funded in part by the state. In either case they are likely to be receiving assistance from external sources. In most developing countries, government family planning expenditures are supplemented by assistance from donor countries provided directly or indirectly through international organizations such as the United Nations' Fund for Population Activities (UNFPA) and the International Planned Parenthood Federations (IPPF) which assists private family planning associations. According to a World Bank Report, by 1984 external aid had accounted for approximately a quarter of all family planning costs in developing countries.[25] Through the receipt of such aid, governments become directly or indirectly vulnerable to external pressure concerning their policies in this area.

In China and some South-east Asian countries policies in the form of economic incentives at family and community level have been introduced to encourage individuals to control their fertility. In China, where the government is promoting the goal of the one-child family, benefits are the largest and most varied. Parents of a one-child family are eligible for better housing, better jobs, an additional monthly stipend, more land and eventually higher pensions.[26]

At the community level, governments throughout Asia encourage private employers to provide incentives to employees who are sterilized or who follow small family norms. In South Korea, businesses are offered specific tax exemptions for this purpose.[27] In Thailand, private sector programmes, organized by Mechai Viravaidya, pioneered income-generating incentives for rural communities, which included low-interest loans and access to direct marketing services for community products made available free or at a discount to family planning users.[28] In some cases, punitive measures have been introduced where individuals have failed to cooperate with government edicts. In China, for each third and subsequent child, a monthly charge is levied; the child's opportunities for education and employment may be threatened and previously paid benefits must be returned.[29]

More indirect measures affecting fertility control have also been enacted. The legal minimum age of marriage has been raised by at least 50 countries over the last two decades. India raised the minimum age for marriage from 18 to 21 for men and from 15 to 18 years for women in 1978.[30] Introducing compulsory education or extending the number of years of existing compulsory education has also proved to be an effective means of delaying and ultimately reducing women's fertility.[31]

LACTATION: A QUESTION OF HEALTH OR FERTILITY CONTROL?

Although governments often perceive the need for fertility regulation in terms of problems of overpopulation, overseas aid agencies may claim that they are introducing and providing measures of fertility control in order to safeguard the health of women and children. Maternal mortality is still high in many areas of the Third World, with the risks increasing in proportion to the number of conceptions experienced. International agencies such as the World Health Organization (WHO) claim that infant mortality and morbidity are related to family size. Although statistics from Third World countries are not reliable, the risk of infant and child mortality does appear to rise with birth order.[32]

International agencies also decree that individuals should have the basic human right to determine their own family size, but their claims regarding the need to limit family size in order to protect maternal health, as well as that of children, sometimes ring false in the light of the policies actually advocated. Perhaps the most famous and controversial of these policies has been the attempt by the WHO to ban the advertisement and distribution of baby milk formulae in Third World countries.[33]

The vigorous campaign against the manufacturers of infant formula products initiated in 1973 and promoted by the WHO is still active today. The controversy generated by the issue of breast milk substitutes continues to cause debate,[34] and provides a striking example of the power that international agencies possess to generate and direct policies concerning fertility by determining the issues that they consider to be of crucial importance in this area. Through the machinery of the UN, the WHO had the contacts, resources and a platform from which it could mobilize an effective campaign against the producers of infant feeding formulae. Not only did this activity result in a legal battle featuring Nestlé SA[35] but it also led to the adoption by the World Health Assembly of an unprecedented international code. The code of marketing breast milk substitutes was the product of meetings held by WHO between 1979 and 1981.[36]

The response to the code has varied. The Commonwealth Secretariat, an international organization based in London, produced a guide to implementing the code for Commonwealth countries and a draft model of legislation. Control of infant formula products has been exercised in a number of different ways. Some countries, such as Malaysia and Singapore, have introduced voluntary codes to deal with this situation. Others, such as Lesotho and Tanzania, are extending and amending existing legislation or introducing new legislation. In 1981, Guyana introduced a ban on the import of infant formula products and Papua New Guinea introduced legislation regulating the supply of bottles and teats and controlling the display of advertisements and the purchase and use of milk substitutes in connection with bottles and teats.[37]

Other governments have done little to implement the code which they approved, and have left the impression that the issue is only a live one at an international level.[38] To dismiss the debate on this basis is shortsighted. It is important because some countries, albeit a minority of those who approved the code, have taken action. They have done so on the basis of expertise presented with the full weight of the authority of international organizations. This expertise is, however, open to question.

The debate between the WHO and Nestlé SA focused primarily on the issue of the dangers posed to child health by the use of breast milk substitutes.[39] Another aspect of this campaign has been the promotion of lactation as a fertility control measure. Policies currently being pursued in Third World countries which promote lactation are viewed as primarily a means of improving maternal and child health and decreasing infant mortality rates, but are also being vigorously pursued because lactation, it is argued, is an effective means of controlling overall population growth. The emphasis on lactation as a 'natural' means of effecting demographic change arose in response to the criticism of policies adopted in the 1960s. The widespread distribution of steroid hormones, whose long-term effects were at the time largely unknown, led to allegations that the Third World was being used as a human laboratory for the large pharmaceutical companies. It is claimed that the multinational pharmaceutical companies have had undue influence on family planning policies because it is cheaper for governments to invest in chemical solutions than in major changes in social infrastructure.[40]

In the West, problems with IUD devices, and the non-acceptability of long-acting injectables such as Depo-Provera, alerted critics to the dangers facing participants in the many family planning programmes which promoted this technology in the underdeveloped nations.[41]

Draconian programmes of compulsory vasectomy, such as those promoted by Sanjay Gandhi in India,[42] drew so much hostile criticism that international agencies were finally forced to look for more acceptable means to achieve their aims. The promotion of lactation appeared to be a solution. Of all the funding agencies, the WHO has been especially active in the encouragement of breastfeeding policies.[43]

The policy of promoting lactation in order to control population growth is based on dubious scientific theory regarding the relationship between lactation and fecundity,[44] and an inadequate statistical model of breastfeeding and birth spacing.[45] The relationship between lactation and fertility is a complex one and maternal nutrition is a variable which also has to be taken into account in promoting such a policy.[46] The biological relationship between nutrition, lactation and fertility is still not fully comprehended; and social and psychological factors are involved, as well as physiological and biochemical mechanisms. There is evidence that policies promoting lactation as a means of population control can lead to negative consequences for both maternal and child health.[47]

The 'Breast is Best' policy involves restrictions on the advertising, distribution and availability of breast milk substitutes. Infant milk formulae are alleged to endanger child health, especially in areas where water supplies are contaminated. Women in the Third World are often thought to be ignorant of the techniques needed to maintain necessary hygiene and, because of widespread illiteracy, unable to follow directions for mixing formulae correctly. In following the International Code of Practice many countries have made it impossible for women to have access to breast milk substitutes and health workers in these countries discourage women from seeking advice about alternatives to breastfeeding.

Social anthropological micro studies reveal that, in fact, a variety of factors other than continuous lactation contribute to limiting family size in underdeveloped countries. Abstinence resulting from postpartum cultural taboo and/or migrant labour, birth trauma and sterility; illness and infertility caused by sexually transmitted diseases, parasitic infection and the widespread incidence of malaria, tuberculosis and bilharzia in Third World countries, as well as the resulting anaemia, have all been implicated. Nothing is known about the rate of spontaneous abortion, little information is available on the number of stillbirths and the statistics of infant mortality are dubious and probably nearly always underestimated. Infanticide is practised in many societies.[48]

Biologists may disagree about the effects of maternal nutrition on female fecundity and the ability to breastfeed but the accumulating evidence from anthropological fieldwork observations points to its importance in explaining at least some aspects of reproductive performance. Anthropologists have also shown that women's nutrition in traditional societies not only depends on the availability of food but also on the social and cultural determinants of eating and feeding behaviour. Breastfeeding is like any other form of eating or feeding behaviour and is equally culturally determined.[49]

In the biological and bioanthropological literature, five lines of argument appear to be current in the discussion relating lactation to fertility and nutrition.[50]

1. Frequent and prolonged lactation stimulates the secretion of high levels of plasma prolactin (PRL), a hormone which inhibits luteinizing hormone (LH) which in turn inhibits ovulation. This thesis is supported by data collected from studies of the !Kung Bushman women in the Kalahari desert,[51] as well as from studies by Wood et al., working with the Gaing in Highland New Guinea,[52] and women studied by Howie in Scotland.[53]

    Roger Short, a reproductive biologist, and an advisor to the WHO with considerable influence on their policies, has been, and continues to be, an active campaigner for the promotion of lactation as a fertility control measure on the strength of this evidence.[54] However data gathered in a traditional community in Central America where women breastfeed continuously and whose PRL levels were comparable to those quoted for the

Gaing and higher than those of Scottish women do not support the thesis.[55]

2. The second hypothesis is that there is a necessary threshold of percentage body fat which must be attained before either menarche or ovulation can be achieved.[56] Howell, working with the same group of !Khung Bushman women as Konner and Worthman on whose data the first hypothesis is based, claims that *her* data demonstrate that the lactational amenorrhoea which Konner claimed was due to frequency of nipple stimulation and the resulting high levels of PRL only persisted while body fat weight was low.[57]

    The data gathered by Fink in Central America support Howell's claims. There *is* a significant negative correlation between the index of body weight and height and the ability to conceive among Mayan women. Menstruation is, however, not affected by this factor, nor are PRL levels.[58]

3. Lunn, Whitehead and others, working in the Gambia, claim that PRL plays an important role not only in the stimulation and secretion of breast milk but also in its metabolism. Women who are poorly nourished secrete, they claim, higher levels of PRL than those who enjoy a better diet, and these resulting high levels of PRL are responsible for inhibiting ovulation.[59] Their observations have not been supported by other investigators.

4. A variation of this argument is that poorly nourished mothers secrete less milk with a lower fat content which is less satisfying to the child, causing it to suckle more often and more vigorously, thus raising PRL levels and prolonging lactational amenorrhoea and conception. Studies conducted in Guatemala among poorly nourished rural peasant women appear to support this thesis.[60] The data in this study are similar to those gathered by Fink in Belize,[61] but can be interpreted in various ways. Delay in the onset of menses and raised levels of PRL are associated in both studies. In neither Guatemala nor Belize, however, are the interbirth intervals as long as those reported for the Gaing in New Guinea or among the !Kung in the Kalahari, although PRL levels are comparable. Other factors such as miscarriage, stillbirth, infanticide and sexual abstinence are possible involved, as well as nutritional status, the sort of food eaten and energy expenditure levels.[62] Contrary to Short's continuing claim,[63] lactational amenorrhoea appears to be no barrier to conception in the village of San Jose in Belize, where Fink has shown only 30 out of 81 women experienced menstrual cycles before conceiving. These data were based on close observation of the women in the course of social anthropological fieldwork investigation carried out over a two-year period.[64]

5. Finally, Warren argues that sympathetic activation such as anxiety may also be a contributory factor in raising energy expenditure. These metabolic perturbations and their possible relation to hormone secretion, nutrition and reproductive regulation have never been investigated. She looks at the data derived from athletes and ballet dancers whose low body fat ratios have also been used in support of Frisch's theory's.[65]

    None of these theories are mutually exclusive and some may be interactive.

Among the Mopan Maya women of San Jose in Southern Belize, Fink found that lactation alone did not serve as an effective method of birth control. Nearly all the infants were fed for 18 months, at frequent intervals during the day and continuously throughout the night. Interbirth intervals were on average 28 months long and completed family size was approaching 9–10 children surviving to adulthood, the maximum number experienced by any society in the world. In the absence of any contraceptive method, birth trauma which causes maternal mortality and sterility and seasonal or ritual sexual abstinence appeared to be more effective factors in limiting population growth than did lactation.[66]

What did appear to be playing an important part in prolonging the period between births was the women's body mass weight as measured by the weight/height ratio which, it must be assumed, is related to the women's nutritional status. In this study infants are described as feeding frequently even when being supplemented with alternative milk products. (Women who supplement before their infants are nine months old have significantly lower weight/height ratios than do women who do not feel they have to supplement at this early stage.)[67]

The fact that the children feed as often as they do even when being supplemented may be the reason why Mopan Maya women do not resume their menstrual cycles as quickly as do Western women. Their raised levels of PRL may also be related to this behaviour but the fact that they do conceive even during the period of lactational amenorrhoea (the length of the delay depending on their weight/height ratio) shows that breastfeeding *alone* cannot delay conception for more than the few months shown for Western women,[68] and that significant delays in conception in traditional societies are more likely to be related to the woman's nutritional status *in conjunction* with her breastfeeding behaviour[69] as well as the many other factors already described.

Children in San Jose persist in breastfeeding even after supplementation has been offered. In the Western developed nations and in the cities of the Third World women report that supplementing stops the child feeding from the breast. In the village of San Jose supplementary foods are rarely satisfying for the child. Infants are given more or less the same foods as adults. These foods are difficult for a young child to handle and competition among siblings for the choicest foodstuffs often leaves the youngest child at a disadvantage. There are no special baby foods, nor do women prepare foods in such a way as to make them easier for an infant to handle or digest. Older children often supplement their own diet with gathered foods. There is a wide variety of nuts available in the village but this important source of protein is not accessible to the young infant.[70]

The lack of suitable baby foods probably accounts for the extended period of frequent breastfeeding found among other groups in rural areas. In Mexico, commercial soft drinks are not only easily available but also very aggressively marketed, even in the most remote villages. In these villages, infants do become more easily weaned from the breast, quickly acquiring a taste for the sweetened drink and rejecting the breast milk.[71]

In Mexico, as long as the infant is less than six months old, infant milk formula is supplied free of charge to women who feel that they cannot feed their infants. This policy has an unintended consequence in that, once acquired, the milk is often used by other children in the family and even by the mother herself, thereby providing a valuable supplement to the family diet. The need to supplement the infant may be only short-term while the mother or infant is unwell, or for a variety of culturally determined reasons which prohibit the mother feeding for a specific time. Attempts by the WHO to persuade the Mexican government to stop supplying this free milk supplement ignored both the reasons for its consumption and the benefits accruing to others in the household.[72]

Jenkins has shown that there are risks to infant health where breastfeeding continues beyond three months without supplementation in areas where women's nutrition is inadequate. In a study conducted in Belize, Jenkins shows that, after three months of age, the growth of rural Mayan infants is stunted and retarded as compared to other groups who have access to appropriate supplementary and alternative milk products.[73] The International Code of Practice which advises countries against allowing rural women access to commercial products for feeding infants, and to which Belize subscribes very diligently, may be held directly responsible for damaging these children's health and growth.

Many women in San Jose also suffer from maternal depletion syndrome. They are universally low in iron and their chronic lack of high energy protein makes them extremely vulnerable to complications in pregnancy. Toxaemia and incompetence of the womb which frequently occur in the village as a result of the women's inadequate diet and the stress of constant childbearing and breastfeeding can, and regularly do, result in maternal mortality.[74] In these conditions it is difficult to accept that 'Breast is Best' for either child or mother.

Perhaps the most reprehensible aspect of the WHO's policy of promoting lactation as a fertility control measure is the assumption that women in the Third World are so stupid and ignorant that they are easily swayed by persuasive advertising and are prepared to risk their children's health because of a glossy picture on a tin. Social anthropologists working closely with women in traditional societies in the Third World have observed that such women are excellent judges of their children's needs and are most unlikely to squander their very meagre disposable income on unnecessary items.[75] Fink observed that women only resorted to supplementing with infant formula or other products, if available, when the baby failed to thrive or when the mother was unable to feed for some reason. Certainly, reasons for not breastfeeding might be culturally, rather than physically determined. In the absence of commercial milk products other substitutes are, and always have been, used worldwide — rice water in India and South-east Asia, corn milk in Central and South America, for example. Fink points out that, in most societies, babies are not put to the breast for the first one to three days because, for a variety of cultural reasons, breast milk at this stage is thought to be dangerous for the child.[76]

In restricting access to infant formula products, agencies such as the WHO are ignoring real needs. In animal populations, as well as in human ones, a percentage of females are unable to lactate.[77] The prevalence of breast infections in tropical conditions, some of which can result in long-term damage to the breast, and the ability to feed must also be taken into account in promoting policies which deny women the right to feed their children with breast milk substitutes. The problem of the inhibition of the milk ejection reflex, which has been estimated to affect up to 15 per cent of all nursing mothers, must also be taken into account.[78]

The questionable relationship between nutrition, lactation and fertility and the complexity of the interaction of the many factors which have been shown to affect fecundity and fertility, as well as the health and well-being of women and children in traditional societies of undeveloped nations, shows how important is the need for careful social anthropological study in conjunction with biological investigation, especially when policies are to be pursued which purport to rely on biological expertise. Such policies must take into account the cultural, social, political, religious and economic diversity of societies in the Third World if they are to be acceptable and effective.

MARRIAGE, KINSHIP AND REPRODUCTIVE BEHAVIOUR

Social anthropologists have always been fascinated by the study of marriage, kinship and social structure. The rules regulating marriage and human reproductive behaviour in traditional societies have been studied intensely from the nineteenth century. For many early scholars the thrust of their enquiries was to demonstrate the universality and evolution of laws regarding marriage and reproductive behaviour from primitive to more 'civilized' societies.[79] Indeed, it was not until the 1970s that the concept of marriage as an organizing principle of traditional society began to be questioned.[80]

Close examination of the rules determining kinship and the regulation of marriage in South-east Asia and South America led social anthropologists such as Lévi-Strauss,[81] Leach,[82] Needham[83] and Rivière[84] to challenge the prevailing view that the function of the institution of marriage was primarily to legitimate children. Theories of marriage and kinship which had been based on the study of societies with strong lineage systems were found to be inadequate in the light of the more recent studies conducted outside Africa and where descent groups were of little importance. Rivière concludes, in his reassessment of the institution of marriage, that it is of no use as an analytic concept since it varies so remarkably from one society to another. Some might argue that, even if marriage is not simply a matter of legitimating children, as a social institution it ensures their well-being; but, among the Trio Amerindians of Surinam with whom Rivière worked, marriage is seen 'as bringing into existence a set of ordered rights and obligations which are mainly for the benefit of the aged'.[85]

Between 1982 and 1984, Griffiths worked with the Kwena, a group related to the Tswana in Botswana – a society for whom Schapera has characterized marriage as the central institution for the study of the family and on which the social structure of that society depends. Schapera found that children of formal marital unions belonged to the family of the woman's husband and, like so many others working in African societies, he saw marriage as ensuring legitimation and ordering of descent groups.[86] However, 50 years later, Griffiths found that the permanent unions as described by Schapera were no longer statistically the normal relationship and, while some women still held to the ideal of a marital union, bearing children was a frequent occurrence outside marriage or indeed any form of 'stable' relationship.[87] While the reasons for this change in reproductive behaviour are not clear, it has been suggested that economic and structural changes in the society have had a profound effect on what Schapera had argued was an inherent, core institution of that society. Griffiths' observations of childbearing among the

Kwena support Rivière's view that changes in social structure can affect changes in institutions such as marriage.

However in *all* societies — whether modern or traditional, developed or undeveloped — regulations, however varied, are imposed on human procreative behaviour. Rules permitting or prohibiting procreation between individuals exist, it has been suggested, for the purpose of maintaining social order. Such rules do not necessarily include sexual relations. The distinction between recreational and procreational sexual relations is an important one, and many biosocial as well as anthropological theories have been proposed to explain so-called incest taboos which derive from prohibitions on procreational sexual relations.

The pursuit of a universal definition of incest has been as futile as the search for a universal definition of marriage. Lévi-Strauss suggests that the incest taboo derives not from any perception of biological dangers, but from the need to regulate access to women — a view to which many other social anthropologists would adhere. What is important for social anthropologists is that rules do exist, whether or not they are primarily concerned with access to women, for their productive and/or reproductive capacities. These rules will reflect the underlying values of the particular society in which they are found and will therefore vary according to that society's system of values. Whether or not these regulations result in more or less children being born in any society is not the present issue. What is important is that the indigenous regulation of procreation is recognized.

CONCLUSION

We have discussed some of those laws, policies and programmes which have been introduced, and often imposed, on the poorer nations of the world by the richer and more powerful ones. The lack of attention paid to the many social anthropological studies of the social regulation of human reproduction in indigenous societies may explain why so many of these policies have failed.

The fact is that the economic, social and political stability of nearly all Third World countries continues to be threatened by their ever increasing populations. 'Natural' disasters, floods, droughts, hurricanes, crop failure, earthquakes, tidal waves and volcanic eruptions are compounded by the huge population losses and shifts which so often accompany these catastrophes.

Massive migration in search of work and food contributes towards elevation of tension and stress along already sensitive national borders — situations which can so easily erupt into full-scale warfare.

At the moment the only effective limits to population growth in much of the Third World appear to be the apocalyptic forces of Famine, Warfare, Pestilence and natural catastrophe.

But we do know, and have witnessed, how effective the introduction of education, particularly for women, healthcare for children, economic stability and *appropriate* social support systems can be in controlling population growth. China, Singapore and Taiwan have been singularly successful and the indications are that in many of the cities of the Third World, especially in Latin America, there is a change in the rate of population growth. The question that now needs to be addressed is why the measures we know to be effective cannot be more quickly implemented in all parts of the world.

NOTES

1. The concept of *pater est quem nuptiae demonstrant* has its origins in Roman Law. It was incorporated into the common law of Scotland and has recently been incorporated into s.5(1)(a) of the Law Reform (Parent and Child) (Scotland) Act 1986. In the case of *Docherty* v. *McGlynn* 1985 SLT 237, blood-test evidence became an issue where an attempt was made to challenge the presumption of paternity by a third party.

2. Among the Mopan Maya of Southern Belize a person will name all the children of him or herself plus all the children of his/her siblings as his or her child. For further discussion of the variety of ways in which societies define parenthood, see Fox, R. (1967), *Kinship and Marriage*, Harmondsworth: Penguin; Needham, R. (1971), 'Remarks on the analysis of kinship and marriage', in R. Needham (ed.), *Rethinking Kinship and Marriage*, London: Tavistock.

3. *R. v. Secretary of State for the Home Office, ex parte Rahman* (unreported) QBD CO/1388/88, 22 November 1988.

4. Social work and adopting agencies are now prepared to help children with information about their family of origin. In Scotland, children, on reaching the age of majority, have always had the right of access to their birth certificate, and this right has recently been extended to children in England, Wales and Northern Ireland.

5. Committee of Inquiry into Human Fertilization and Embryology (Warnock Committee), Cmnd 9314/1984.

6. Human Fertilization and Embryology Act 1990.

7. Goody, E. (1982), *Parenthood and Social Reproduction, Fostering and Occupational Roles in West Africa*, Cambridge University Press: Cambridge, p. 348.

8. Evans Pritchard, E. E. (1951), *Kinship and Marriage among the Nuer*, Oxford: Clarendon Press.

9. This practice is based on the story that the prophet Mohammed, who was born to a city-dwelling merchant family, was given to a desert woman to be wet-nursed, the milk of such a woman being considered to be more strength-inducing than that of his city-bred mother! cf. El Saadawi, N. (1980), *The Hidden Face of Eve: women in the Arab world*, London: Zed Press.

10. Ott, S. (1981), *The Circle of Mountains: A Basque Shepherding Community*, Oxford: Clarendon Press, p. 201.

11 Goody, op. cit., note 7 above.
12 In the Mopan Maya Amerindian community of San Jose in the Toledo District of Southern Belize, children are often sent to live in the childless homes of elderly relatives. It is these kin who teach the child the skills necessary for survival. The economic, social and psychological interdependence of such households is an important feature of the total social structure of the community: cf. Fink, A. E. (1988), *Food, Family and Ideology: some determinants of social and biological reproduction among the Mopan Maya of Southern Belize*, D. Phil. thesis, Oxford: Bodleian Library.
13 Shorter, E. (1973), *The Making of the Modern Family*, London: Fontana Books, pp. 35–7.
14 Nutini, H. G. and Bell, B. (1970), 'The structure and historical development of the *compradzgo* system in rural Tlaxcala', *Ritual Kinship*, **1**.
15 Macura, M. (1974), 'Population policies in socialist countries of Europe', *Population Studies*, part 3, pp. 369–79.
16 Heitlinger, A. (1976), 'Pro-natalist population in Czechoslovakia', *Population Studies*, Part 1, pp. 123–35; for further discussion, see chapter 4.
17 Population Reports (1984) Series E, no. 7, *Law and Policy*, Maryland: Johns Hopkins University, pp. 105–6.
18 Finkel, J. L. and Crane, B. B. (1975), 'The politics of Bucharest: population development and the new international economic order', *Population and Development Review*, **2(1)**, p. 87.
19 Gould, K. H. (1976), 'The twain never met: Sheruper, India and the family planning program', in J. Marshall and S. Polgar (eds), *Culture, Natality and Family Planning*, Chapel Hill: Carolina Population Center.
20 Fink, A. E. (1982), 'Aspects of Infant Nutrition in Two Mexican Rural Communities', unpublished M.Phil. thesis, Oxford University.
21 Massiah, J. (1983), *Women as Heads of Households in the Caribbean: family structure and feminine status*, Paris: UNESCO.
22 Epstein, T. S. (1973), *South India: yesterday, today and tomorrow*, London: Macmillan.
23 Population Reports (1984), E121–125, op. cit., note 17 above.
24 Ibid., E115–117.
25 World Bank (1984), *Development Report*, New York: Oxford University Press, p. 286.
26 Chen, P-C, and Kols, A. (1982), 'Population and birth planning in the People's Republic of China', *Population Reports*, Series J, **(25)**, p. 44.
27 International Labor Organization (1982), *Inter-Country Seminar on Incentives for Family Planning: family welfare in industrial sectors*; Puncak: ILO, p. 65.
28 David, H. P. (1982), 'Incentives, reproductive behaviour and integrated community development in Asia', *Studies in Family Planning*, **13(5)**, p. 159.
29 Chen, P-C., Tian, X-Y. and Tuan, C-H. (1982), '11m. Chinese opt for "one child glory certificate" ', *People*, **9(4)**, p. 12.
30 Child Marriage Restraint (Amendment) Act 1978 (India).
31 Harrison, D. (1981), 'The effect of education and wages on fertility: some evidence from Malaysia', *Department of Economics Seminar Papers No. 15/81*, Population Association of American Meetings, Melbourne: Monash University, p. 3.
32 Population Reports (1981), Series J, **(24)**, *Breast Feeding, Fertility and Family Planning*, J525–75.
33 Dobbing, J. (ed.) (1988), *Infant Feeding: anatomy of a controversy 1973–1984*, Berlin: Springer-Verlag.
34 'Nestlé Boycott', *298 British Medical Journal*, 1989, p. 702.
35 *Audienz des Gerichtspresidenten VIII von Bern. Forsetzung der Hauptverhandlung*

wegen Ehrverletzung, 22–24 June 1976. (Libel Proceedings Verbatim Record Bern 1976), tr. by G. J. Ebrahim.

36 In May 1980 the World Health Assembly endorsed the recommendation that there should be an international code of marketing infant formula and other products used as breast milk substitutes in Resolution WHA 31.47. In May 1981 the World Health Assembly adopted the code in resolution WHA 34.22.

37 *Action Guide: on implementing the International Code of Marketing Breastmilk Substitutes*, drawn up by the Commonwealth Secretariat, UNICEF, New York, in Association with WHO, 1983–84.

38 Dobbing, *Infant Feeding*, op. cit., note 33 above, p. vii.

39 Ibid.

40 Djerassi, C. (1975), 'Problems of manufacture and distribution. The manufacture of steroidal contraceptives: technical versus political aspects', *Proceedings of the Royal Society of London*, B195, p. 175.

41 Population Reports (1975) Series K, no. 1, *Injectables and Implants*, K1–16.

42 Gwatkin, D. R. (1979), 'Political will and family planning: the implication of India's emergency experience', *Population and Development Review*, **5(1)**, p. 29.

43 World Health Organization (1981), *International Code of Marketing of Breastmilk Substitutes*, Geneva: WHO.

44 Short, R. (1976), 'The Evolution of Human Reproduction', *Proceedings of the Royal Society of London*, **195(118)**, p. 3; Short, R. (1984), 'Breastfeeding', *Scientific American*, **250**, p. 23; Short, R. (1988), 'Breastfeeding, birth spacing and their effects on child survival', *335 Nature*, p. 679.

45 Bongaarts, J. (1980), 'A comment on the determinants of !Kung fertility', in W. P. Handwerker (ed.) (1985), *Culture and Reproduction: an anthropological critique of demographic transition theory*, New York: Population Council.

46 Fink (1988), op. cit., note 12 above.

47 Hodgson, C. S. (1981), 'Using and misusing ethnographic data: lactation as "nature's contraceptive" ', *Medical Anthropology*, **16**, p. 36; Jenkins, C. L. (1981), 'Patterns of growth and malnutrition among preschoolers in Belize', *American Journal of Physical Anthropology*, **56**, p. 169.

48 Wilmsen, E. N. (1988), 'Biological determinants of fecundity and fecundability: an application of Bongaart's model to forager fertility', in Handwerker, op. cit., note 45 above; Hodgson, op. cit., note 47 above; Shostak, M. (1981), *Nisa: the life and words of a !Kung woman*, London: Allen Lane; Marshall, L. (1976), *The !Kung of Nyae Nyae*, Cambridge, Mass: Harvard University Press.

49 Fink, A. E. (1985), 'Nutrition, Lactation and Fertility in two Mexican Rural Communities', *Social Science and Medicine*, vol. 20, no. 12, pp. 1295–1305.

50 Ibid., p. 1296–7.

51 Konner, M. and Worthman, C. (1980), 'Nursing frequency, gonadal function and birth spacing among !Kung hunter gatherers', *207 Science*, p. 790.

52 Wood, J. W. et al. (1985), 'Lactation and birth spacing in highlands New Guinea', *Journal of Biosocial Science*, Supplement 9, p. 159.

53 Howie, P. W. et al. (1981), 'Effect of supplementary food on suckling patterns and ovarian activity during lactation', *British Medical Journal*, **283**, p. 757.

54 Short (1984 and 1988), cited in note 44 above.

55 Fink (1988), op. cit., note 12 above, pp. 282–3.

56 Frisch, R. (1984), 'Body fat, puberty and fertility', *Biological Review*, **59**, p. 161.

57 Howell, N. (1979), *Demography of the Dobe !Kung*, New York: Academic Press.

58   Fink (1988), op. cit., note 12 above, pp. 274–6, 282–3.
59   Lunn, R. G. *et al.* (1980), 'Influence of maternal diet on plasma prolactin levels during lactation', *Lancet*, **1**, p. 623; Lunn, R. G. *et al.* (1984), 'The effects of improved nutrition on plasma prolactin concentrations and post-partum infertility in lactating Gambian women', *American Journal of Clinical Nutrition*, **39**, p. 227.
60   Delgado, H. L. *et al.* (1982), 'Nutrition, lactation and birth interval components in rural Guatemala', *The American Journal of Clinical Nutrition*, p. 1468.
61   Fink (1988), op. cit., note 12 above, pp. 274–6, 282–3.
62   Hodgson, op. cit., note 47 above; Wilmsen, op. cit., note 48 above.
63   Short (1988), op. cit., note 44 above.
64   Fink (1988), op. cit., note 12 above, p. 281.
65   Warren, M. P. (1982), 'The effects of altered nutritional states, stress and systemic illness on reproduction in women', in J. L. Vaitukatitis (ed.), *Clinical Reproductive Neuroendocrinology*, Elsevier Science Publishing Co. Inc.; Warren, M. P. (1988), 'The effects of undernutrition on reproductive function in the human', *Endocrine Reviews*, **4**, p. 364.
66   Fink (1988), op. cit., note 12 above, pp. 265–6.
67   Ibid., p. 281.
68   Howie, *et al.*, op. cit., note 53 above.
69   Fink (1988), op. cit., note 12 above, pp. 280–2.
70   Ibid., pp. 245–6.
71   Fink, op. cit., note 49 above.
72   Fink (1982), fieldwork notes, op. cit., note 20 above.
73   Jenkins, op. cit., note 47 above.
74   Fink (1988), op. cit., note 12 above, p. 265.
75   Raphael, D. and Davis, F. (1985), *Only Mothers Know Patterns of Infant Feeding in Traditional Cultures*, Westport, Conn.: Greenwood Press.
76   Fink, op. cit., note 49 above.
77   In San Jose, Fink found that three women out of a total of 97 who were observed feeding during the fieldwork period were totally unable to feed, although there may have been others in the village who were then past childbearing. The percentage is small, but the children of these women were unnecessarily put at risk because of their mothers' inability to obtain an appropriate milk substitute. In fact, two died during the fieldwork as a result of malnutrition. Another child survived because local missionaries supplied the mother with infant formula for four weeks during which time she persisted in trying to breastfeed, and indeed eventually succeeded in so doing. The child continued to need supplementation and thrived on the combination; Fink (1988), op. cit., note 12 above, pp. 270–1.
78   Jelliffe, D. B. and Jelliffe, E. F. P. (1978), *Human Milk in the Modern World*, Oxford: Oxford University Press.
79   Morgan (1887), p. 47.
80   Rivière, P. 'Marriage: a reassessment', in Needham, op. cit., note 2 above.
81   Lévi-Strauss, C. (1969), *The Elementary Structures of Kinship*, London: Eyre and Spottiswoode.
82   Leach, E. R. (1961), *Rethinking Anthropology*, London: Athlone Press.
83   Needham, op. cit., note 2 above; Needham, R. (1971), 'Remarks on the analysis of kinship and marriage', in Needham, op. cit., note 2 above.
84   Rivière, in ibid.,
85   Ibid., p. 60.
86   Schapera, I. (1938), *A Handbook of Tswana Law and Custom*, London.
87   Griffiths, A. (1989), 'Women, Status and Power: The Negotiation of Family

Disputes in Botswana', *Cornell International Law Journal*, 3, pp. 575–622, New York: Ithaca.

BIBLIOGRAPHY

Barnard, A. and Good, A. (1984), *Research Practices in the Study of Kinship*, Academic Press: London.

Bongaarts, J. (1980), *The Fertility–Inhibiting Effect of the Intermediate Fertility Variables*, Centre for Policy Studies Working Paper No. 57, Population Council: New York.

Bongaarts, J. (1985), 'A Comment on the Determinants of !Kung Fertility', in Handwerker, W. P. (ed.), *Culture and Reproduction: An Anthropological Critique of Demographic Transition Theory*, Population Council: New York.

British Medical Journal (1989), Nestle Boycott, vol. 298, p. 702.

Chen, P.-C. and Kols, A. (1982), 'Population and Birth Planning in the People's Republic of China', *Population Reports*, no. 25, Series J., p. 44.

Chen, P.-C., Tian, X.-Y and Tuan, C.-H (1982), '11m.Chinese opt for "one child glory certificate" ', *People*, **9**, (4), pp. 12–15.

David, H. P. (1982), 'Incentives, Reproductive Behaviour and Integrated Community Development in Asia', *Studies in Family Planning*, **13** (5), pp. 159–73.

Delgado, H. L., Martorell, R. and Klein, R. E. (1982), 'Nutrition, Lactation and Birth Interval Components in Rural Guatemala', *The American Journal of Clinical Nutrition*, pp. 1468–76.

DHSS (1987), *Human Fertilisation and Embryology: A Framework for Legislation*.

Djerassi, C. (1976), 'Problems of Manufacture and Distribution. The Manufacture of Steroidal Contraceptives: Technical versus Political Aspects', *Proceedings of the Royal Society of London*, **195**, pp. 175–86.

Dobbing, J. (ed.) (1988), *Infant Feeding: Anatomy of a Controversy 1973–1984*, Springer-Verlag: Berlin.

El Saadawi, N. (1980), *The Hidden Face of Eve: Women in the Arab World*, Zed Press: London.

Epstein, T. S. (1973), *South India: Yesterday, Today and Tomorrow*, Macmillan: London.

Evans Pritchard, E. E. (1951), *Kinship and Marriage among the Nuer*, Clarendon Press: Oxford.

Fink, A. E. (1982), 'Aspects of Infant Nutrition in Two Mexican Rural Communities', unpublished M.Phil thesis: Oxford University.

Fink, A. E. (1985), 'Nutrition, Lactation and Fertility in Two Mexican Rural Communities', *Social Science and Medicine*, vol. 20, no. 12, pp. 1295–1305.

Fink, A. E. (1988), *Food, Family and Ideology: Some Determinants of Social and Biological Reproduction Among the Mopan Maya of Southern Belize*, D.Phil Thesis, Bodleian Library: Oxford.

Finkel, J. L. and Crane, B. B. (1975), 'The Politics of Bucharest: Population, Development and the New International Economic Order', *Population and Development Review*, vol. 11, no. 1., pp. 87–114.

Fox, R. (1967), *Kinship and Marriage*, Penguin Books Ltd: Harmondsworth.

Frisch, R. (1984), 'Body Fat, Puberty and Fertility', *Biological Review*, **59**, pp. 161–88.

Goody, E. (1982), *Parenthood and Social Reproduction. Fostering and Occupational Roles in West Africa*, Cambridge University Press: Cambridge.

Gould, K. H. (1976), 'The Twain Never Met: Sheruper, India and the Family

Planning Program', in Marshall, J. and Polgar, S. (eds), *Culture, Natality, and Family Planning*, Carolina Population Center: Chapel Hill, North Carolina.

Griffiths, A. (1989), 'Women, Status and Power. The Negotiation of Family Disputes in Botswana', *Cornell International Law Journal*, 3, pp. 575–622, Ithaca: New York.

Gwatkin, D. R. (1979), 'Political Will and Family Planning: The Implication of India's Emergency Experience', *Population and Development Review*, vol. 5, no. 1, pp. 29–59.

Harrison, D. (1981), *The Effect of Education and Wages on Fertility: Some Evidence from Malaysia*, Department of Economics Seminar Papers, no. 15/81, Population Association of America Meetings, Monash University Melbourne: Australia.

Heitlinger, A. (1976), 'Pro-natalist Population in Czechoslavakia', *Population Studies*, pt. 1, pp. 123–35.

Hodgson, C. S. (1985), 'Using and Misusing Ethnographic Data: Lactation as "Nature's Contraceptive" ', *Medical Anthropology*, **16**, pp. 36–41.

Howell, N. (1979), *Demography of the Dobe !Kung*, Academic Press: New York.

Howie, P. W., McNeilly, A. S., Houston, M. J., Cook, A. and Boyle, H. (1981), 'Effect of Supplementary Food on Suckling Patterns and Ovarian Activity during Lactation', *British Medical Journal*, **283**, pp. 757–63.

International Labor Organization (1982), 'Inter-country Seminar on Incentives for Family Planning: Family Welfare in Industrial Sector', Puncak: Indonesia I.L.O.

Jelliffe, D. B. and Jelliffe, E. F. P. (1978), *Human Milk in the Modern World*, Oxford University Press: Oxford.

Jenkins, C. L. (1981), 'Patterns of Growth and Malnutrition among Preschoolers in Belize', *American Journal of Physical Anthropology*, **56**, pp. 169–78.

Konner, M. and Worthman, C. (1980), 'Nursing Frequency, Gonadal Function and Birth Spacing among !Kung Hunter Gatherers', *Science*, **207**, pp. 790–1.

Leach, E. R. (1961), *Rethinking Anthropology*, Athlone Press: London.

Levi-Strauss, C. (1969), *The Elementary Structures of Kinship*, Eyre and Spottiswoode (Publishers) Ltd.: London.

Lunn, R. G., Prentice, A. M., Austin, S. and Whitehead, R. G. (1980), 'Influence of Maternal Diet on Plasma Prolactin Levels during Lactation', *Lancet*, **1**, pp. 623–5.

Lunn, R. G., Austin, S., Prentice, A. M. and Whitehead, R. G. (1984), 'The Effect of Improved Nutrition on Plasma Prolactin Concentrations and Post-Partum Infertility in Lactating Gambian Women', *American Journal of Clinical Nutrition*, **39**, pp. 227–35.

Macura, M. (1974), 'Population Policies in Socialist Countries of Europe', *Population Studies*, pt. 3, pp. 369–79.

Marshall, L. (1976), *The !Kung of Nyae Nyae*, Harvard University Press: Cambridge Mass.

Massiah, J. (1983), *Women as Heads of Households in the Caribbean: Family Structure and Feminine Status*, UNESCO: Paris.

Needham R. (ed.) (1971a), *Rethinking Kinship and Marriage*, Tavistock Publications: London.

Needham, R. (ed.) (1971b), 'Remarks on the Analysis of Kinship and Marriage', in Needham, R. (ed.) (1971a), *Rethinking Kinship and Marriage*, Tavistock Publications: London, pp. 1–34.

Nutini, H. G. and Bell, B. (1970), 'The Structure and Historical Development of the Compradzgo System in Rural Tlaxcala,' *Ritual Kinship*, vol. 1.

Ott, S. (1981), *The Circle of Mountains: A Basque Shepherding Community*, Clarendon Press: Oxford.

Population Report (1975), Series K, no. 1, *Injectables and Inplants*.

Population Report (1981), Series J, no. 24, *Breast-Feeding, Fertility and Family Planning*.
Population Report (1984), Series E, no. 7, *Law and Policy*, The Johns Hopkins University: Baltimore, Maryland.
Raphael, D. and Davis, F. (1985), *Only Mothers Know Patterns of Infant Feeding in Tradtional Cultures*, Greenwood Press: Westport, Connecticut.
Rivière, P. (1971), 'Marriage: A Reassessment', in Needham, R. (ed.) (1971a), *Rethinking Kinship and Marriage*, Tavistock Publications: London, pp. 57–74.
Schapera, I. (1938), *A Handbook of Tswana Law and Custom*, London.
Short, R. (1976), 'The Evolution of Human Reproduction', *Proceedings of the Royal Society of London*, vol. 195, no. 118, pp. 3–24.
Short, R. (1984), 'Breastfeeding', *Scientific American*, **250**, pp. 23–41.
Short, R. (1988), 'Breast Feeding, Birth Spacing and their Effects on Child Survival', *Nature*, vol. 335, pp. 679–82.
Shorter,E. (1975), *The Making of the Modern Family*, Fontana Books: London.
Shostak, M. (1981), *Nisa: The Life and Words of a !Kung Woman*, Allen Lane: London.
Warnock, M. (1984), *Report of the Committee of Inquiry into Human Fertilisation and Embryology*, HMSO: London, Cmnd 9314.
Warren, M. P. (1982), 'The Effects of Altered Nutritional States, Stress and Systemic Illness on Reproduction in Women', in Vaitukatitis, J. L. (ed.), *Clinical Reproductive Neuroendocrinology*, Elsevier Science Publishing Co. Inc.
Warren, M. P. (1983), 'The Effects of Undernutrition on Reproductive Function in the Human', *Endocrine Reviews*, **4**, pp. 364–77.
Wood, J. W., Lai, D., Johnson, L., Campbell, K. L. and Maslar, I. A. (1985), 'Lactation and Birth Spacing in Highland New Guinea', *Journal of Biosocial Science*, supplement 9, pp. 159–73.
WHO (1979), *Report on Breastfeeding*, Geneva.
WHO (1981), *Report: International Code of Marketing of Breast-Milk Substitutes*, Geneva.
Wilmsen, E. N. (1985), 'Biological Determinants of Fecundity and Fecundability: An Application of Bongaarts' Model to Forager Fertility', in Handwerker, W. P. (ed.), *Culture and Reproduction: An Anthropological Critique of Demographic Transition Theory*, pp. 59–89.
World Bank Development Report (1984), Oxford University Press: New York.

Index